Bladder Biopsy Interpretation

Bladder Biopsy Interpretation

David G. Bostwick, M.D.
Professor of Pathology and Urology
Mayo Clinic
Rochester, Minnesota (USA)

and

Antonio Lopez-Beltran, M.D.
Professor of Pathology
University of Cordoba
Cordoba, Spain

© United Pathologists Press 1999
ISBN 1-883477-27-1
Library of Congress CIP 98-85142
Printed in Korea

TABLE OF CONTENTS

PREFACE

The bladder is prone to develop an unique and extraordinarily diverse array of inflammatory, metaplastic, and neoplastic abnormalities. Cancer of the bladder accounts for the fifth most common cancer in the human body, with more than 50,000 new urothelial carcinomas diagnosed annually in the United States. Many patients with cancer have prolonged survival, resulting in numerous follow-up cystoscopic biopsies and urine cytology specimens. This has generated a great diagnostic burden for the pathologist.

The objective of *Bladder Biopsy Interpretation* is to describe and selectively illustrate the pathologic conditions that afflict the bladder and urothelium. We are pleased to incorporate international standards that were established in 1998 for classification and grading of flat and papillary urothelial lesions of the bladder. After 3 years of preparation of this text, final publication was purposely delayed to include these important changes and update all references. The nomenclature and diagnostic criteria for these new and consistent standards were developed by an international team of more than 35 pathologists, including the authors of this book, representing the World Health Organi-

zation and International Society of Urologic Pathologists. The standards provide, for the first time, a framework on which diagnostic features can be compared, evaluated, and integrated.

This bladder biopsy interpretation book was prepared with the practicing pathologist as the foremost consideration. It reflects the contemporary practice of urologic pathology at two busy centers (Mayo Clinic and University of Cordoba). We hope that this text and collection of tables and photomicrographs will materially aid in continuing efforts to recognize, understand, and accurately interpret the light microscopic findings in bladder biopsy specimens. This book is not intended to replace comprehensive textbooks of urologic pathology, urinary tract cytology, or other original sources of information, but rather to complement them as a practical aid.

We are indebted to many individuals who have been involved in the preparation of this book. Ms. Patti Wolf of Wolf Publications, Inc., and her staff provided expert and invaluable editorial assistance throughout this project. Elizabeth Rafferty of United Pathologists Press was a tireless champion of this effort. Mr. Ray Howe was instrumental in optimizing the cover

design and book production. The encourage-
ment and cooperation of our colleagues in the
Division of Anatomic Pathology at Mayo Clinic
Rochester are sincerely appreciated. To our
families, we owe a particular debt of gratitude
for their understanding and patience.

We earnestly solicit constructive criticism
from colleagues so that the utility of this text
can be expanded and improved in subsequent
editions to its maximum potential.

David G. Bostwick M.D., Rochester, MN (USA)
Antonio Lopez-Beltran, M.D., Cordoba, Spain
January, 1999

1
NORMAL ANATOMY AND HISTOLOGY

1.1 EMBRYOLOGY

Early in fetal life, when cloacal dilation first appears and the hindgut ends in a blind sac, an ectodermal depression develops under the root of the tail. This depression, known as the *proctodeum,* deepens until only a thin layer of tissue remains between the gut and the outside of the body; this tissue layer is known as the *cloacal membrane.* The division of the cloaca results from development of the urorectal fold, which closes caudally toward the cloacal membrane. As the urorectal fold cuts progressively deeper into the cloaca, a wedge-shaped mass of mesenchyme accompanies it and forms a dense septum between the urogenital sinus anteriorly and the rectum posteriorly. This separation of the cloaca is completed before the cloacal membrane ruptures so that its two parts open independently. When it first opens to the outside, the urogenital sinus, which is the ventral division of the cloaca, is tubular and continuous with the allantois. At this stage, it can be divided into a ventral or pelvic portion, which will become the bladder proper, and a urethral portion, which receives the mesonephric and fused müllerian ducts and later becomes the prostatic and membranous urethra in the male and the entire urethra in the female (Tanagho, 1992).

After 8 weeks, the ventral part of the urogenital sinus expands to form an epithelial sac, the apex of which tapers into an elongated narrowed urachus. The splanchnic mesoderm surrounding both segments differentiates as interlacing bands of smooth muscle fibers and an outer fibroconnective tissue coat. By 12 weeks, the layers of the adult urethra and bladder can be recognized. This sequence of events indicates that the detrusor muscle and the urethral musculature have the same origin, constituting one uninterrupted structure (Tanagho, 1992). This arrangement is easily observed in the female, in which the bladder and urethra form one tubular unit with expansion of the upper part. However, in the male, the structure is complicated by simultaneous development of the prostate gland. The developmental sequence is the same in both sexes, and the structural arrangement in the male is only slightly more complex than that in the female (Tanagho, 1992).

1.2 ANATOMY

1.2.1 Gross Anatomy

The bladder is a hollow muscular organ whose main function is that of a reservoir. When empty, the adult bladder lies behind the symphysis pubis and is largely a pelvic organ. In infants and children, it is more cephalad than in adults. When full, the bladder rises above the symphysis and can readily be palpated or percussed. When overdistended, as in acute and chronic urinary retention, it may cause the lower abdomen to visibly bulge and is easily palpable in the suprapubic region (Chevallier, 1994; Tanagho, 1992). The empty bladder has an apex (superior surface), two infralateral or anterolateral surfaces, a base (posterior surface), and a neck. The apex extends a short distance above the pubic bone and ends as a fibrous cord derivative of the urachus. This fibrous cord extends from the apex of the bladder to the umbilicus between the peritoneum and the transversalis fascia. It raises a ridge of peritoneum called the median umbilical ligament. There is a peritoneal covering at the apex in both sexes that also covers a small part of the base in males (Chevallier, 1994; Tanagho, 1992).

The apex of the bladder is apposed to the uterus and ileum in the female and the ileum and pelvic portion of the colon in the male. The base of the bladder faces posteriorly and is separated from the rectum by the uterus and vagina in the female and by the vasa deferentia, seminal vesicles, and ureters in the male. The anterolateral surface on each side of the bladder is apposed to the pubic bone, levator ani, and obturator internus muscles, but the central anterior bladder is separated from the pubic bone by the retropubic space, which contains abundant fat and venous plexuses. The neck of the bladder, its most inferior part, connects with the urethra. When the bladder is distended with urine, the neck remains fixed and stationary, whereas the dome rises above the pelvic cavity into the lower abdomen, touching the posterior aspect of the lower anterior abdominal wall and the small and large bowel (Chevallier, 1994).

Beneath the urothelial lining of the inner bladder, there is loose connective tissue that permits considerable stretching of the mucosa.

As a result, the urothelial mucosal lining is wrinkled when the bladder is empty but smooth and flat when the bladder is distended (de Groat, 1993). This arrangement exists throughout the bladder except at the trigone, where the mucous membrane is firmly adhered to the underlying muscle; consequently, the trigone is always smooth, regardless of the level of distension (Fig 1.1).

1.2.2 Blood Supply and Lymphatic Drainage

The bladder is supplied by the superior, middle, and inferior vesical arteries, all of which are branches of the anterior division of the hypogastric artery. Between the bladder wall proper and the outer adventitial layer, there is a rich plexus of veins that converge in several main trunks and ultimately terminate in the hypogastric veins (Tanagho, 1992).

The bladder lymphatics drain into the external iliac, hypogastric, and common iliac lymph nodes. There is a rich lymphatic anastomosis between the pelvic and genital organs (Poggi et al, 1995; Ravery et al, 1993; Scelsi et al, 1996).

1.2.3 Nerve Supply

The bladder is innervated by divisions of the autonomic nervous system (de Groat, 1993; Tanagho, 1992). Sympathetic nerves originate from the lower thoracic and upper lumbar segments, mainly T11-12 and L1-2. These sympathetic fibers descend into the sympathetic trunk and the lumbar splanchnic nerves, connecting with the superior hypogastric plexus, an inferior extension of the aortic plexus. The latter separates into the right and left hypogastric nerves, which extend inferiorly to join the pelvic plexus of the pelvic parasympathetic nerves. Parasympathetic nerves arise from sacral segments S2-4, which form the pelvic parasympathetic plexus. This plexus joins the sympathetic hypogastric plexus, and vesical branches emerge from this plexus toward the bladder

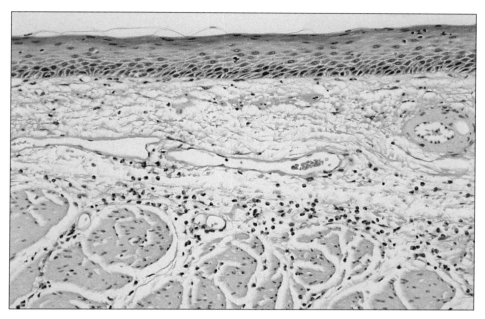

Figure 1.1 Normal trigone in a woman during the reproductive years. Note the squamous mucosa and closely packed underlying muscle.

base, innervating the bladder and urethra (de Groat, 1993).

1.3 NORMAL HISTOLOGY

1.3.1 Urothelium (Transitional Epithelium)

The urothelium is a unique stratified epithelium of variable thickness (Fig 1.2). The number of cell layers depends on the degree of distension of the bladder, usually varying from three to seven layers. When distended, the bladder appears to be at least three cell layers thick, although the typical biopsy contains five to seven layers. For practical purposes, urothelium composed of more than seven cell layers is considered abnormal (Ayala & Ro, 1989). In addition, the urothelium is thought to be monoclonal in origin, with some features of mosaicism (Tsai et al, 1995).

The normal urothelium contains a layer of large superficial cells that are frequently multinucleated and often referred to as *umbrella cells*.

These cells have abundant eosinophilic cytoplasm, with large nuclei whose long axes are perpendicular to that of the smaller cells of the underlying basal and intermediate cell layers. The superficial cells vary in size and configuration according to the degree of bladder distension and angle of tissue section; they may appear cuboidal in the distended bladder. In addition, superficial cells are loosely attached to the underlying cells and may be absent from otherwise normal urothelium in routine biopsies. Superficial cells may persist on the surface of a low-grade papillary urothelial carcinoma, a finding of some importance in the pathologic grading of bladder cancer (Lopez-Beltran et al, 1992) (Chapter 9).

Basal and intermediate cells are located between the basal lamina and the superficial cells. These cells are morphologically identical to each other and are distinguished only by their position in the mucosa. They are regularly arranged, with distinct cell boundaries and oval, round, or fusiform nuclei with occasional prominent nuclear grooves (Ayala & Ro, 1989). The nuclei

(a)

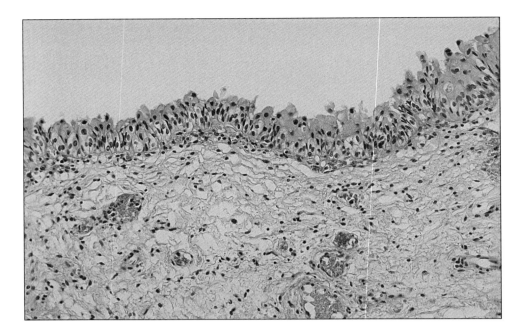

(b)

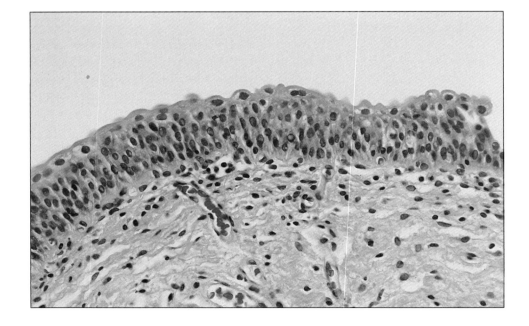

(c)

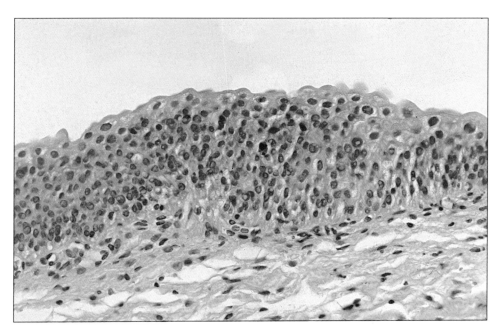

Figure 1.2 Normal urothelium. **(a):** This section is no thicker than 3 cells, with prominent superficial cells. Compare with **(b)**, showing a thicker mucosa with less distinct superficial cells. **(c):** In this preparation, the urothelium is up to 7 cells in thickness, with cells whose long axis is often perpendicular to the mucosal surface.

are centrally located in the cells and contain finely granular chromatin that often accentuates the nuclear borders. Nucleoli are usually small and difficult to detect, and mitotic figures are rare in the normal urothelium. The long axis of the basal and intermediate cells is perpendicular to the basal lamina. The basement membrane is visible in routine hematoxylin and eosin or periodic acid-Schiff stained sections. Basement membrane markers such as laminin and type IV collagen may be useful diagnostically in select cases but are not routinely employed (Wilson et al, 1995).

1.3.2 Bladder Wall

The lamina propria, located beneath the basement membrane, consists of a compact layer of fibrovascular connective tissue (Fig 1.3). It contains an incomplete muscularis mucosa composed of thin delicate smooth muscle fibers that may be mistaken for muscularis propria in biopsy specimens (Anderstrom et al, 1980; Dixon & Gosling, 1983; Keep et al, 1989; Ro et al, 1987; Younes et al, 1990). Proper diagnosis of the muscularis mucosa is a potential pitfall in evaluating bladder carcinoma because the management of cancer invading the muscularis propria is different from that of tumors limited to the lamina propria and surrounding the muscularis mucosa. Therefore, it is important for pathologists to be aware of the existence of delicate muscle bundles within the lamina propria (Ro et al, 1987). In biopsy specimens, these smooth muscle fibers may appear as a continuous layer, as a discontinuous or interrupted layer, or as scattered thin bundles of smooth muscle fibers that do not form an obvious layer (Ro et al, 1987). The muscle fibers lie parallel to the mucosal surface, midway between the epithelium and the underlying muscularis propria. Large blood vessels are a constant feature, running

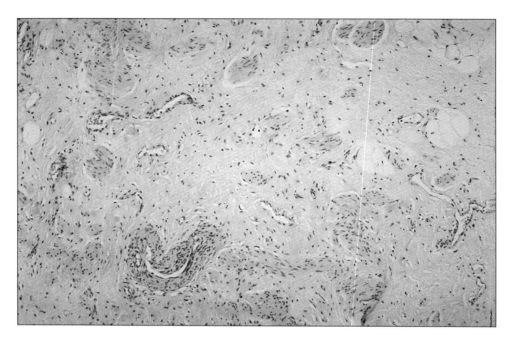

Figure 1.3 Normal lamina propria. The muscularis mucosa consists of scant delicate muscle bands interspersed with blood vessels and connective tissue stroma.

parallel to the surface urothelium in close association with the fibers of the muscularis mucosa. To avoid overstaging bladder cancer, it is important for the pathologist to be aware of the existence of fat within the lamina propria and the muscularis propria (Bochner et al, 1995).

The muscle proper of the bladder, the muscularis propria, is moderately thick and consists of an inner longitudinal layer, a middle circular layer, and an outer longitudinal layer. It spirals around each ureteral orifice and increases in thickness around the internal urethral orifice, forming the internal sphincter of the bladder. The muscularis is surrounded by a coat of fibroelastic connective tissue, the adventitia, and perivesical fat (Ayala & Ro, 1989; Chevallier et al, 1994; Tanagho, 1992).

1.3.3 Paraganglionic Tissue

Paraganglia are rarely found in routine sections of the urinary bladder (Honma, 1994). Their presence in a bladder biopsy may be confused with neoplasm. Distinguishing features that are useful include the distinctive arrangement of cell nests, a sinusoidal vascular pattern, monotonous benign cytology of the cells, and the absence of a stromal reaction (Young, 1989).

1.4 THE URACHUS

The urachus is an intra-abdominal embryonic remnant. It contains the allantois, which connects the apex of the urinary bladder to the body wall at the umbilicus. The allantois originates in the portion of the yolk sac that gives rise to the cloacal portion of the hindgut. As the embryo grows, the urachus elongates to maintain its connection with the bladder dome and the body wall. At birth, the dome of the bladder and the umbilicus are closely apposed, and the urachus is only 2.5–3 mm long, with a diameter of 1 mm throughout most of its course and 3 mm where it joins the bladder (Begg, 1930). The urachus lies in a space anterior to the peritoneum, bounded anteriorly and posteriorly by the umbilicovesical fascia. Laterally, it is bounded by the two umbilical arteries, which, in turn, are surrounded by umbilicovesical fascia. Inferiorly, the umbilicovesical fascial layers cover the surface of the dome of the bladder. This space, the space of Retzius, is roughly pyramidal, and fascial planes separate it from the peritoneum and other structures. At the junction with the urinary bladder, the adult urachus is 4–8 mm wide, narrowing to about 2 mm at its superior end.

The urachus has three segments, including the supravesical, intramural, and intramucosal segments (Begg, 1930). Tubular urachal remnants are found within the wall of the urinary bladder in approximately one-third of adults and are evenly distributed between men and women (Fig 1.4). There are three architectural patterns of intramural urachal canals (Schubert et al, 1982), varying from simple tubular canals to complex branching canals (Fig 1.5). The mucosal portion of the urachus may have a wide diverticular opening, papilla, or a small opening flush with the mucosal surface. The major-

ity (70%) of intramural urachal remnants are lined by urothelium; the remainder are lined by columnar epithelium, occasionally with small papillae, or, rarely, with mucous goblet cells or mucus-secreting columnar epithelium (Eble, 1989; Schubert et al, 1982; Tyler, 1964).

1.5   THE RENAL PELVIS AND URETERS

The ureter and renal pelvis develop from the ampullary bud, which arises from the distal mesonephric duct during the 4th week of development. As the ureter elongates, there is a period of luminal obliteration followed by recanalization in the 5th week. Recanalization begins in the middle of the ureter and extends proximally and distally with the ureteropelvic and ureterovesical junctions, which are the last segments to recanalize. The mesonephric duct distal to the ampullary bud (the common nephric duct) is incorporated into the developing urogenital sinus, whereas the ureteral orifice migrates to the trigone and contributes to the prostatic urethra in the male.

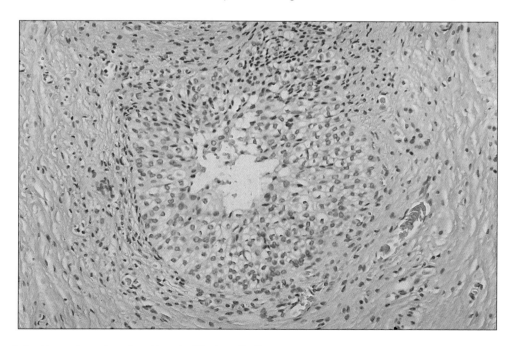

Figure 1.4   Normal urachus lined by stratified urothelium.

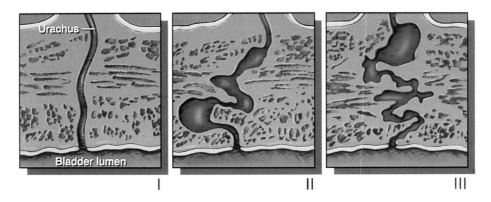

Figure 1.5 Patterns of intramural urachal canals. Type I: tubular canal without complexity; Type II: tubular canal with marked segmental dilatation and variable curvature; Type III: tubular canal with marked tortuosity and distortion, including segmental dilatation.

Concomitant development of the male and female reproductive tract forms the mesonephric (wolffian) and müllerian ducts, respectively, and division of the cloaca into the bladder and hindgut occurs as the ureter and kidney develop. As a consequence, multiple malformations in these areas often occur together.

The lumen of the renal pelvis and ureter is lined by urothelium that rests on a basement membrane. The urothelium is composed of three to five layers of cells in the pelvis and four to seven layers of cells in the ureter. The pelvis and ureter have a continuous muscular wall that originates in the fornices of the minor calyces as small interlacing fascicles of the smooth muscle cells. The muscularis propria is not divided into distinct layers. Near the bladder, the ureter acquires an external sheath from the detrusor muscle and the muscle fascicles become oriented longitudinally. The longitudinal fibers continue through the wall of the bladder and into the submucosa, where they surround the ureteral orifice and contribute to the trigone muscle.

1.6 THE URETHRA

The epithelium of the urethra is derived from the urogenital sinus, which is formed when the endodermal cloaca divides into the rectum dorsally and the urogenital sinus ventrally, separated by the urorectal septum. In females, the epithelium of the urethra is derived from endoderm of the urogenital sinus, while the surrounding connective tissue and smooth muscle arise from splanchnic mesenchyme. In males, the epithelium also is derived from the urogenital sinus except in the fossa navicularis, where it is derived from ectodermal cells migrating from glans penis. As in females, the connective tissue and smooth muscle surrounding the male urethra are derived from splanchnic mesenchyme.

In men, the urethra is 15–20 cm long and divided in three anatomic segments. The prostatic urethra begins at the internal urethral orifice at the bladder neck and extends through the prostate to the prostatic apex. In the central part of the urethral crest is an eminence called the *verumontanum*. The verumontanum contains a slitlike opening that leads to an epithelium-lined sac called the *prostatic utricle*, a müllerian vestige. The ejaculatory ducts empty into the urethra on either side of the prostatic utricle. The membranous urethra extends from the prostatic apex to the bulb of the penis. Cowper's glands are located on the left and right sides of the membranous urethra, and their ducts empty into it. The penile urethra extends from the lower surface of the urogenital diaphragm to the urethral meatus in the glans penis. Bulbourethral glands are located in the proximal (bulbous) portion of the penile urethra. In addition, scattered mucus-secreting periurethral glands (Littre's glands) are present at the periphery of the penile urethra except anteriorly.

The female urethra is approximately 4 cm long; at its periphery are paraurethral Skene's glands. The type of epithelium lining of the urethra varies along its length. In general, urothelium lines the prostatic urethra, pseudostratified columnar epithelium lines the membranous segment and most of the penile urethra, and nonkeratinized stratified squamous epithelium lines the fossa navicularis and external urethral orifice. In females, the proximal one-third of the urethra is lined by urothelium and the distal two-thirds by nonkeratinized stratified squamous epithelium.

1.7 IMMUNOHISTOCHEMICAL FINDINGS

The urothelium has a characteristic immunophenotype. It expresses cytokeratins of both low and high molecular weights, including keratins 7, 8, 13, and 19; keratin 18 is present in the su-

perficial cells. This pattern of expression differs from that of normal stratified squamous epithelium, which shows predominantly high–molecular-weight keratin immunoreactivity, and from endometrium, endocervix, colorectum, and prostate, which demonstrate a preponderance of low–molecular-weight keratin. High–molecular-weight keratin immunoreactivity is restricted to the basal cell layer of the urothelium and squamous mucosa of the trigone. This cell layer can also be readily stained with anti-keratin antibody (MAC387). Other epithelial markers such as epithelial membrane antigen (EMA), carcinoembryonic antigen (CEA), and CD15 are found on the surface of the urothelium. The normal urothelium synthesizes blood group isoantigens A, B, and H (O), as well as Lewis blood group antigens (Witjes et al, 1995). Prostate-specific antigen (PSA, or human glandular kallikrein 3), prostatic acid phosphatase, prostate-specific membrane antigen, and human glandular kallikrein 2 are not produced by the urothelium.

1.8 BLADDER SAMPLING AND REPORTING

The most common bladder specimens are obtained from endoscopic biopsies and transurethral resections (TURB), both of which sample

Table 1.1 Evaluation of bladder biopsies

Macroscopic findings	Microscopic findings
Cold-cup: record the number of pieces, dimensions (mm), and presence of papillary growth	Evaluation of epithelial surface (intact, ulcerated, denuded)
Transurethral resection of the bladder (TURB): proportion of tissue embedded	Presence or absence of muscularis propria
Total weight of resected tissue fragments	Histologic diagnosis (urothelial carcinoma, adenocarcinoma)
A minimum of 6 g or 3 cassettes should be submitted	Pattern of growth (papillary, flat, nodular)
	Pathologic grade
	Extent (depth) of invasion (pathologic stage)
	Vascular/lymphatic invasion
	Pattern of infiltration (tentacular, broad, mixed)
	Findings in the adjacent mucosa
	Comment on biopsy artifact if it compromises evaluation

9

Table 1.2 Handling and reporting of bladder cold-cup biopsies

Macroscopic findings	*Microscopic findings*
Record the number of specimens	Diagnosis of pathologic abnormalities
Measure the largest and smallest specimen and record greatest dimensions of each	Type, grade, depth of invasion (lamina propria / submucosa, muscularis propria), the presence of microvascular invasion of neoplasm
Fix in a Bouin's-type solution, such as Hollandes's, or in zinc formalin; either is preferable to phosphate-buffered formalin	Associated conditions such as granulomas, inflammation, ulcers
Sectioning at multiple levels may be helpful	A comment on thermocoagulation artifact only if this impedes diagnostic evaluation

Note: for associated intraepithelial abnormalities (carcinoma in situ, dysplasia), if the intraepithelial abnormality is adjacent to a papillary or invasive tumor, record as a flat component of that tumor. If the intraepithelial abnormality is not contiguous, record as a separate diagnosis.

Table 1.3 Handling and reporting of transurethral resection specimens

Macroscopic findings	*Microscopic findings*
Weigh specimen	Include all diagnostic findings
Record dimensions of largest and smallest pieces (aggregate dimensions are less reliable than a combination of weight and measurement)	With cancer, record histologic type, pattern of growth (papillary, flat, mixed), grade, depth of invasion, pattern of invasion (broad, tentacular, mixed), and the presence of angiolymphatic invasion
Sample generously; in most cases, the entire specimen can be embedded in less than 10 cassettes. Up to 6 grams or 3 cassettes should be processed in their entirety	Record the presence of muscularis propria (detrusor muscle) and whether invaded by the neoplasm; avoid confusion with muscularis mucosa
Bouin's-type fixatives may not be optimal for large specimens; zinc Formalin is preferred by some, but buffered Formalin is most widely used	Record the presence of inflammation and granulomas
	Comment on thermocoagulation artifact only if it compromises microscopic evaluation

subepithelial tissue of varying depth (Tables 1.1–1.3). Other specimens can be obtained from a cystectomy, cystoprostatourethrectomy, pelvic exenteration, resection of diverticulae, and partial cystectomy; for example, surgical excision of a urachal carcinoma usually includes the bladder dome, urachus, and umbilicus (Hermanek & Sobin, 1992; Parkinson & Fisher, 1991).

A bladder biopsy is usually performed to exclude carcinoma. It also provides information to assess risk factors for recurrence, progression, and response to treatment, including tumor extent (Coloby et al, 1994; Friedell et al, 1980;

Gephardt & Baker, 1995; Kiemeney et al, 1994a, 1994b).

1.8.1 Biopsy and Transurethral Resection

Small noninvasive papillary neoplasms are often excised by biopsy using cold-cup forceps such as Storz, diathermy forceps, or a small diathermy loop. Excellent biopsy results are obtained in the urinary bladder using a computerized tomography–guided transmural needle with a 1.2-mm cutting needle (Malmstrom et al, 1993). To avoid tissue distortion, these specimens should be transferred to fixative with minimal handling (Table 1.2). Larger neoplasms are often sampled by TURB using a diathermy loop that produces strips of tissue 6 mm in diameter and of variable length. Resection or biopsy of the muscle base may produce a specimen that allows complete evaluation of the site (Murphy, 1994; Parkinson & Fisher, 1991). All hyperemic or velvety areas of urothelium are sampled to exclude carcinoma in situ; random biopsies are commonly taken from macroscopically normal urothelium distant from the tumor site to determine the extent of involvement (Mufti & Singh, 1992). Ideally, random samples should be obtained from predetermined sites in four vesical quadrants (Parsons et al, 1980; Sakamoto et al, 1993; Soloway et al, 1978; Vicente-Rodriguez et al, 1994; Wallace et al, 1979). Some urologists also submit biopsy specimens of the urethra and prostate to assess other areas of the urothelium, particularly in patients with high-grade papillary urothelial carcinoma or carcinoma in situ

(Coloby et al, 1994; Kunze et al, 1994; Sakamoto et al, 1993).

1.8.2 Tissue Artifacts

Pathologists should alert surgeons when important tissue artifacts are encountered, including mechanical distortion that occurs when tissues are transferred from biopsy forceps to fixative with the aid of a gauze swab and thermal distortion that occurs when tissue is overheated by the diathermy loop (Fig 1.6). The epithelium of carcinoma in situ is particularly delicate and prone to partial or complete detachment from the lamina propria. Occasionally, carcinoma in situ is identified in Brunn's nests, even when the overlying urothelium is denuded. Denuding cystitis is another source of concern (Chapter 3). Tissue may be fixed in formalin or formol-saline, but picric acid–based fixatives may provide bet-

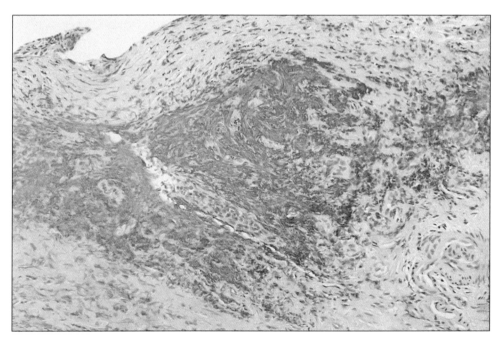

Figure 1.6 Cold-cup biopsy of the bladder markedly distorted by thermal artifact. This finding is uninterpretable, and an additional biopsy is recommended.

ter tissue preservation of bladder biopsies (Murphy et al, 1993).

1.8.3 Reporting

Pathology reports of cold-cup biopsies should include the number, size, and classification of epithelial proliferations (Table 1.2). Transurethral resections should be weighed in aggregate; we recommend complete submission of the specimen for histopathologic examination, but some laboratories prefer to submit only representative samples. In partially sampled specimens, effort should be made to select those fragments that contain muscle; also, the proportion of the specimen processed for examination should be stated if only partially sampled. When there is no evaluable muscularis propria in the sample, all of the tissue should be processed (Manyak & Nochomovitz, 1992; Murphy, 1994; Parkinson & Fisher, 1991).

The biopsy report should record which tissues are present. In patients with urothelial malignancy, a report of "denuded biopsy" is significantly different from one stating that "no tumor is seen" (Parkinson & Fisher, 1991). Similarly, invasion of the lamina propria may have different implications depending on the presence of attached muscularis propria. Care must be taken to distinguish the thin and often incomplete muscularis mucosa within the lamina propria from the muscularis propria (Ro et al, 1987). Routine reporting of muscle in the specimen when there is no cancer present may be useful for surgical quality control, but it is not uniformly included by all pathologists; we consider this a useful statement to include in the report.

Other important biopsy features include pathologic grade and stage of tumor, microvascular invasion, and the pattern of tumor invasion (broad or tentacular) (Larsen et al, 1990; Raghavan et al, 1990). Biopsies submitted separately, including random biopsies, should receive separate diagnoses. The depth of muscle invasion is often impossible to assess in TURB specimens, and the only reasonable statement may be "stage T2 at least" (Parkinson & Fisher, 1991). The presence of adipose tissue in biopsy specimens is not a clear indication of extravesical sampling because fat may be present within the lamina propria or the muscle layers (Bochner et al, 1995; Murphy, 1994; Parkinson & Fisher, 1991).

Recently, the Association of Directors of Anatomic and Surgical Pathology (Murphy et al, 1996) and the College of American Pathologists (Hammond & Henson, 1996) provided recommendations for the reporting of urinary bladder specimens and those from the ureter, renal pelvis, and urethra (Tables 1.1–1.3).

REFERENCES

Anderstrom C, Johansson S, Nilsson S. The significance of lamina propria invasion on the prognosis of patients with bladder tumors. *J Urol.* 1980;124: 23–26.

Ayala AG, Ro JY. Premalignant lesions of the urothelium and transitional cell tumors. In: Young RH, ed. *Pathology of the urinary bladder.* New York: Churchill Livingstone;1989.

Begg RC. The urachus: its anatomy, histology and development. *J Anat.* 1930;64:170–185.

Bochner BH, Nichols PW, Skinner DG. Overstaging of transitional cell carcinoma: clinical significance of lamina propria fat within the urinary bladder. *Urology.* 1995;45:528–531.

Chevallier JM. The bladder. Surgical anatomy. Cystectomy. *Soins Chirurgie.* 1994;159:41–43.

Coloby PJ, Kakizoe T, Tobisu K, et al. Urethral involvement in female bladder cancer patients: mapping of 47 consecutive cysto-urethrectomy specimens. *J Urol.* 1994;152:1438–1442.

de Groat WC. Anatomy and physiology of the lower urinary tract. *Urol Clin N Am.* 1993;20: 383–401.

Dixon JS, Gosling JA. Histology and fine structure of the muscularis mucosae of the human urinary bladder. *J Anat.* 1983;136:265–271.

Eble JN. Abnormalities of the urachus. In: Young RH, ed. *Pathology of the urinary bladder.* New York: Churchill Livingstone;1989.

Friedell GH, Parja GC, Nagy GK, et al. The pathology of human bladder cancer. *Cancer.* 1980;45:1823–1831.

Gephardt GN, Baker PB. Interinstitutional comparison of bladder carcinoma surgical pathology report adequacy. A College of American Pathologists Q-Probes study of 7234 bladder biopsies and curettings in 268 institutions. *Arch Pathol Lab Med.* 1995;119:681–685.

Hammond EH, Henson DE. Practice protocol for the examination of specimens removed from patients with carcinoma of the urinary bladder, ureter, renal pelvis, and urethra. *Arch Pathol Lab Med.* 1996;120:1103–1110.

Hermanek P, Sobin LH, eds. *TNM classification of malignant tumours* (4th ed, 2nd vers). Berlin: Springer-Verlag;1992.

Honma K. Paraganglia of the urinary bladder: an autopsy study. *Zentralblatt Pathologie.* 1994;139:465–469.

Keep JC, Piehl M, Miller A, et al. Invasive carcinomas of the urinary bladder. Evaluation of tunica muscularis mucosae involvement. *Am J Clin Pathol.* 1989;91:575–579.

Kiemeney LA, Witjes JA, Heijbroek RP, et al. Dysplasia in normal-looking urothelium increases the risk of tumour progression in primary superficial bladder cancer. *Eur J Cancer.* 1994a;30A:1621–1625.

Kiemeney LA, Witjes JA, Heijbroek RP, et al. Should random urothelial biopsies be taken from patients with primary superficial bladder cancer? A decision analysis. Members of the Dutch South-East Co-Operative Urological Group. *Br J Urol.* 1994b;73:164–171.

Kunze E, Weidhase A, Schulz H. Incidence and morphology of concurrent primary carcinomas of the urinary bladder and prostate in transurethral resection specimens. *Zentralblatt Pathologie.* 1994;140:113–122.

Larsen MP, Steinberg GD, Brendler CB, et al. Use of Ulex europaeus agglutinin I (UEA I) to distinguish vascular and "pseudovascular" invasion in transitional cell carcinoma of bladder with lamina propria invasion. *Mod Pathol.* 1990;3:83–88.

Lopez-Beltran A, Croghan GA, Croghan I, et al. Prognostic factors in survival of bladder cancer. *Cancer.* 1992;70:799–807.

Malmstrom PU, Lonnemark M, Busch C, et al. Staging of bladder carcinoma by computer tomography-guided transmural core biopsy. *Scand J Urol Nephrol.* 1993;27:193–198.

Manyak MJ, Nochomovitz LE. Cystourethroscopy, biopsy, tissue preparation. In: Nochomovitz LE, ed. *Bladder biopsy interpretation.* New York: Raven Press;1992.

Mufti GR, Singh M. Value of random mucosal biopsies in the management of superficial bladder cancer. *Eur Urol.* 1992;22:288–293.

Murphy WM. ASCP survey on anatomic pathology examination of the urinary bladder. *Am J Clin Pathol.* 1994;102:715–723.

Murphy WM, Ramsey J, Soloway MS. A better nuclear fixative for diagnostic bladder and prostate biopsies. *J Urol Pathol.* 1993;1:79–87.

Murphy WM, Crissman JD, Johansson SL, et al. Recommendations for the reporting of urinary bladder specimens that contain bladder neoplasms. *Mod Pathol.* 1996;9:796–798.

Parkinson MC, Fisher C. Gross examination of bladder specimens. *J Clin Pathol.* 1991;44:890–895.

Parsons KF, Scott AG, Traer S, et al. Endoscopic biopsy in the diagnosis of peripheral denervation of the bladder. *Br J Urol.* 1980;52:455–459.

Poggi P, Marchetti C, Tazzi A, et al. The lymphatic vessels and their relationship to lymph formation in the human urinary bladder. *Lymphology.* 1995;28:35–40.

Raghavan D, Shipley WU, Garnick MD, et al. Biology and management of bladder cancer. *N Engl J Med.* 1990;322:1129–1138.

Ravery V, Chopin DK, Abbou CC. Surgical anatomy of the lymphatic drainage of the bladder. *Ann Urol.* 1993;27:9–11.

Ro JY, Ayala AG, el-Naggar A. Muscularis mucosa of urinary bladder: importance for staging and treatment. *Am J Surg Pathol.* 1987;11:668–673.

Sakamoto N, Tsuneyoshi M, Naito S, et al. An adequate sampling of the prostate to identify prostatic involvement by urothelial carcinoma in bladder cancer patients. *J Urol.* 1993;149:318–321.

Scelsi R, Scelsi L, Gritti A, et al. Structure of the lymphatic microcirculation in the human urinary bladder with different intraluminal pressure and distension. *Lymphology.* 1996;29:60–66.

Schubert GE, Pavkovic MB, Bethke-Bedürftig BA. Tubular urachal remnants in adult bladders. *J Urol.* 1982;127:40–42.

Soloway MS, Murphy W, Rao MK, et al. Serial multiple-site biopsies in patients with bladder cancer. *J Urol.* 1978;120:57–59.

Tanagho EA. Anatomy of the urinary tract. The urinary bladder. In: Walsh PC, Reznick AB, Stamey TA, Vaughan ED, eds. *Cambell's urology.* Philadelphia: W.B. Saunders;1992.

Tsai YC, Simoneau AR, Spruck CH, et al. Mosaicism in human epithelium: macroscopic monoclonal patches cover the urothelium. *J Urol.* 1995;153:1697–1700.

13

Tyler DE. Epithelium of intestinal type in the normal urachus: a new theory of vesical embryology. *J Urol.* 1964;92:505–509.

Vicente-Rodriguez J, Laguna P, Salvador B, et al. Endoscopic biopsy in the staging of infiltrating tumor of the bladder. *Arch Esp Urol.* 1994;47:24–30.

Wallace DM, Hindmarsh JR, Webb JN, et al. The role of multiple mucosal biopsies in the management of patients with bladder cancer. *Br J Urol.* 1979; 51:535–540.

Wilson CB, Leopard J, Nakamura RM, et al. Selective type IV collagen defects in the urothelial basement membrane in interstitial cystitis. *J Urol.* 1995;154:1222–1226.

Witjes JA, Umbas R, Debruyne FM, et al. Expression of markers for transitional cell carcinoma in normal bladder mucosa of patients with bladder cancer. *J Urol.* 1995;154:2185–2189.

Younes M, Sussman J, True LD. The usefulness of the level of the muscularis mucosae in the staging of invasive transitional cell carcinoma of the urinary bladder. *Cancer.* 1990;66:543–548.

Young RH. Non-neoplastic epithelial abnormalities and tumorlike lesions. *Contemp Issues Surg Pathol.* 1989;13:1–64.

2

CONGENITAL DISORDERS
AND PEDIATRIC PATHOLOGY

2.1 URINARY BLADDER

2.1.1 Exstrophy

Complete failure of bladder development results in agenesis (Metoki et al, 1986; Palmer & Russi, 1969), and incomplete closure of the bladder produces exstrophy (Ives et al, 1980). Exstrophy affects about 1 in 30,000 to 50,000 births (Higgins, 1962). It is usually accompanied by other urinary tract defects, particularly epispadias. The common coexistence of exstrophy and epispadias is collectively designated the *exstrophy–epispadias complex* (Culp, 1964). Exstrophy may also be associated with cloacal anomalies.

Bladder exstrophy may be incomplete or complete. Both types are recognizable at birth as a mucocutaneous defect in the midline of the infraumbilical region. The macroscopic abnormality results from exposure of the posterior bladder wall without its anterior investiture of mesoderm-derived tissue. Typically, the mucosa is irregular, nodular, and thickened, with a fibrotic wall containing mucin-filled cysts. Urothelial abnormalities result from exposure to the external environment; consequently, sur-

gical repair is recommended early to avoid these changes (Dehner, 1987). Proliferative changes are present in virtually all cases, including cystitis cystica and glandularis, and squamous metaplasia occurs in about 25% of cases (Beynon et al, 1985; De Reise & Warmbold, 1986; Parker, 1970). Prominent lymphoid hyperplasia in the lamina propria may impart a finely nodular appearance macroscopically. Initially, the lamina propria is edematous and contains a variable amount of acute and chronic inflammation, but eventually fibrosis develops.

Bladder exstrophy is considered an important risk factor for malignancy and is associated with adenocarcinoma (Carter et al, 1974), squamous cell carcinoma, urothelial carcinoma, and rhabdomyosarcoma (Semerdjian et al, 1972).

A less frequent form of exstrophy, cloacal exstrophy or vesicointestinal fissure, consists of an exstrophied portion of intestine from which a distal intestinal segment emerges into a blind rectal pouch. Males and females are equally prone to cloacal exstrophy, unlike the male predominance with bladder exstrophy (3:1 ratio). Cloacal exstrophy is a more severe deformity and usually has a coexistent exstrophic bladder with an exposed hemibladder along the lateral border of the exstrophic intestine.

Urothelial abnormalities in the hemibladder are similar to those in uncomplicated bladder exstrophy (Diamond & Jeffs, 1985; Jeffs, 1978).

2.1.2 Duplication and Diverticulum

Duplication is rare, characterized by incomplete or complete partitioning of the bladder (Cheng & Maizels, 1996; Dunetz & Bauer, 1985; Feins & Cranley, 1986; Kapoor & Saha, 1987; Vaage et al, 1985).

A bladder diverticulum is classified as congenital or acquired, which includes iatrogenic cases (Livne & Gonzales, 1985). Most congenital diverticula are incidentally discovered without other urologic anomalies. Acquired diverticula in children are usually discovered as a complication of bladder neck obstruction, which may be congenital or associated with a neurogenic bladder in patients with meningomyelocele (Peterson et al, 1973). Acquired diverticula are the most common form in adults and are frequently associated with inflammation, urothelial dysplasia, and carcinoma (Cheng & Maizels, 1996; Rajan et al, 1996).

2.1.3 Fistula and Cysts

A congenital fistula between the bladder and the anterior abdominal wall may form a superior or inferior vesical fissure and is considered a less severe form of exstrophy than typical exstrophy.

A congenital prepubic sinus is a midline sinus from the skin immediately superior to the pubis that may communicate with the anterior bladder wall. Microscopically, the sinus tract is lined by urothelium and surrounded by a smooth muscle sheath. The sinus is considered a urethral duplication rather than a variant of exstrophy (Chatterjee & Sarkar, 1973; Herlihy & Barnes, 1985).

A trigonal cyst is a developmental anomaly, lined by unremarkable urothelium, located at or near the trigone.

2.1.4 Megacystis

An enlarged bladder may result from any distal anatomic obstruction, often at the bladder neck or urethral valves, or as a manifestation of a syndrome complex such as the prune-belly syndrome in which bilateral cryptorchidism is associated with urologic malformations and absence of the abdominal wall musculature. Some authors do not consider it strictly within the category of a congenital malformation (Carter et al, 1974; Inamdar et al, 1984). Megacystis is one component of the syndrome of megacystis–microcolon–intestinal hypoperistalsis.

2.1.5 Congenital Bladder Obstruction (Marion's Disease)

Congenital bladder obstruction is an obstructive condition that results in recurrent urinary tract infections in children. Histologically, there is concentric fibromuscular hypertrophy and elastosis of the bladder wall, often with chronic inflammation.

2.2 URACHUS

2.2.1 Patent Urachus

A patent urachus may be complete or incomplete (Fig 2.1). In its complete form, a patent urachus results in urine flow from the umbilical stump or umbilicus as a result of patency of the lumen from the bladder to the umbilicus at birth (Nix et al, 1958). It occurs at any age and is twice as likely to occur in males than in females. The umbilicus is often swollen and inflamed. Most patients have no other developmental anomaly, but some may have a congenital deficiency of the abdominal musculature as part of the prune-belly syndrome.

There are multiple incomplete forms of a patent urachus in which the lumen is closed at

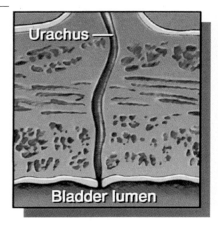
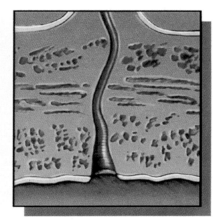
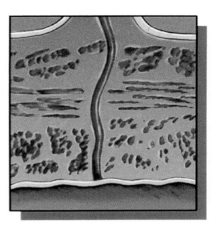
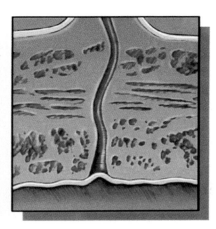

Figure 2.1 Urachal openings into the bladder. Top left: patent urachus with mucosal papilla; top right: patent urachus with wide opening; bottom left: imperforate urachus with mucosal covering; bottom right: imperforate urachus with mucosal depression.

least focally, resulting in an umbilicourachal sinus, vesicourachal sinus, or diverticulum. In the blind variant, the urachus is closed at both ends but remains patent in the middle segment. Rarely, calculi form in the cavities of urachal malformations. In patients with a vesicourachal sinus, the stone is chemically similar to typical vesical calculi. The surgical pathologist rarely encounters biopsy or tissue specimens of a patent urachus.

2.2.2 Urachal Remnants and Cysts

A patent urachus usually presents at birth, but other urachal remnants may present during late childhood or adulthood (Berman et al, 1988; Sterling & Goldsmith, 1953). The most common problems with urachal remnants are infection and cyst formation (Eble, 1989; Newman et al, 1986). Patients present with abdominal pain and symptoms of urinary tract infection; this latter

17

symptom is particularly common when there is communication of the urachal remnant with the bladder or umbilicus. Severe cases may present with rupture of an infected urachal cyst in the peritoneal cavity with resultant peritonitis (Nair, 1987). The most common organism cultured in urachal cyst fluid is *Staphylococcus aureus*.

A urachal cyst may occur at any level of the urachus and may be small and incidental or large and compressive (Fig 2.2). The cyst may be intramural and unilocular or multilocular. Smaller cysts are commonly lined by urothelium or cuboidal cells, but columnar epithelium may also be seen (Nair, 1987). Larger cysts are usually lined by flattened atrophic epithelium (Fig 2.3). When infected, the cyst lining may be lost, and the wall replaced with granulation and scar tissue. Large urachal diverticula such as those in prune-belly syndrome may require resection because of urethral obstruction. The urachus and its remnants may also be involved in tuberculosis, echinococcus, and actinomycosis.

2.3 INFLAMMATORY AND RELATED CONDITIONS IN CHILDREN

Inflammatory and reactive conditions in the bladder of children are encountered most frequently by the pathologist at postmortem examination. Often, these children have an indwelling catheter or have undergone instrumentation. The catheter tip may traumatize the mucosa in the trigone and posterior bladder wall, producing ulceration and secondary epithelial proliferation with atypia and other changes typical of proliferative cystitis. The catheter may act as a conduit for the introduction of bacteria and other organisms.

Cystitis in a child is histologically identical to that occurring in the adult, and all forms of cystitis have been encountered (Geist & Antolak, 1970). Inflammation of the bladder is more common in children than would be ex-

pected given the small number of bladder biopsies submitted for histologic examination. The indications for bladder biopsy are similar to those in an adult, including unexplained hematuria, voiding difficulties, or a lower abdominal mass (Yadin, 1994). Often, the biopsy reveals nonspecific inflammation and reactive mucosal changes. Nonspecific histologic changes in the bladder of children include edema, focal hemorrhage, vascular ectasia, and variable amounts of acute and chronic inflammation. The inflammation is often less impressive than the other findings.

Hemorrhagic cystitis is an uncommon form of acute cystitis characterized by hemorrhage, fibrin deposition, and necrosis (Numazaki et al, 1968). Occasionally, this may be caused by adenovirus type II (Chang, 1970; Goldman & Warner, 1970; Mufson et al, 1973). It is often difficult to identify intranuclear inclusions characteristic of the organism because of mucosal sloughing (Hashida et al, 1976). The lamina propria contains aggregates of lymphocytes surrounded by erythrocytes, reminiscent of follicular cystitis. Hemorrhagic cystitis may also be caused by cytomegalovirus, with typical intranuclear and cytoplasmic inclusions within endothelial cells and macrophages (Chang, 1970; Cos et al, 1982). Hemorrhagic cystitis may also result from cyclophosphamide and its metabolites with direct cytotoxic changes within the mucosa (Berkson et al, 1973). About 8% of children who receive cyclophosphamide weekly for acute lymphocytic leukemia or other diseases develop sterile hematuria. Macroscopically, the bladder wall is thick and boggy, with blood clots in the lumen and diffusely hemorrhagic, friable, and ulcerated mucosa. Numerous ectatic blood vessels are present in the lamina propria, some with fibrin thrombi or evidence of necrosis. There may be a striking paucity of inflammatory cells, but eosinophils and atypical multinucleated cells may be ob-

(a)

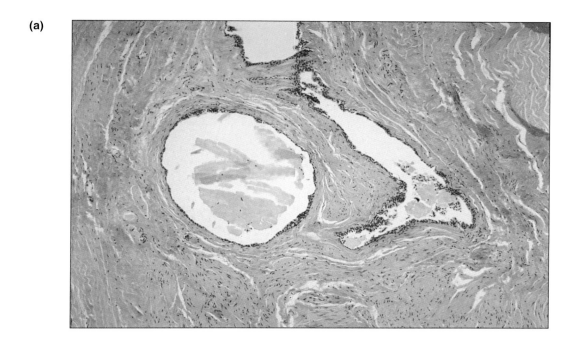

(b)

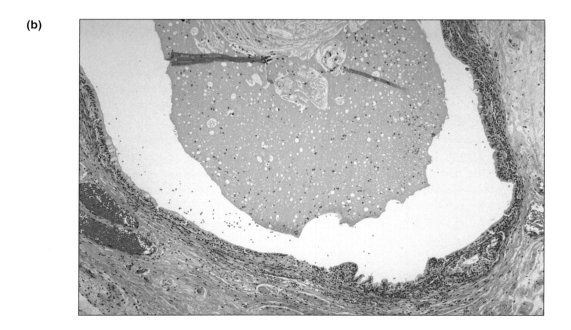

Figure 2.2 Urachal cyst. **(a):** This intramural segment of urachus with mild cystic dilatation was an incidental finding at autopsy. Compare with **(b)**, a symptomatic urachal cyst with marked dilatation.

19

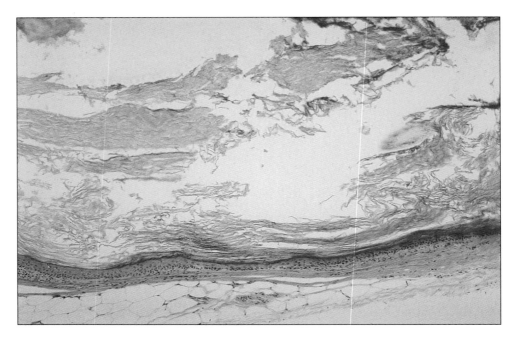

Figure 2.3 This large cyst in the dome of the bladder is lined by keratinizing squamous epithelium. Clinically, it was thought to be urachal in origin.

served. The urothelium often displays marked cytologic abnormalities thought to be regenerative and not neoplastic. A late finding is the presence of interstitial fibrosis within the wall.

Children may also develop eosinophilic or follicular cystitis, usually with no specific causative agent (Sutphin & Middelton, 1984). Eosinophilic cystitis may result from Toxocara, but the typical necrotizing eosinophilic granulomas of toxocariasis are absent in the bladder (Perlmutter et al, 1968).

Interstitial cystitis (Hunner's ulcer) most often occurs in middle-aged women, but it has been occasionally observed in children, usually with the same clinical manifestations.

Granulomatous cystitis in children is rare, and patients should be evaluated for the possibility of mycobacterial, fungal, or parasitic infection (Ehrlich & Lattimer, 1971; Wishahi et al, 1984). In endemic regions, where *Schis-tosoma haematobium* exposure occurs in children in a large percentage of the population, bilharziosis results (Johnson et al, 1967). The ova are typically deep in the bladder wall, and a superficial biopsy may be negative.

Chronic granulomatous disease in childhood may include chronic cystitis with characteristic palisading necrotizing granulomas and central collections of neutrophils (Cyr et al, 1973). Some cases are associated with prominent bullous cystitis.

Crohn's disease may occur in children or young adults, involving the bladder by contiguous spread of fistulas and inflammatory tracts from the adjacent bowel mucosa. Endoscopy reveals polypoid masses in the dome, and biopsies reveal acute inflammation and edema of the lamina propria with scattered epithelioid histiocytes. Rarely, there may be a terminal ileal stricture.

Malacoplakia is uncommon in children.

2.4 RUPTURE AND CALCULI IN CHILDREN

Rupture of the bladder is rare in children. It usually results from blunt trauma with or without pelvic fracture. Although most ruptures occur into the extraperitoneal space in adults, intraperitoneal rupture with disruption of the dome is more common in children. Rarely, rupture presents as neonatal urinary ascites secondary to spontaneous perforation of the bladder. The presence of posterior urethral valves creates increased intravesical pressure in the majority of such patients.

Bladder calculi in children in the United States and Europe are very uncommon (Carson & Malek, 1982; Dalens et al, 1982). Causative factors include foreign body, *Proteus mirabilis* infection, exstrophy, proliferative cystitis, and neurogenic bladder. Most stones consist of calcium oxalate or a mixture of oxalate and calcium phosphate.

2.5 PEDIATRIC NON-NEOPLASTIC EPITHELIAL AND POLYPOID LESIONS

Children are prone to an uncommon and heterogeneous group of lesions that sometimes form a mass, occasionally with exophytic growth. Proliferative cystitis is one of these lesions, resulting from chronic irritation, exstrophy, or unknown factors. The spectrum of proliferative cystitis includes Brunn's nests, cystitis cystica, and cystitis glandularis (Aabech & Lien, 1982). These changes may be limited to the trigone but, when large, may resemble sarcoma botryoides, although they usually are small. Girls with chronic urinary tract infection are most likely to have proliferative cystitis, particularly cystitis cystica, with a frequency ranging from 2.5% to 22%.

Squamous metaplasia is rare in children, but some of the most dramatic examples reported occurred in children with exstrophy or schistosomiasis (Morgan & Cameron, 1980).

Nephrogenic metaplasia is an uncommon finding in children and usually follows manipulation, instrumentation, or trauma of the bladder (Oliva & Young, 1995). Patients present with hematuria, urgency, dysuria, and secondary enuresis. Interestingly, it is found exclusively in the bladder in children, but the histologic findings are otherwise similar to those in the adult (Schumacher et al, 1997). Transurethral resection is the treatment of choice.

Very few cases of hamartoma of the urinary bladder and prostatic-type polyps have occurred in children (Nuovo et al, 1986; Remik & Kumar, 1984). One interesting case arose in a 4-year-old girl with Peutz–Jeghers syndrome–like lesions in the colon, and two other cases occurred in brothers (Sommerhaug & Mason, 1970). A fibroepithelial polyp is a distinct entity that usually arises in the proximal ureter and even more uncommonly in the bladder (Davides & King, 1976; Eilenberg et al, 1977; Van Poppel et al, 1986). In one case, the fibroepithelial polyp of the bladder neck arose in an infant with Beckwith–Wiedemann syndrome. Most polyps measure less than 2 cm in diameter and have a smooth surface of normal urothelium and supporting stroma of hypocellular fibrous connective tissue. In small biopsies, this lesion may be mistaken for embryonal rhabdomyosarcoma, particularly if the submucosal stromal cells are prominent and condensed in the subepithelial area. However, the stromal cells of a fibroepithelial polyp appear benign, although exceptionally they have a pseudosarcomatous appearance. Adenomatous polyp also rarely occurs in children (Rubin et al, 1981).

Inflammatory myofibroblastic tumor (inflammatory pseudotumor) of the bladder is another rare lesion that is more common in adults than children (Dehner, 1987; Hojo et al, 1995; Lopez-Beltran et al, 1995; Nochomovitz & Orenstein, 1985; Varsano et al, 1975). When the bladder is involved, the differential diagnostic considerations include postoperative spindle cell nodule, myogenic tumor, and sarcoma. The tumor often presents as a large intramural or exophytic mass in the bladder. Microscopically, the spindle cell proliferation is variably cellular with chronic inflammation composed chiefly of lymphocytes and plasma cells with prominent edema and a focally prominent vascular network. Some mitotic figures may be identified, but no atypical forms are present. Ultrastructurally, the spindle cells have the same features as myofibroblasts elsewhere in the body. These cells are immunoreactive for vimentin and muscle-specific actin but do not stain for desmin or myoglobin. We find the inflammatory infiltrate to be diagnostically useful, and embryonal rhabdomyosarcoma is an important diagnostic consideration, but this tumor usually has small neoplastic cells that are uniform, with densely hyperchromatic nuclei, and intensely eosinophilic cytoplasm, often with a cambium layer. Immunohistochemistry and electron microscopy may be of value in difficult cases.

2.6 PEDIATRIC NEOPLASMS

2.6.1 Benign Pediatric Neoplasms

Most benign tumors in children involving the bladder arise in the soft tissue (Table 2.1). The most common is a hemangioma, which usually arises in the first two decades of life. More than 30% of children with a hemangioma have a similar lesion elsewhere in the body (Van Dessel & Michielsen, 1978). Hemangioma appears as a solitary polypoid lesion in the dome or trigone but rarely presents as a diffuse multilobular vasoformative proliferation within the wall of the bladder with involvement of the bowel, mesentery, and retroperitoneum. The vascular spaces are variable in appearance but usually appear as small crowded capillary masses. Cavernous hemangioma consists of large vascular spaces, often with thrombi (Lee et al, 1995). An epithe-

lioid hemangioma is rare in childhood, as is diffuse lymphangiomatosis (Caro & Brown, 1976).

The second most common soft tissue tumor of childhood is neurofibroma. This tumor is more common in boys than girls and is an expression of Recklinghausen's neurofibromatosis (Clark et al, 1977). These children often have other sites of genitourinary tract involvement. Grossly, the bladder is enlarged and contains multiple glistening nodules in the wall accompanied by broad polypoid masses protruding into the lumen. Microscopically, the lamina propria shows diffuse replacement by nodules of neurofibroma (Kramer et al, 1981). Plexiform bundles of neurofibromatous tissue are characteristic and may separate and compress the smooth muscle of the muscularis propria. Another less common histologic pattern of genitourinary neurofibromatosis is extensive ganglioneuromatosis similar to that in the intestinal tract.

Primary paraganglioma of the bladder is very rare (Rahman et al, 1995). Other rare tumors of the bladder include leiomyoma (Mutchler & Gorder, 1972), granular cell tumor, and dermoid cyst (Bhargava et al, 1977).

2.6.2 Malignant Pediatric Neoplasms

2.6.2.1 Rhabdomyosarcoma

Seventy-five percent of malignant tumors of the bladder in children are rhabdomyosarcoma

Table 2.1 Bladder tumors in childhood (in descending order of frequency)

Rhabdomyosarcoma (> 75%)
Hemangioma
Neurofibroma
Urothelial carcinoma
Leiomyoma
Leukemia/lymphoma (secondary)
Others

(Fleischmann et al, 1981; Geary et al, 1994). The average age at diagnosis is 5 years, and there is a predominance of boys to girls (3:2 ratio). The urinary bladder was the primary site in only 5% of cases submitted to the Intergroup Rhabdomyosarcoma Study (Hartley et al, 1993; Heyn et al, 1993; Raney et al, 1993). Bladder neck obstruction with or without hematuria is the usual presenting symptom. Because of the limited anatomic space in the pelvis and the juxtaposition of anatomic structures, it is sometimes difficult to determine whether the sarcoma originated in the prostate and extended superiorly into the bladder neck or, alternatively, whether it arose in the retroperitoneum and invaded the bladder and vagina (Geary et al, 1994). When the tumor presents as multiple polypoid masses in the lumen of the bladder, there is no difficulty in assignment of the primary site of origin. Long-term survival for genitourinary rhabdomyosarcoma is 55%–80% (Dehner, 1987).

Microscopically, rhabdomyosarcoma of the bladder may have the appearance of sarcoma botryoides, consisting of multiple glistening polypoid masses containing condensed rhabdomyoblasts immediately beneath the epithelium and an edematous stroma with dispersed malignant stromal cells (Fig 2.4). Another pattern of rhabdomyosarcoma consists of a large solitary mass that bulges into the bladder and may replace the wall. In such cases, this sarcoma has a more variable histology with typical embryonal rhabdomyosarcoma alternating with spindle and alveolar-like areas (Fleischmann et al, 1981; Leuschner et al, 1993). Recently, a new international rhabdomyosarcoma classification has been reported (Newton et al, 1995). Histologically recognizable types are assigned to one of three prognostic groups (Table 2.2) (Coffin, 1997).

Microscopically, the different patterns of rhabdomyosarcoma may merge with each other and appear diffuse. Ultrastructural and immunohistochemical studies are useful as confirmatory tests of the diagnosis but may not be necessary in typical classic cases. Rare cases of rhabdomyosarcoma contain well-differentiated rhabdomyoblasts with deceptively low-grade cytologic features, striking eosinophilic cytoplasm, and well-formed cross-striations. Such tumors may resemble rhabdomyoma, but this tumor has not been reported to date in the childhood bladder, and these are considered well-differentiated embryonal rhabdomyosarcoma. Similar findings can be encountered after a full course of chemotherapy, with residual sarcoma cells appearing as large rhabdomyoblasts or rhabdomyocytes.

Differential diagnostic considerations for rhabdomyosarcoma include leiomyosarcoma and inflammatory pseudotumor. Leiomyosarcoma can be effectively excluded because it virtually never occurs in the first two decades of life (Borzi & Frank, 1994; Weitzner, 1978). Furthermore, the histologic findings should be useful in making this distinction; in difficult cases, ancillary studies may be of value.

2.6.2.2 Urothelial Carcinoma in Children

Urothelial carcinoma is very uncommon in children, and the majority of such cases appear between 15 and 20 years of age (Benson et al, 1983). Most cases arise as solitary papillary lesions in the trigone or lateral wall (Curtis et al, 1996; Hoenig et al, 1996). With rare exceptions, urothelial tumors in children are low-grade carcinoma or papilloma occasionally associated with lymphangiectasia (Bruce, 1982; Punjani, 1983; Refsum & Refsum, 1975; Waaler et al, 1975; Williams et al, 1986; Yanase et al, 1991). The differential diagnostic considerations include papillary hyperplasia, polypoid cystitis, and inverted papilloma (Francis, 1979). Occasionally, urothelial carcinoma may be associated with the epidermal nevus syndrome. Isolated examples of inverted papilloma have also been reported in children (DeMeester et al, 1975; Lorentzen & Rohr, 1979).

(a)

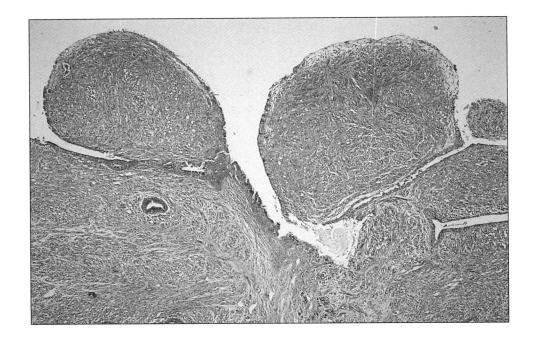

(b)

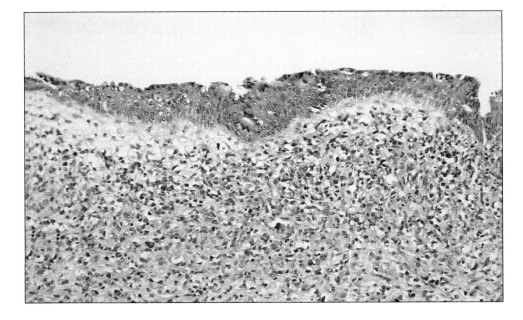

(c)

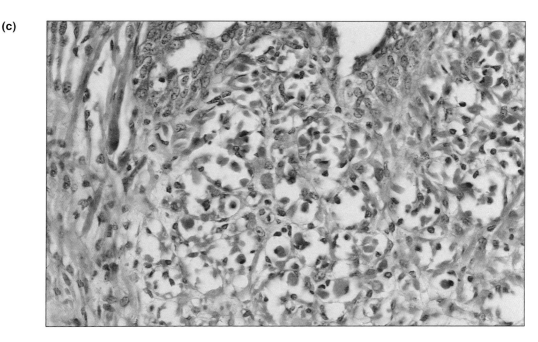

Figure 2.4 Rhabdomyosarcoma of the bladder. **(a):** Polypoid masses of tumor, characteristic of a botryoides growth pattern; **(b):** intact urothelium with underlying cambium layer of malignant spindle cells; **(c):** diagnostic malignant rhabdomyoblasts are present.

2.6.2.3 Other Bladder Carcinomas in Children

Squamous cell carcinoma and adenocarcinoma of the bladder are even less common than urothelial carcinoma in children (Brumskine et al, 1977; Castellanos et al, 1975; Chandy et al, 1975; Gupta & Gupta, 1976; Nielsen & Nielsen, 1983; Raghavaiah & Reddy, 1976). Germ cell tumors of the bladder in children are rare, with reported cases of dermoid cyst (Bhargava et al, 1977) and endodermal sinus tumor (yolk sac tumor) (Taylor et al, 1983). The childhood bladder may also be a rare site for involvement by leukemia and lymphoma (Givler, 1971; Grooms et al, 1973; Lewis et al, 1983). Very rarely, there may be metastases to the bladder, including Wilms' tumor (Candia & Zegel, 1982; Taykurt, 1972).

2.6.2.4 Endodermal Sinus Tumor (Yolk Sac Tumor) of the Bladder

Yolk sac tumor of the bladder is extremely rare. One case arose in a 1-year-old boy as a polypoid, hemorrhagic, gelatinous, necrotic mass (Taylor et al, 1983). Histologically, it contained solid and cystic areas with cuboidal and columnar cells displaying eosinophilic to clear cytoplasm. Schiller-Duval bodies and hyaline globules were present. He underwent a partial cystectomy, pelvic lymph node dissection, and chemotherapy and, at 4 months after all treatment, showed no evidence of recurrence (Taylor et al, 1983). Another case, in a 2-year-old boy, arose in apparent urachal remnants and was entirely removed; the boy was tumor-free after 3 years (D'Alessio et al, 1994).

Table 2.2 International classification of rhab-domyosarcoma

I. Superior prognosis
   A. Botryoid rhabdomyosarcoma
   B. Spindle cell rhabdomyosarcoma
II. Intermediate prognosis
   A. Embryonal rhabdomyosarcoma
III. Poor prognosis
   A. Alveolar rhabdomyosarcoma
   B. Undifferentiated sarcoma
IV. Subtypes whose prognosis is not presently evaluable
   A. Rhabdomyosarcoma with rhabdoid features

2.6.2.5 *Rhabdoid Tumor of the Bladder*

Fewer than five cases of primary rhabdoid tumor have been described in the bladder, including one with coexistent urothelial carcinoma (Carter et al, 1989; Harris et al, 1987).

2.7 RENAL PELVIS AND URETER

Duplication, ectopia, ureteral agenesis (Brannan & Henry, 1973), ureterocele, and obstructive lesions are the most common types of ureteral malformations. More than one abnormality may be present, resulting in a complex anomaly. Ureteral duplication is most likely to be partial and unilateral. Ureteral ectopia with or without duplication is a common cause of vesico-ureteral reflux. The ectopic insertion may be located in the rectum, vagina, urethra, or abnormally situated in the bladder. Ureteral agenesis virtually always accompanies renal agenesis. Ureterocele is a marked dilatation of the intravesical portion of the distal ureter at its orifice. Ureteral obstruction may involve any portion of the urinary tract but is most frequent at the ureteropelvic junction. Inflammatory lesions of the renal pelvis and ureter are generally an extension of pyelonephritis or reflux nephropathy (Le Guillou et al, 1980). Neoplastic lesions of the upper urinary tract are exceedingly uncommon in children (Werth et al, 1981). Fibroepithelial polyp is an uncommon benign lesion of the ureter (Crawford et al, 1979; Naucler et al, 1983; Van Poppel et al, 1986). Rhabdomyosarcoma and urothelial carcinoma may rarely be found in the ureter (Punjani, 1983).

2.8 URETHRA

Duplication of the urethra may occur with complex rectal and urogenital malformations. Obstructive lesions of the lower urinary tract include posterior urethral valves, urethral stenosis, or atresia (Presman et al, 1972). Benign tumors of the lower urinary tract are infrequent in children. Inflammatory or fibrovascular polyps are noted occasionally in the urethra. Other tumors include leiomyoma, neurofibroma, and paraganglioma (Boyle et al, 1996). Malignant tumors of the urethra in children are very rare.

REFERENCES

Aabech HS, Lien EN. Cystitis cystica in childhood: clinical findings and treatment procedures. *Acta Paediatr Scand.* 1982;71:247–252.

Benson RC Jr, Tomera KM, Kelalis PP. Transitional cell carcinoma of the bladder in children and adolescents. *J Urol.* 1983;130:54–55.

Berkson BM, Lome LG, Shapiro I. Severe cystitis induced by cyclophosphamide. Role of surgical management. *JAMA.* 1973;225:605–606.

Berman SM, Tolia BM, Laor E, et al. Urachal remnants in adults. *Urology.* 1988;31:17–21.

Beynon J, Zwink R, Chow W, et al. The late presentation of adenocarcinoma in bladder exstrophy. *Br J Surg.* 1985;72:989–995.

Bhargava SK, Pal V, Lakhtakia HS, et al. Dermoid cyst of the urinary bladder. *Ind Pediatr.* 1977;14:161–162.

Borzi PA, Frank JD. Bladder leiomyosarcoma in a child: a 6 year follow-up. *Br J Urol.* 1994;73:219–220.

Boyle M, Gaffney EF, Thurston A. Paraganglioma of the prostatic urethra. A report of three cases and a review of the literature. *Br J Urol.* 1996;77:445–448.

Brannan W, Henry HH II. Ureteral ectopia: report of 39 cases. *J Urol.* 1973;109:192–195.

Bruce PT. Bladder papilloma in young patients. *Med J Aust.* 1982;1:43–45.

Brumskine W, Dragan P, Sanvee L. Transitional cell carcinoma and schistosomiasis in a 5-year-old boy. *Br J Urol.* 1977;49:540–546.

Candia A, Zegel HG. The occurrence of Wilms' tumor in 2 patients with exstrophy of the bladder. *J Urol.* 1982;128:589–590.

Caro DJ, Brown JS. Hemangioma of bladder. *Urology.* 1976;7:479–481.

Carson CC III, Malek RS. Observations on lower urinary tract calculi in children. *J Urol.* 1982;127:977–978.

Carter RL, McCarthy KP, Al-Sam SZ, et al. Malignant rhabdoid tumor of the bladder with immunohistochemical and ultrastructural evidence suggesting histologic origin. *Histopathology.* 1989;14:179–190.

Carter TC, Tomskey GR, Ozog LS. Prune-belly syndrome. Review of ten cases. *Urology.* 1974;3:279–282.

Castellanos RD, Wakefield PB, Evans AT. Carcinoma of the bladder in children. *J Urol.* 1975;113:261–263.

Chandy PC, Pai MG, Budihal MR, et al. Carcinoma of the bladder in young children: report of 2 cases. *J Urol.* 1975;113:264–265.

Chang SC. Urinary cytologic diagnosis of cytomegalic inclusion disease in childhood leukemia. *Acta Cytol.* 1970;14:338–343.

Chatterjee SK, Sarkar SK. Retrovesical cysts in boys. *J Urol.* 1973;109:107–110.

Cheng EY, Maizels M. Complete duplication of the bladder and urethra in the coronal plane: case report. *J Urol.* 1996;155:1414–1415.

Clark SS, Marlett MM, Prudencio RF, et al. Neurofibromatosis of the bladder in children: case report and literature review. *J Urol.* 1977;118:654–656.

Coffin CM. The new international rhabdomyosarcoma classification, its progenitors, and consideration beyond morphology. *Adv Anat Pathol.* 1997;4:1–16.

Cos LR, Rabinowitz R, Bryson MF, et al. Hereditary hemorrhagic telangiectasia of bladder in a child. *Urology.* 1982;20:302–304.

Crawford DB, Levinson ED, Henken EM, et al. Fibroepithelial ureteric polyps. *Br J Radiol.* 1979;52:913–916.

Culp DA. The histology of the exstrophied bladder. *J Urol.* 1964;91:538.

Curtis M, Schned A, Hakim S, et al. Papillary transitional cell carcinoma of the bladder with lymphangiectasia in an 8-year-old boy. *J Urol.* 1996;156:202–204.

Cyr WL, Johnson H, Balfour J. Granulomatous cystitis as a manifestation of chronic granulomatous disease of childhood. *J Urol.* 1973;110:357–360.

Dalens B, Vanneuville G, Vincent L, et al. Congenital polyp of the posterior urethra and vesical calculus in a boy. *J Urol.* 1982;128:1034–1035.

D'Alessio A, Verdelli G, Bernardi M, et al. Endodermal sinus (yolk sac) tumor of the urachus. *Eur J Pediatr Surg.* 1994;4:180–181.

Davides KG, King LM. Fibrous polyps of the ureter. *J Urol.* 1976;115:651–653.

Dehner LP. Lower genitourinary system. In: *Pediatric surgical pathology* (2nd ed). Chapter 10. Baltimore, MD: Williams & Wilkins;1987:693–711.

DeMeester LJ, Farrow GM, Utz DC. Inverted papillomas of the urinary bladder. *Cancer.* 1975;36:505–513.

De Reise W, Warmbold H. Adenocarcinoma in exstrophy of the bladder: a case report and review of the literature. *Int Urol Nephrol.* 1986;18:159–162.

Diamond DA, Jeffs RD. Cloacal exstrophy: a 22-year experience. *J Urol.* 1985;133:779–782.

Dunetz GN, Bauer SB. Complete duplication of bladder and urethra. *Urology.* 1985;25:179–181.

Eble JN. Abnormalities of the urachus. In: Young RH, ed. *Pathology of the urinary bladder.* New York: Churchill Livingstone;1989:213–243.

Ehrlich RM, Lattimer JK. Urogenital tuberculosis in children. *J Urol.* 1971;105:461–465.

Eilenberg J, Seery W, Cole A. Multiple fibroepithelial polyps in the pediatric age group: case report. *J Urol.* 1977;117:793–795.

Feins NR, Cranley W. Bladder duplication with one exstrophy and one cloaca. *J Pediatr Surg.* 1986;21:570–572.

Fleischmann J, Perinetti EP, Catalona WJ. Embryonal rhabdomyosarcoma of the genitourinary organs. *J Urol.* 1981;126:389–392.

Francis RR. Inverted papilloma in a 14-year-old male. *Br J Urol.* 1979;51:327–329.

Geary ES, Gong MC, Shortliffe LM. Biology and treatment of pediatric genitourinary tumors. *Curr Op Oncol.* 1994;6:292–300.

Geist RW, Antolak SJ Jr. Interstitial cystitis in children. *J Urol.* 1970;104:922–925.

Givler RL. Involvement of the bladder in leukemia and lymphoma. *J Urol.* 1971;105:667–670.

Goldman RL, Warner NE. Hemorrhagic cystitis and cytomegalic inclusions in the bladder associated with cyclophosphamide therapy. *Cancer.* 1970;25:7–11.

Grooms AM, Morgan SK, Turner WR Jr. Hematuria and leukemic bladder infiltration. *JAMA.* 1973;223:193–194.

Gupta S, Gupta IM. Ectopia vesicae complicated by squamous cell carcinoma. *Br J Urol.* 1976;48:244–247.

Harris M, Eyden BP, Joglekar VM. Rhabdoid tumor of the bladder: a histological, ultrastructural and immunohistochemical study. *Histopathology.* 1987;11:1083–1092.

Hartley AL, Birch JM, Blair V, et al. Patterns of cancer in the families of children with soft tissue sarcoma. *Cancer.* 1993;72:923–930.

Hashida Y, Gaffney PC, Yunis EJ. Acute hemorrhagic cystitis of childhood and papovavirus-like particles. *J Pediatr.* 1976;89:85–87.

Herlihy RE, Barnes WF. Neonatal vesical necrosis and perforation secondary to posterior urethral valves. *J Urol.* 1985;133:476–477.

Heyn R, Haeberlen V, Newton WA, et al. Second malignant neoplasms in children treated for rhabdomyosarcoma: Intergroup Rhabdomyosarcoma Study Committee. *J Clin Oncol.* 1993;11:262–270.

Higgins CC. Exstrophy of the bladder: report of 158 cases. *Ann Surg.* 1962;28:99–110.

Hoenig DM, McRae S, Chen SC, et al. Transitional cell carcinoma of the bladder in the pediatric patient. *J Urol.* 1996;156:203–205.

Hojo H, Newton WA Jr, Hamoudi AB, et al. Pseudosarcomatous myofibroblastic tumor of the urinary bladder in children: a study of 11 cases with review of the literature. An intergroup rhabdomyosarcoma study. *Am J Surg Pathol.* 1995;19:1224–1236.

Inamdar S, Mallouh C, Ganguly R. Vesical gigantism or congenital megacystis. *Urology.* 1984;24:601–603.

Ives E, Coffey R, Carter CO. A family study of bladder exstrophy. *J Med Genet.* 1980;17:139–141.

Jeffs RD. Exstrophy and cloacal exstrophy. *Urol Clin N Am.* 1978;5:127–140.

Johnson HW, Elliott GD, Israels S, et al. Granulomatous cystitis of children, bilharzia-like, occurring in British Columbia. *Pediatrics.* 1967;40:808–815.

Kapoor R, Saha MM. Complete duplication of the bladder, urethra and external genitalia in a neonate: a case report. *J Urol.* 1987;137:1243–1244.

Kramer SA, Barrett DM, Utz DC. Neurofibromatosis of the bladder in children. *J Urol.* 1981;126:693–694.

Lee KW, Rodo J, Margarit J, et al. Cavernous haemangioma of the bladder in a child. *Br J Urol.* 1995;75:799–801.

Le Guillou M, Richard F, L'Henaff F, et al. Bilateral ureteral necrosis in a child with dermatomyositis. *Eur Urol.* 1980;6:190–191.

Leuschner I, Newton WA Jr, Schmidt D, et al. Spindle cell variants of embryonal rhabdomyosarcoma in the paratesticular region: a report of the Intergroup Rhabdomyosarcoma Study. *Am J Surg Pathol.* 1993;17:221–230.

Lewis RH, Mannarino FG, Worsham GF, et al. Burkitt's lymphoma presenting as urinary outflow obstruction. *J Urol.* 1983;130:120–124.

Livne PM, Gonzales ET Jr. Congenital bladder diverticula causing ureteral obstruction. *Urology.* 1985;25:273–276.

Lopez-Beltran A, Lopez-Ruiz J, Vicioso L. Inflammatory pseudotumors of the urinary bladder. *Urol Int.* 1995;55:173–176.

Lorentzen M, Rohr N. Urinary bladder tumours in children. Case report of inverted papilloma. *Scand J Urol Nephrol.* 1979;13:323–327.

Metoki R, Orikasa S, Ohta, et al. A case of bladder agenesis. *J Urol.* 1986;136:662–664.

Morgan RJ, Cameron KM. Vesical leukoplakia. *Br J Urol.* 1980;52:96–100.

Mufson MA, Belshe RB, Horrigan TJ, et al. Cause of acute hemorrhagic cystitis in children. *Am J Dis Child.* 1973;126:605–609.

Mutchler RW Jr, Gorder JL. Leiomyoma of the bladder in a child. *Br J Radiol.* 1972;45:538–540.

Nair KP. Mucous metaplasia and rupture of urachal cyst as a rare cause of acute abdomen. *Br J Urol.* 1987;59:281–282.

Naucler J, Johansson SL, Nilson AE, et al. Fibroepithelial polyp of the ureter. *Scand J Urol Nephrol.* 1983;17:379–383.

Newman BM, Karp MP, Jewett TC, et al. Advances in the management of infected urachal cysts. *J Pediatr Surg.* 1986;21:1051–1054.

Newton WA Jr, Gehan EA, Webber BL. Classification of rhabdomyosarcomas and related sarcomas: pathologic aspects and proposal for a new classification—an Intergroup Rhabdomyosarcoma study. *Cancer.* 1995;76:1073–1085.

Nielsen K, Nielsen KK. Adenocarcinoma in exstrophy of the bladder: the last case in Scandinavia? A case report and review of literature. *J Urol.* 1983;130:1180–1182.

Nix JT, Menville JG, Albert M, et al. Congenital patent urachus. *J Urol.* 1958;79:264–269.

Nochomovitz LE, Orenstein JM. Inflammatory pseudotumor of the urinary bladder: possible relationship to nodular fasciitis. Two case reports, cytologic observations, and ultrastructural observations. *Am J Surg Pathol.* 1985;9:366–373.

Numazaki Y, Shigeta S, Kumasaka T, et al. Acute hemorrhagic cystitis in children. Isolation of adenovirus type II. *N Engl J Med.* 1968;278:700–704.

Nuovo GJ, Nagler HM, Fenoglio JJ Jr. Arteriovenous malformation of the bladder presenting as gross hematuria. *Hum Pathol.* 1986;17:94–97.

Oliva E, Young RH. Nephrogenic adenoma of the urinary tract: a review of the microscopic appearance of 80 cases with emphasis on unusual features. *Mod Pathol.* 1995;8:722–730.

Palmer JM, Russi MF. Persistent urogenital sinus with absence of the bladder and urethra. *J Urol.* 1969;102:590–594.

Parker C. Cystitis cystica and glandularis: a study of 40 cases. *Proc R Soc Med Engl.* 1970;63:239–242.

Perlmutter AD, Edlow JB, Kevy SV. Toxocara antibodies in eosinophilic cystitis. *J Pediatr.* 1968;73:340–344.

Peterson LJ, Paulson DF, Glenn JF. The histopathology of vesical diverticula. *J Urol.* 1973;110:62–64.

Presman D, Ross LS, Nicosia SV. Fibromuscular hyperplasia of the posterior urethra: a cause for lower urinary tract obstruction in male children. *J Urol.* 1972;107:149–153.

Punjani HM. Transitional cell papilloma of the ureter causing hydronephrosis in a child. *Br J Urol.* 1983;55:572–573.

Raghavaiah NV, Reddy CR. Adenocarcinoma of the bladder in a boy. *J Urol.* 1976;116:526–528.

Rahman SI, Matthews LK, Shaikh H, et al. Primary paraganglioma of the bladder in a 14-year-old boy. *Br J Urol.* 1995;75:682–683.

Rajan N, Makhuli ZN, Humphrey DM, et al. Metastatic umbilical transitional cell carcinoma from a bladder diverticulum. *J Urol.* 1996;155:1700–1702.

Raney B Jr, Heyn R, Hays DM, et al. Sequeale of treatment in 109 patients followed for 5 to 15 years after diagnosis of sarcoma of the bladder and prostate: a report from the Intergroup Rhabdomyosarcoma Study Committee. *Cancer.* 1993;71:2387–2394.

Refsum S Jr, Refsum SB. Bladder papilloma in a child. Case report. *Scand J Urol Nephrol.* 1975;9:285–288.

Remick DG Jr, Kumar NB. Benign polyps with prostatic-type epithelium of the urethra and the urinary bladder. A suggestion of histogenesis based on histologic and immunohistochemical studies. *Am J Surg Pathol.* 1984;8:833–839.

Rubin J, Khanna OP, Damjanov I. Adenomatous polyp of the bladder: a rare cause of hematuria in young men. *J Urol.* 1981;126:549–550.

Schumacher K, Heimbach D, Bruhl P. Nephrogenic adenoma in children. Case report and review of literature. *Eur J Pediatr Surg.* 1997;7:115–117.

Semerdjian HS, Texter JH, Yawn DH. Rhabdomyosarcoma occurring in repaired exstrophied bladder: a case report. *J Urol.* 1972;108:354–356.

Sommerhaug RG, Mason T. Peutz-Jeghers syndrome and ureteral polyposis. *JAMA.* 1970;211:120–122.

Sterling JA, Goldsmith R. Lesions of the urachus which appear in the adult. *Ann Surg.* 1953;137:120–132.

Sutphin M, Middelton AW. Eosinophilic cystitis in children: a self-limited process. *J Urol.* 1984;132:117–119.

Taykurt A. Wilms' tumor at lower end of the ureter extending to the bladder: case report. *J Urol.* 1972;107:142–143.

Taylor G, Jordan M, Churchill B, et al. Yolk sac tumor of the bladder. *J Urol.* 1983;129:591–594.

Vaage S, Foerster A, Gerhardt PG, et al. A complete pyelo-uretero-vesical duplication. *Scand J Urol Nephrol.* 1985;19:309–313.

Van Dessel J, Michielsen JP. The haemangioma of the bladder. Case report and review of the literature. *Acta Urol Belg.* 1978;46:369–377.

Van Poppel H, Nuttin B, Oyen R, et al. Fibroepithelial polyps of the ureter. Etiology, diagnosis, treatment and pathology. *Eur Urol.* 1986;12:174–179.

Varsano I, Savir A, Grunebaum M, et al. Inflammatory processes mimicking bladder tumors in children. *J Pediatr Surg.* 1975;10:909–912.

Waaler G, Schistad G, Serck-Hanssen A. Papillary urothelial tumor of the bladder in a child. *J Pediatr Surg.* 1975;10:841–842.

Weitzner S. Leiomyosarcoma of urinary bladder in children. *Urology.* 1978;12:450–452.

Werth DD, Weigel JW, Mebust WK. Primary neoplasms of the ureter. *J Urol.* 1981;125:628–631.

Williams JL, Cumming WA, Walter RD III, et al. Transitional cell papilloma of the bladder. *Pediatr Radiol.* 1986;16:322–323.

Wishahi MM, el-Sherbeni E, el-Baz H. Granulomatous cystitis: a reversible lesion in children. *Eur Urol.* 1984;10:368–369.

Yadin O. Hematuria in children. *Pediatr Ann.* 1994;23:474–478.

Yanase M, Tsukamoto T, Kumamoto Y, et al. Transitional cell carcinoma of the bladder or renal pelvis in children. *Eur Urol.* 1991;19:312–314.

3
INFLAMMATION

A wide variety of non-neoplastic inflammatory conditions may involve the bladder primarily or secondarily (Table 3.1).

3.1   ACUTE AND CHRONIC CYSTITIS

Most cases of acute and chronic cystitis result from infection with gram-negative coliform bacteria such as *Escherichia coli* (Fukushi et al, 1979; Parsons & Mulholland, 1978). The most common portal of entry is the urethra. Predisposing factors include structural abnormalities of the urinary bladder; systemic illnesses such as diabetes, diverticuli, and calculi; and any process or lesion that causes outflow obstruction. Infectious causes of cystitis include bacterial, viral, fungal, and protozoal agents. Irritative agents that cause cystitis include trauma from instrumentation and catheterization, radiation therapy, chemotherapy, bladder calculi, and chemical irritants such as formalin, turpentine, and ether (chemical cystitis) (Menon & Tan, 1992; O'Neill, 1994). Some cases of cystitis are of unknown etiology. Other forms of cystitis include interstitial, eosinophilic, and follicular cystitis (Marsh et al, 1974).

In early acute bacterial cystitis, there is vascular dilatation and congestion, erythematous

Table 3.1   Inflammatory conditions of the bladder and urothelium

Acute and chronic cystitis
   Polypoid
   Follicular
   Interstitial
   Eosinophilic
   Encrusted
   Emphysematous
   Gangrenous
   Hemorrhagic
   Viral
   Cystitis with atypical giant cells
   Denuding
Granulomatous cystitis
   Postsurgical
   Suture
   BCG-induced
   Schistosomiasis
   Malacoplakia
   Tuberculosis
   Xanthoma
   Other
Other infectious cystitides
   Fungal
   Actinomycosis
   Miscellaneous

and hemorrhagic mucosa, and moderate to severe edema. With time, polypoid or bullous cystitis may develop, sometimes with ulceration. The urothelium may be hyperplastic or metaplastic and, when ulcerated, is often covered by a fibrinous membrane with neutrophils and bacterial colonies. Stromal edema and chronic inflammation gradually become more pronounced, particularly in the lamina propria. If the acute inflammation persists, chronic cystitis usually develops, sometimes with prominent mural fibrosis.

In chronic cystitis, the mucosa may be thin, hyperplastic, or ulcerated, often with changes of reactive atypia (Fig 3.1). Granulation tissue is typically conspicuous in the early stages and may be replaced by dense scarring, particularly in the late healing stages. This process may be transmural and involve perivesicular tissue.

Recurrent lower urinary tract infections are common after menopause and occur in greater than 10% of women over 60 years of age. Urogenital atrophy is a late manifestation of menopause and is often underdiagnosed and undertreated. Postmenopausal cystitis results from a rise in vaginal pH and alteration of normal vaginal flora; however, not all postmenopausal cystitis is bacterial (Cardozo, 1996).

3.1.1 Polypoid Cystitis (Papillary Cystitis; Bullous Cystitis)

Polypoid cystitis may be clinically and microscopically mistaken for papillary urothelial carcinoma (Algaba, 1991; Buck, 1984). The designation *papillary cystitis* is used when thin, finger-like papillae are present, and *polypoid cystitis* refers to lesions with edematous and broad-based papillae (Fig 3.2). In both cases, there is typically abundant chronic inflammation in the stroma accompanied by prominent and often ectatic blood vessels. Sometimes the inflammation is not prominent, and the appearance varies from papillary or polypoid cystitis to bullous cystitis depending on the amount of stromal edema. In bullous cystitis, the lesion is wider than in polypoid and papillary cystitis (Young, 1988).

Exophytic growth of polypoid and papillary cystitis is most often confused with carcinoma (Algaba, 1991; Young, 1988). Occasionally, these cystitides may be associated with metaplastic changes in the overlying or adjacent urothelium. Less commonly, florid polypoid cystitis may suggest an inverted papilloma (Young, 1988). Two clinical settings suggest that an exophytic bladder lesion is reactive or inflammatory: (1) patients with an indwelling catheter (Milles, 1965), and (2) those with a vesical fistula (Young, 1988). Polypoid and bullous lesions are usually less than 0.5 cm in diameter, but larger macroscopically visible lesions may involve the dome or posterior wall. The entire bladder is sometimes involved when a catheter has been present for more than 6 months (Ekelund et al, 1983; Johnson et al, 1991; Young, 1988). Long-standing cases of polypoid cystitis may have a fibrous rather than edematous stroma. The mucosal changes associated with vesical fistula may have the characteristics of polypoid and papillary cystitis.

Polypoid cystitis should be differentiated from low-grade papillary urothelial carcinoma (Algaba, 1991). Important distinguishing features include the clinical history of catheterization and the presence of broad fronds in polypoid cystitis. Of greater diagnostic difficulty are the thin papillae of papillary cystitis, although the urothelium is usually not as thick as in carcinoma and umbrella cells are more common. The fibrovascular cores of the papillae of urothelial carcinoma typically have less inflammation and edema than polypoid cystitis, but exceptions have been observed (Grignon & Sakr, 1995). The urothelium adjacent to papillary carcinoma is often hyperplastic, and significant cytologic abnormalities within a papillary lesion or the adjacent urothelium favors the diagnosis of carcinoma (Young, 1988).

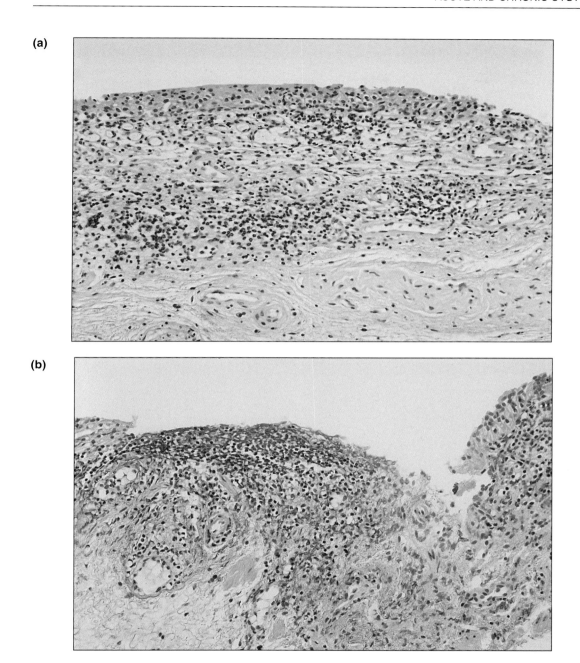

Figure 3.1 Chronic nonspecific cystitis. **(a):** The mucosa is intact but thinned, and the lamina propria contains a mixed chronic inflammatory infiltrate; **(b):** chronic cystitis with mucosal erosion.

(a)

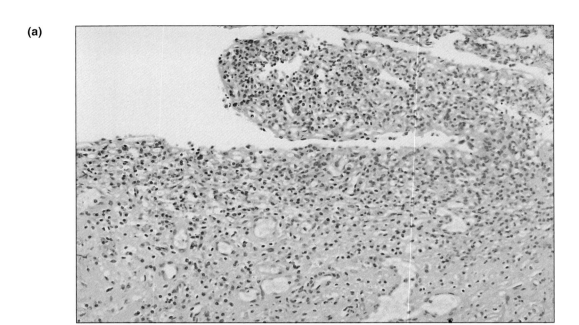

(b)

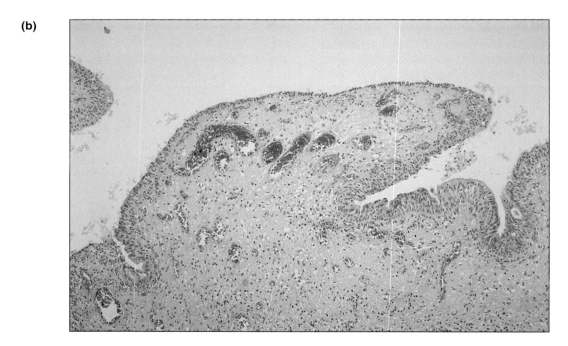

(c)

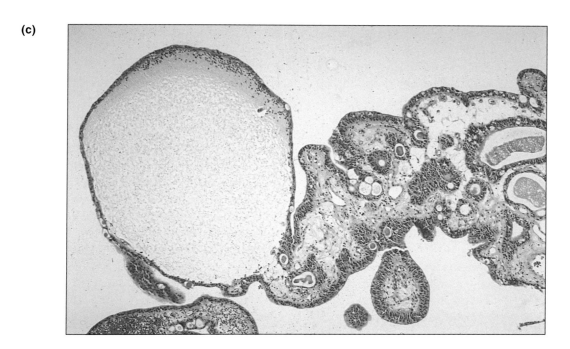

(d)

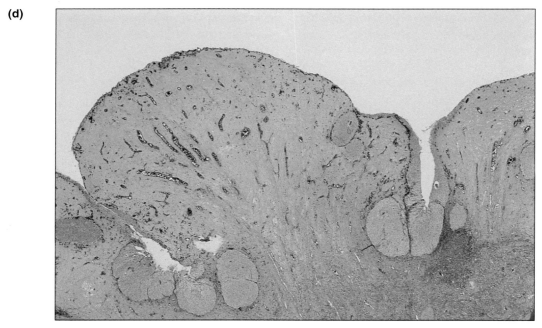

Figure 3.2 Polypoid cystitis. **(a):** The urothelium is partially preserved, and the lamina propria contains dense chronic inflammation and granulation tissue; **(b):** a broad frond of mucosa with prominent blood vessels and benign urothelial lining; **(c):** polypoid cystitis with focal bullous formation; **(d):** broad polypoid growth, which had a cobblestone appearance cytoscopically.

3.1.2 Follicular Cystitis (Cystitis Follicularis)

Follicular cystitis is present at least focally in 40% of patients with bladder cancer and in 35% of those with urinary tract infection (Sarma, 1970; Schlomovitz, 1942). Macroscopically, it typically consists of one or more small nodules of pink, white, or gray tissue, often with erythema, and may be mistaken for urothelial carcinoma. Microscopically, there are numerous lymphoid follicles within the lamina propria, usually with germinal centers, often slightly elevating the overlying intact urothelium (Fig 3.3) (Santamaria et al, 1988).

Malignant lymphoma is the most important differential diagnostic consideration for follicular cystitis, particularly in small biopsy specimens. However, patients usually have a history of lymphoma elsewhere, and the infiltrate in lymphoma is usually massive. Immunohistochemical studies are useful in distinguishing difficult cases.

3.1.3 Interstitial Cystitis

Interstitial cystitis is a chronic idiopathic inflammatory bladder disease of unknown cause and pathogenesis (Erickson et al, 1994; Hukanen et al, 1996; Koziol, 1994; MacDermott et al, 1991; Ratliff et al, 1994, 1995; Speights et al, 1995). The diagnosis is based on a combination of symptoms, cystoscopic findings, and clinical findings that exclude other bladder diseases; biopsy is useful but often not necessary. Patients with interstitial cystitis suffer from urgency, frequency, and bladder-associated pain. At least 90% of the patients are women (Aabeck & Lien, 1982; de la Serna & Alarcon-Segovia, 1981; Fall et al, 1985; Holm-Bentzen & Lose, 1987; Holm-Bentzen et al, 1987; Warren, 1994). The pathogenesis and potential role of neurogenic inflammation was recently reviewed (Elbadawi, 1997).

High–pressure cystoscopy (up to 80 cm H_2O) reveals two patterns of cases: ulcer (classic) and nonulcer (early) interstitial cystitis. Ulcer pa-

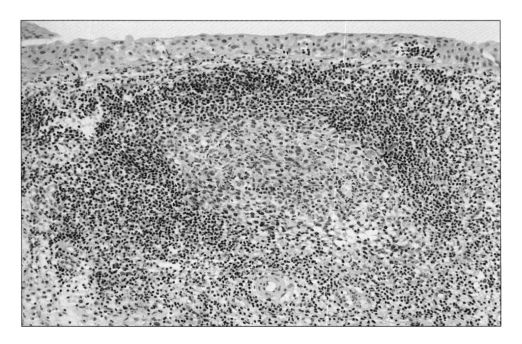

Figure 3.3 Follicular cystitis. A thin urothelium overlies a large benign lymphoid follicle.

tients have Hunner's ulcer (Hunner, 1914), whereas nonulcer patients have multiple strawberry-like petechial hemorrhages referred to as *glomerulations*. The trigone is usually not involved in interstitial cystitis (Messing & Stamey, 1978).

The utility of a bladder biopsy in patients with interstitial cystitis is controversial (Hofmeister et al, 1997). Some authors contend that the histopathologic findings are nonspecific and of limited value except to rule out carcinoma in situ (Maloney et al, 1974; Utz & Zincke, 1974; Van de Merwe et al, 1993). Others believe that the histopathologic findings are useful in confirming the diagnosis (Lynes et al, 1987). In situ and invasive carcinoma of the bladder may be mistaken clinically for intersti-

tial cystitis (Lamm & Gittes, 1977; Utz & Zincke, 1974).

The majority of patients with the ulcer pattern of interstitial cystitis have ulcerations, marked inflammation, and granulation tissue (Table 3.2; Fig 3.4). The inflammatory changes are almost always limited to the lamina propria (Bohne et al, 1962; Hand, 1949). The ulcerations are wedge-shaped and frequently filled with fibrin. Adjacent tissue may show marked chronic inflammation composed principally of lymphocytes and plasma cells, often with germinal centers. The urothelium is frequently denuded, detached, or floating above the surface. Mucosal denudation is more common in ulcer-type interstitial cystitis than nonulcer interstitial cystitis but is rare in patients without cystitis (Lynes

Table 3.2   Histologic findings in interstitial cystitis (Messing & Stamey, 1978)

Classification of interstitial cystitis	No. patients	Ulcer	Granulation tissue	Mucosal hemorrhage	Mucosal rupture	Mononuclear infiltrate				Perineural infiltrate
						±	+	++	+++	
Ulcer (classic)	146	96%	89%	86%	0	0	11%	48%	41%	81%
Nonulcer (early)	64	0	0	89%	83%	77%	14%	9%	0	0

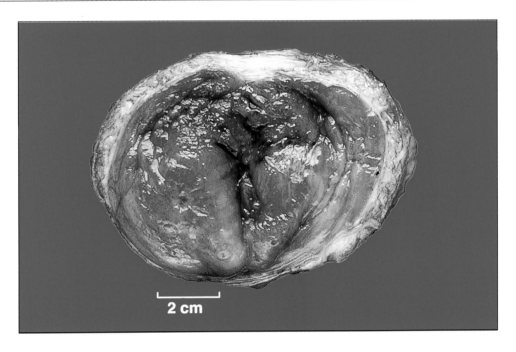

2 cm

(b)

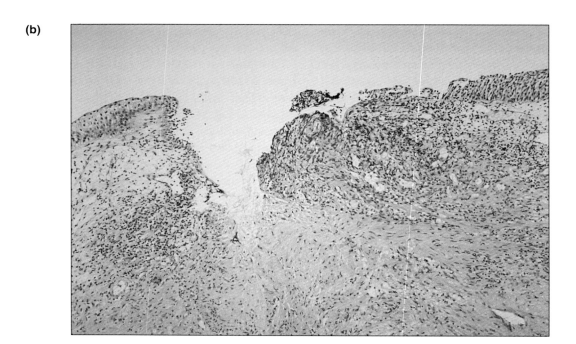

(c)

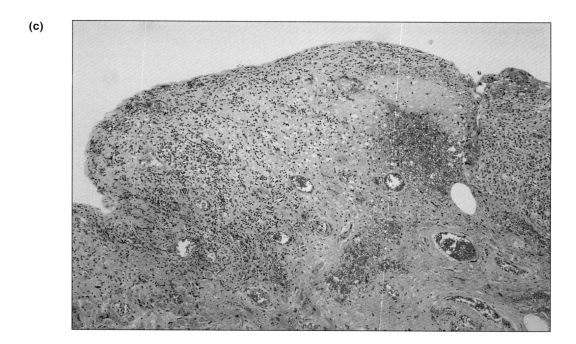

Figure 3.4 Interstitial cystitis, ulcer pattern. **(a):** Grossly, there are scattered mucosal erosions and erythema; **(b):** note wedge-shaped erosion with adjacent inflammation; **(c):** the erosion is accompanied by prominent hemorrhage in the lamina propria. This young woman had clinical features typical of interstitial cystitis.

et al, 1987). Denudation probably results from instrumentation, but the urothelium in interstitial cystitis is particularly fragile, perhaps resulting from a type IV collagen defect in the urothelial basement membrane (Wilson et al, 1995). The lamina propria is edematous and contains dilated venules. In about one-third of cases, abundant neutrophils in the venules show margination and involvement of the wall of the vein. Hemorrhage of the lamina propria is more marked in ulcer patients than in nonulcer patients. Eighty percent of patients have perineural inflammation, but this is also frequently seen in those with bladder cancer and is not specific for interstitial cystitis (Johansson & Fall, 1994). Granulation tissue probably results from rupture of the bladder mucosa during normal filling, with formation of reparative tissue. Significant fibrosis of the detrusor muscle is present in only 10% of cases but is virtually never seen in nonulcer patients. One report described fibrosis with collagen distribution in a characteristic fashion within the muscle fascicles in interstitial cystitis, but this finding has not been confirmed (Larsen et al, 1982).

In contrast with ulcer interstitial cystitis, nonulcer interstitial cystitis shows very mild histopathologic changes (Fig 3.5). About 90% of cases display some urothelial hemorrhage corresponding to the glomerulations (Johansson & Fall, 1994). This hemorrhage is usually focal but may be extensive, sometimes extending into the urothelium. Up to 83% of cases have mucosal rupture that only superficially involves the lamina propria and is not associated with inflammation; rupture is associated with suburothelial hemorrhage and probably represents a defect in the urothelial lining (Johansson & Fall, 1994). The majority of nonulcer cases have little or no inflammation, although edema and vascular congestion are frequently seen.

Mast cells are considered by some as a marker for interstitial cystitis (Sant & Theo-

harides, 1994), but this has been refuted by others (Johansson & Fall, 1994; Lynes et al, 1987). One study suggested that 28 mast cells per square millimeter in the detrusor muscle was diagnostic of interstitial cystitis (Larsen et al, 1982); however, other researchers found that control patients without interstitial cystitis had higher values (Johansson & Fall, 1994; Lynes et al, 1987). Conventional toluidine blue and Giemsa stains are not adequate for identifying all mast cells, according to some investigators, and they contend that it is necessary to fix tissues in iso-osmotic formaldehyde/acetic acid (Christmas & Rode, 1991). This action prevents initial aldehyde blocking, and subsequent staining with conventional or 5-day toluidine blue reveals a second population of mast cells, the so-called *mucosal mast cells* (Johansson & Fall, 1994). In ulcer-type interstitial cystitis, mast cell numbers are significantly increased in the lamina propria and the detrusor muscle (Feltis et al, 1987; Johansson & Fall, 1994; Pang et al, 1995). This type of interstitial cystitis is associated with characteristic microscopic changes that are helpful in diagnosis. Large transurethral resection specimens are preferred to cold-cup biopsies. Tamm-Horsfall protein is deposited in the epithelium and submucosa in patients with interstitial cystitis, indicating a barrier defect in this disease (Bushman et al, 1994; Neal et al, 1991; Wilson et al, 1995).

3.1.4 Eosinophilic Cystitis

Eosinophilic cystitis is classified as allergic or nonallergic, depending on the likelihood of allergic etiology (Rubin & Pincus, 1974). Other causative factors include atopic diseases, parasitic infection, systemic and topical agents such as mitomycin C (Ulker et al, 1996), and food allergy. Allergic eosinophilic cystitis occurs at any age, although more than 30% of patients are children. It is twice as likely in females. Patients typically have episodes of frequency, dys-

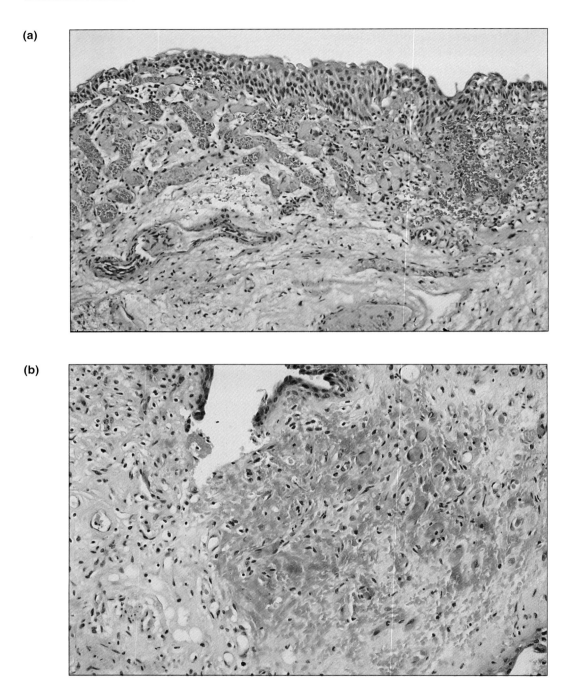

Figure 3.5 Interstitial cystitis, non-ulcer pattern. **(a):** The urothelium is reactive, and there is prominent vascular congestion; **(b):** glomerulation of the submucosa. Both cases had clinical features typical of interstitial cystitis.

uria, and hematuria; many have a history of asthma or other allergic diseases, often with peripheral eosinophilia (Gregg & Utz, 1974). However, eosinophils are not always present in significant numbers in the urine or blood. The striking polypoid growth may be cystoscopically mistaken for carcinoma (Constantinides et al, 1994) or, in a child, for sarcoma botryoides pattern of rhabdomyosarcoma (Barry & Jafri, 1994; Goldstein, 1971; Hansen & Kristensen, 1993; Ladocsi et al, 1995; Littleton et al, 1982; Rosenberg et al, 1994). Nodular and sessile growth with or without ulceration may also occur (Peterson, 1985). Multiple deep biopsies should be obtained to exclude differential diagnostic considerations. Microscopically, the lamina propria is typically edematous and chronically inflamed with numerous eosinophils. Giant cells and granulomatous inflammation are occasionally present (Antonakopoulous & Newman, 1984; Brown, 1960; Ladocsi et al, 1995). The eosinophilic infiltrate is often transmural. Giemsa stain is useful for quantitating eosinophils.

In nonallergic eosinophilic cystitis, patients often have a history of transurethral resection with or without topical chemotherapy, but no history of allergy (Choe et al, 1995). The typical patient is an elderly man with another urologic disorder such as prostatic nodular hyperplasia or bladder cancer who sustains bladder injury from instrumentation (Castillo et al, 1988; Mitas & Thompson, 1985). The cystoscopic findings are similar to those in allergic eosinophilic cystitis, and the histologic pattern may be identical (Fig 3.6). Microscopically, necrosis and fibrosis of muscle are more common than in the allergic form (Hellstrom et al, 1979).

3.1.5 Encrusted Cystitis

This uncommon condition occurs when urea-splitting organisms alkalinize the urine, creating superficial deposits of inorganic salts (Estorc

et al, 1992). Encrusted cystitis is more common in women and is associated with inflammatory or traumatic urothelial damage. Patients usually complain of urinary frequency, dysuria, and, commonly, hematuria often associated with the passage of gritty material, blood, mucus, and pus in the urine. In extensive cases in which salts are rich in calcium, encrusted cystitis may be detected radiographically (Estorc et al, 1992).

Macroscopically, there are single or multiple discrete exophytic or flat mineral deposits that are characteristically gritty. Deposits are most common at the bladder base. In rare instances, encrusted cystitis may mimic a neoplasm.

Microscopically, calcified deposits are mixed with fibrin and necrotic debris on the mucosal surface or submucosa; muscle involvement is uncommon (Fig 3.7). In early lesions, there may be prominent chronic inflammation, but the infiltrate is usually scant and there is a variable amount of fibrosis. Encrustation may also occur on the surface of a necrotic tumor or on necrotic tissue after a tumor has been fulgurated and sometimes masks the neoplasm, a critical factor in evaluating such cases (Young, 1989). Encrusted cystitis may be found in combination with malacoplakia (Berney et al, 1996).

3.1.6 Emphysematous Cystitis

Emphysematous cystitis is an uncommon condition characterized by the presence of gas-filled vesicles that are visible cystoscopically or on gross examination (Bailey, 1961; Lund et al, 1939). It is more common in women than men, and 50% of patients are diabetic. Emphysematous cystitis is associated with a wide variety of infectious agents, including bacteria such as *Escherichia coli* or *Aerobacter aerogenes*, and, occasionally, the fungus *Candida albicans* (Bartkowski & Lanesky, 1988; Maliwan, 1979). Macroscopically, there are small, thin-walled vesicles measuring between 0.5 cm and 3 cm in diameter that easily rupture. Microscopically,

(a)

(b)

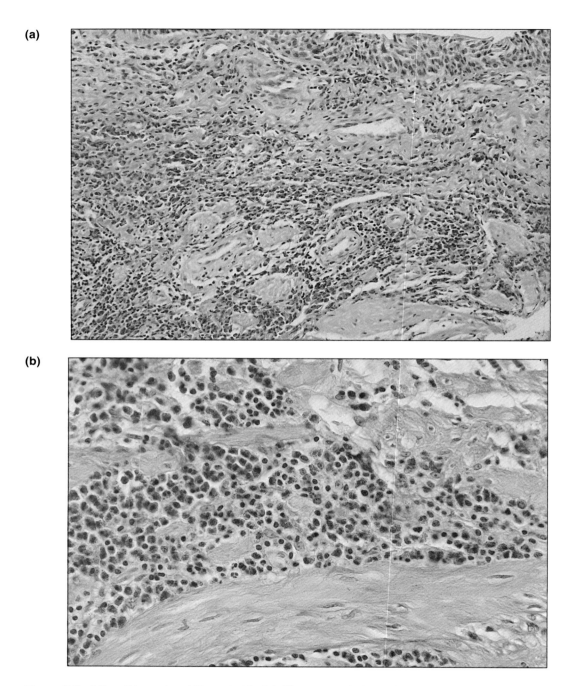

Figure 3.6 Idiopathic eosinophilic ureteritis. **(a):** The mucosa is intact, but there is dense inflammation in the submucosa with an abundance of eosinophils; **(b):** the muscular wall is involved.

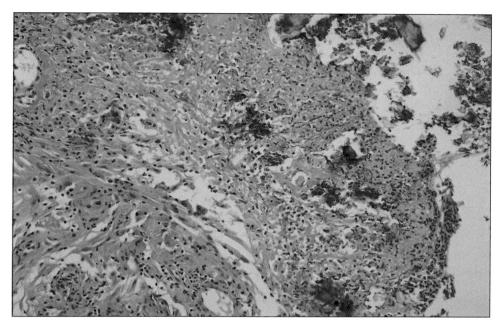

Figure 3.7 Encrusted cystitis. The biopsy is distorted by mineralized debris.

these small vesicular cysts are surrounded by thin connective tissue septa in the lamina propria that may extend into the muscularis propria (Hawtrey et al, 1974).

3.1.7 Gangrenous Cystitis

This uncommon type of cystitis is typically found in elderly or debilitated patients, including those with compromised circulation and systemic infection (Cristol & Greene, 1945; Moncada et al, 1994). There is often a urinary tract infection that progresses to diffuse gangrenous cystitis. No specific pathogen has been consistently identified, and the most likely cause is ischemia of variable severity or duration in combination with infection (Dao, 1994; Devitt & Sethia, 1993). Virtually all of the bladder urothelium is necrotic and ulcerated, with blood clot and fibrinopurulent debris forming a membranous cast of the bladder lumen. The depth of necrosis into the bladder wall is variable but often involves the muscularis propria. Necrosis of blood vessels

results in intramural and intraluminal hemorrhage (Stirling & Hopkins, 1934).

3.1.8 Hemorrhagic Cystitis

The classic cause of hemorrhagic cystitis is cyclophosphamide irritation. This chemotherapeutic agent was introduced in 1957 for the treatment of select types of leukemia but is now widely used for numerous malignancies as well as autoimmune disorders and organ transplantation (Cox, 1979; deVries & Freiha, 1990; George, 1963; Marshall & Klinefelter, 1979; Stillwell & Benson, 1988). Other causes include adenovirus type II and papovavirus, particularly in children (Ambinder et al, 1986; Arthur et al, 1986; Numazaki et al, 1968; Shindo et al, 1986).

Patients note sudden onset of dysuria and hematuria that is occasionally massive and intractable. There is no sex or age predominance, and it appears to be independent of the administered dose of cyclophosphamide. The histologic changes in hemorrhagic cystitis include severe edema, vascular telangiectasia, and hemorrhage within the lamina propria, usually associated with mucosal ulceration. Intramural fibrosis is present in 25% of cases examined at autopsy. Reversible cytologic abnormalities of the urothelial cells may be mistaken for malignancy, and a history of cyclophosphamide exposure is useful in avoiding this pitfall.

3.1.9 Viral Cystitis

3.1.9.1 Human Papillomavirus Infection and Condyloma Acuminatum

Occasional cases of viral cystitis are associated with human papillomavirus infection (Shibutani et al, 1992), but in our experience, this is extremely uncommon (Lopez-Beltran & Munoz, 1995).

The result of papillomavirus infection, condyloma acuminatum of the bladder, is more common in females than males (2:1 ratio) and affects patients of all ages, although most are younger than 50 years (Farrow, 1992). It usually arises in patients with condylomata of the urethra, vulva, vagina, anus, or perineum, but isolated bladder involvement has been reported. Some cases are associated with human immunodeficiency virus infection (Asvesti et al, 1991; Jimenez Lasanta et al, 1997). At cystoscopy, condyloma acuminata typically consists of a solitary lesion, but diffuse involvement has been reported (Bruske et al, 1997). It usually occurs in the region of the bladder neck and trigone as an exophytic papillary mass, and the major differential diagnostic consideration is papillary urothelial carcinoma. Microscopically, it has similar features to its counterpart in other organs, including the presence of koilocytotic cells with abundant clear cytoplasm and hyperchromatic wrinkled nuclei with perinuclear halos (Fig 3.8) (Keating et al, 1985). Condylomata within the bladder, as elsewhere, may undergo malignant transformation (Libby et al, 1985), and this transformation may be predicted by the type of human papillomavirus involved in its etiology (Lopez-Beltran & Munoz,

1995). Urothelial carcinoma may contain foci of koilocytosis, but this is very uncommon (Fig 3.8). Although condyloma acuminatum is considered by one author to be synonymous with squamous papilloma (Murphy, 1989), we and most others do not agree and consider these to be separate entities, similar to counterpart lesions in many other organs in the body. The differential diagnosis of condyloma includes squamous papilloma, papillary urothelial carcinoma with squamous differentiation, and verrucous carcinoma.

3.1.9.2 Viruses other than Human Papillomavirus

A variety of RNA and DNA viruses have been identified in bladder specimens. Patients are usually immunosuppressed or suffer from herpes genitalis (Mininberg et al, 1982). The most commonly isolated viruses include adenovirus and papovavirus (hemorrhagic cystitis), herpes simplex virus type 2, herpes zoster, and cytomegalovirus, particularly in immunosuppressed children (Goldman & Warner, 1970; Masukawa et al, 1972). Polyomavirus infection may mimic high-grade urothelial carcinoma of the bladder (Seftel et al, 1996). Despite the frequency of viruria in patients with systemic viral infections or infection involving other organs, clinically significant viral infections of the bladder are rare and histologic descriptions are sparse (Hanash & Pool, 1970).

3.1.10 Cystitis with Atypical Giant Cells

Giant cell cystitis should not be considered as a distinct type of inflammation, but merely as cystitis with a noticeable number of stromal giant cells (Fig 3.9). Atypical mononucleated or multinucleated stromal cells are common in the lamina propria of the bladder, particularly in patients after instrumentation (Wells, 1938). These cells are also common in routine biopsies without obvious evidence of cystitis and, when present in large numbers, may cause di-

(a)

(b)

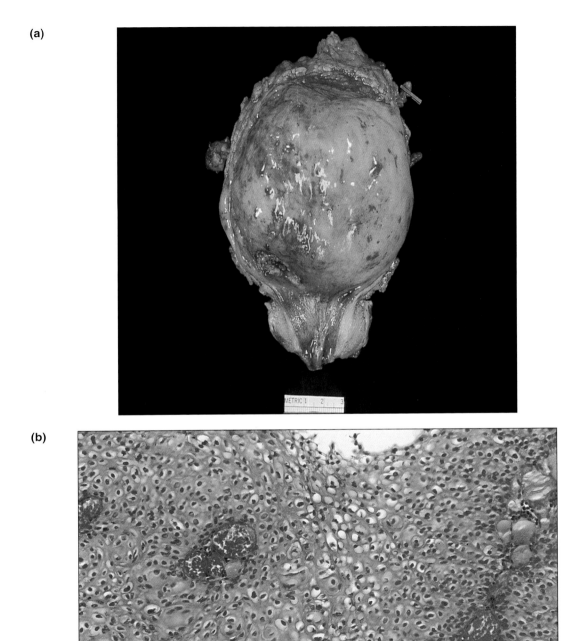

Figure 3.8 **(a):** Condyloma of the bladder at bottom left of bladder lumen. **(b):** Focal koilocytotic change in otherwise typical low-grade papillary urothelial carcinoma.

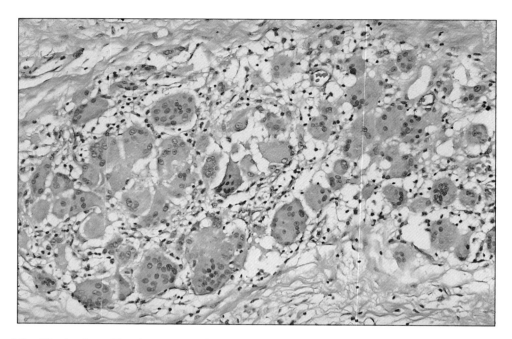

Figure 3.9   Giant cell cystitis after transurethral resection of the bladder for low-grade papillary carcinoma.

agnostic difficulty (Grignon & Sakr, 1995). The atypical cells may be stellate or elongate, with tapering eosinophilic cytoplasmic processes that simulate smooth and skeletal muscle cells. The nuclei are typically hyperchromatic and often irregular in size and shape, but mitotic figures are not present. Similar cells are seen in patients treated with chemotherapeutic agents or radiation (Gowing, 1960).

3.1.11   Denuding Cystitis

Denuding cystitis refers to urothelial carcinoma in situ of the bladder in which there is extensive loss of the surface epithelium. Denuded epithelium also frequently occurs in association with many inflammatory conditions, including interstitial cystitis (Elliot et al, 1977). Recognition of this pattern of carcinoma in situ is important and should be considered in the differential diagnosis of any urinary bladder biopsy in which the urothelium is absent (Grignon & Sakr, 1995).

3.2   GRANULOMATOUS CYSTITIS

3.2.1   Granuloma after Transurethral Resection (Postsurgical Necrobiotic Granuloma)

Necrotizing palisading granuloma resembling a rheumatoid nodule and foreign-body–type granuloma commonly occurs after biopsy or transurethral resection of the bladder, with a reported frequency in second resection specimens of 13% (Spagnolo & Waring, 1986). The frequency with which granuloma occurs increases with the number of surgical procedures. Necrotizing granuloma may be oval, linear, or serpiginous, often with a prominent infiltrate of eosinophils (Fig 3.10) (Eble & Banks, 1990). Granuloma may extend from the overlying ulcerated mucosa into the muscularis propria, eventually resulting in fibrous scarring and occasional dystrophic calcification (Spagnolo & Waring, 1986). Diathermy may induce antigenic

(a)

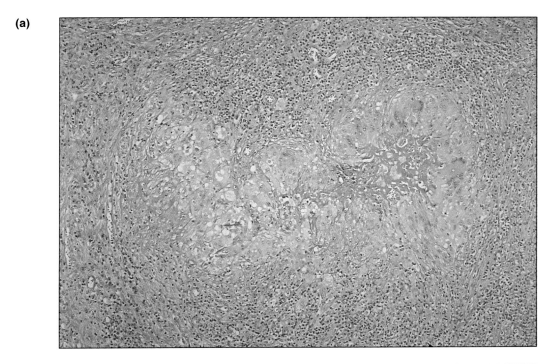

(b)

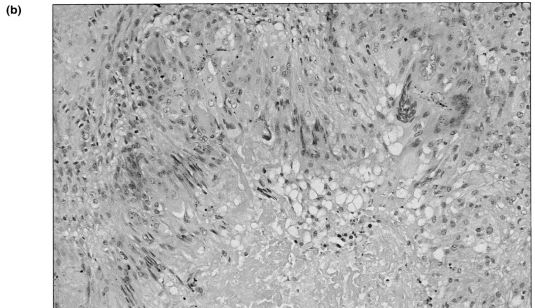

(c)

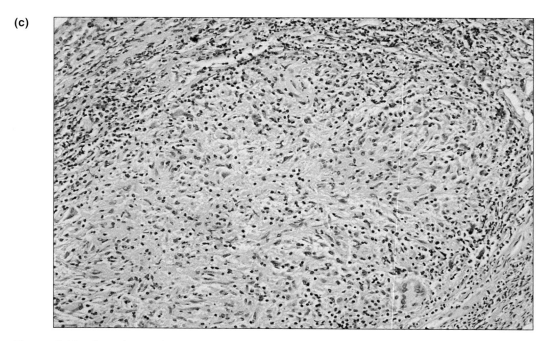

Figure 3.10 Granuloma after transurethral resection. The granulomas may be tightly cohesive **(a, b)** or poorly defined **(c)**, invariably mixed with adjacent inflammation.

changes in the collagen of the subepithelial connective tissue, eliciting the granulomatous host response (Eble & Banks, 1990).

3.2.2 Suture Granuloma

Granuloma occasionally arises in response to silk sutures introduced at the time of herniorrhaphy or other surgical procedure, producing a mass in or adjacent to the bladder (Fig 3.11) (Helms & Clark, 1977). In most cases, the herniorrhaphy was complicated by wound infection. The interval between herniorrhaphy and the appearance of the bladder mass was as long as 11 years in one case (Helms & Clark, 1977). Bladder neoplasm is the clinical impression in most of these cases, and the patients presented with urinary symptoms, including hematuria, frequency, and dysuria (Pearl & Someren, 1980). The process primarily involves the bladder wall and perivesical tissue, producing an intraluminal mass visible at cystoscopy. Microscopically,

there is a predominantly histiocytic reaction to the suture with foreign-body giant cells and varying degrees of fibrosis and chronic inflammation. We have observed a case with prominent fibrosis associated with a silk suture granuloma following diverticulectomy (Fig 3.11).

3.2.3 BCG-Induced Granulomatous Cystitis

Bacillus Calmette-Guérin (BCG), an attenuated strain of tubercle bacilli, is an effective topical therapeutic agent for noninvasive bladder cancer (Bassi et al, 1992). The mechanism of action is unclear but may result from creation and maintenance of chronic inflammation in the lamina propria rather than activation of the immune system. Indications for the use of BCG are similar to those for topical drugs, but this regimen is especially beneficial in patients with carcinoma in situ. Complications are more frequent than with topical drugs and rarely in-

(a)

(b)

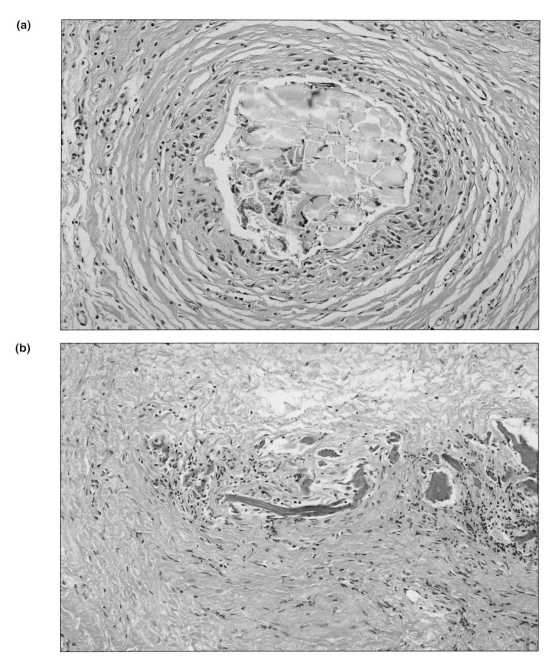

Figure 3.11   (a, b): Suture granluoma, with residual foreign material eliciting a granulomatous response.

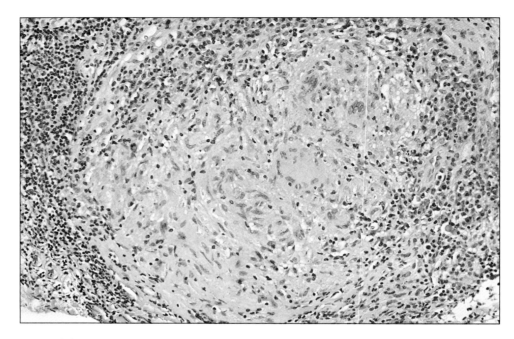

Figure 3.12 BCG-induced granuloma.

clude systemic infections with tubercle bacilli (Betz et al, 1993). The pathologic changes associated with BCG are similar to those of tuberculous cystitis, including superficial ulceration with acute and chronic inflammation surrounding noncaseating granulomas (Fig 3.12). A granulomatous reaction apparently correlates with BCG activity and may be an important indicator for potential tumor response.

3.2.4 Schistosomiasis (Bilharziasis)

Schistosomal disease of the urinary bladder induces a wide spectrum of cytoscopic and histologic changes, including urothelial polyposis, ulceration, hyperplasia, metaplasia, dysplasia, and carcinoma (Fig 3.13; Tables 3.3 and 3.4) (Khafagy et al, 1972; Nash et al, 1982; Raziuddin et al, 1993; Rosin et al, 1994a, 1994b; Smith & Christie, 1986). Schistosomal polyposis consists of multiple large inflammatory pseudopolyps resulting from heavy localized egg deposition during active disease. These lesions usually re-

gress in the inactive stage of the disease. When polypoid, they may obstruct the urethral or ureteral orifices, or may bleed, producing large obstructive clots and anemia. Approximately 30% of schistosomal polyps are found in inactive disease (Table 3.4) and appear as fibrocalcific outgrowths representing the remains of granulomatous polyps (Von Lichtenberg et al, 1971). Five percent of schistosomal polyps are composed of hyperplastic epithelium. However, almost 60% of polypoid lesions of the urinary bladder in patients with schistosomiasis are a result of causes other than the parasite, including nonspecific cystitis and edema (polypoid or bullous cystitis).

In the schistosomal bladder, ulcers occur in the active and chronic stages. Those that form during the early active stage are rare, occurring when a necrotic polyp sloughs into the urine. Those that form in the chronic stage are more common, producing constant, deep, "hard" pelvic pain that is the sequela of heavy infection (greater than 250,000 eggs/g of bladder tissue). Chronic ulcers

(a)

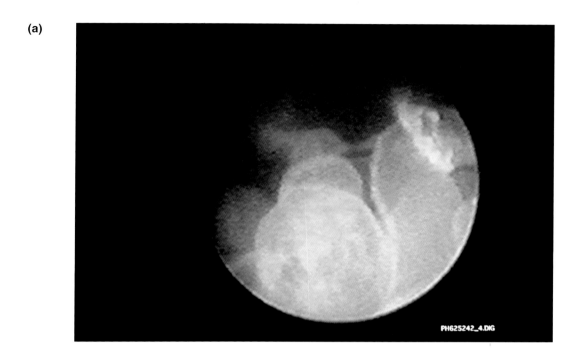

PH625242_4.DIG

(b)

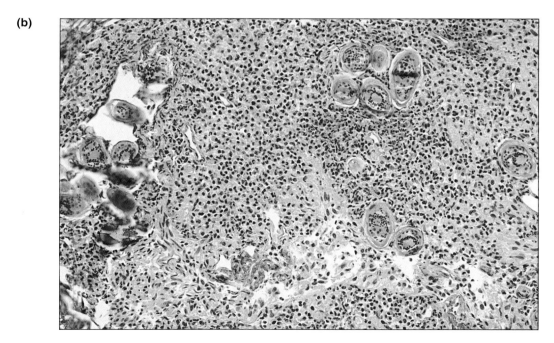

Figure 3.13 Schistosomiasis of the bladder. **(a):** Cystoscopic appearance of urothelial polyposis in a 9-year-old boy. **(b):** Characteristic eggs are present in association with prominent chronic inflammation.

Table 3.3 Histopathologic grading of schistosomal urinary bladder disease

Grade	Criteria
I	Occasional eggs in lamina propria
II	Lamina propria filled with eggs; no involvement of detrusor muscle
IIIa	Lamina propria filled with eggs; involvement of superficial third of detrusor muscle
IIIb	Lamina propria filled with eggs; involvement of external two-thirds of detrusor muscle

are located at or near the posterior midsagittal line of the bladder and may be stellate or ovoid. They usually occur in younger patients with a mean age of 29 years, suggesting that they result from the rapid accumulation of eggs.

The spectrum of urothelial proliferation includes hyperplastic squamous epithelium that is often keratinized. Hyperplasia associated with severe urinary schistosomiasis is seen in all stages of disease, although most commonly in the late stages. Dysplastic changes may accompany squamous metaplasia similar to the uterine cervix, but this is inconsistent.

Urinary schistosomiasis may also cause bladder cancer. In endemic regions, schistosomiasis-induced bladder cancer is the most common malignant tumor. This cancer is found in a younger age group than other forms of bladder cancer (mean age: 46 years), is more common in women than men, and is rare in the trigone (Koraitim et al, 1995). Gross hematuria is less frequent than in patients with typical bladder cancer. Irritative symptoms are common, and white flakes of keratin may be passed in the urine; bladder calcification is sometimes seen on radiographs. These patients have a higher frequency of squamous cell carcinoma and adenocarcinoma than those without schistosomiasis; the remainder of patients who do not have squamous cell carcinoma or adenocarcinoma have urothelial or undifferentiated carcinoma. Squamous cell carcinoma in these patients is usually low grade, may be verrucous, and has a better prognosis than nonschistosomiasis-induced squamous cell carcinoma, which is often high grade (Koraitim et al, 1995).

3.2.5 Malacoplakia

Malacoplakia is an uncommon inflammatory condition that usually affects the urinary tract, with a predilection for the urinary bladder (Dubey et al, 1988; Long & Althausen, 1989). *Malacoplakia*, derived from the Greek, means "soft plaque." Urinary tract malacoplakia primarily affects women (75% of cases) with a peak incidence in the fifth decade; in men, it peaks in the seventh decade. There is a strong association with infection by coliform organisms, particularly *E. coli*, with impairment of the intracellular

Table 3.4 Comparison of active and inactive schistosomiasis

Feature	Active	Inactive
Adult worm pairs	+	−
Oviposition	+	−
Urinary egg excretion	+	−
Granulomatous host response	+	−
Polypoid lesions	+ (Possibly obstructive)	Very rare
Sandy patches	+ (In late active)	+ (Possibly obstructive)
Cause of obstructive uropathy	Polypoid lesions	Sandy patches
Schistosomal ulceration	Uncommon	Common
Treatment	Chemotherapy	Surgical repair

− = absent; + = present

capacity of mononuclear cells to kill bacteria (Callea et al, 1982). Patients with vesicular malacoplakia present with symptoms and signs of urinary tract infection, and hematuria is also common. Occasionally, it appears in patients receiving immunosuppressive therapy (Biggar et al, 1981). Urine cultures most often yield *E. coli*, but *Proteus vulgaris*, *A. aerogenes*, alpha-hemolytic *Streptococci*, *Klebsiella pneumoniae*, and other organisms have also been isolated. Intracellular bacilliform organisms have been found by transmission electron microscopy (Abdou et al, 1977; McClurb et al, 1973).

Macroscopically, malacoplakia consists of multiple soft yellow or yellow-brown plaques, nodules, or papillary or polypoid masses, usually measuring less than 2 cm in diameter. Central umbilication and a hyperemic rim are common. When large and necrotic, malacoplakia may be mistaken for carcinoma (Baniel et al, 1987).

Microscopically, it is characterized by submucosal accumulation of macrophages with eccentric nuclei and granular eosinophilic cytoplasm (Hansemann cells) (Feldman et al, 1980). Diagnostic intracytoplasmic inclusion bodies,

Michaelis-Gutmann bodies, consist of round 5 to 8 micron diameter targetoid ("bull's eye") calcospherites. Frequently, these bodies are basophilic, but sometimes they are pale and difficult to see in routine preparations. Michaelis-Gutmann bodies are brilliantly positive with periodic acid-Schiff stain (Fig 3.14) and resistant to diastase stain and contain calcium and frequently iron salts; consequently, they give a positive reaction with the von Kossa technique and Perls' Prussian blue stain (Damjanov & Katz, 1981). Michaelis-Gutmann bodies are not always conspicuous, particularly in the early stages of malacoplakia, and aggregates of macrophages without Michaelis-Gutmann bodies may represent a prediagnostic phase. In some cases, there is granulation tissue, extensive fibrosis, and marked acute inflammation that may obscure the histiocytic nature of the process (Baniel et al, 1987). Malacoplakia may also contain foreign-body or Langhans-type giant cells and lymphoid follicles at the edge (Callea et al, 1982). The main differential diagnostic considerations are carcinoma with inflammatory stroma and xanthogranulomatous cystitis (Lamm & Gittes, 1977; Skudowitz & Weintraub, 1977). Malacoplakia

(a)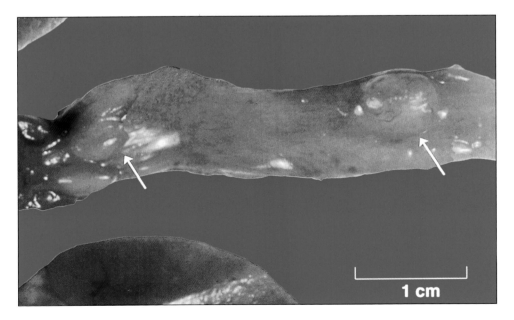

(b)

(c)

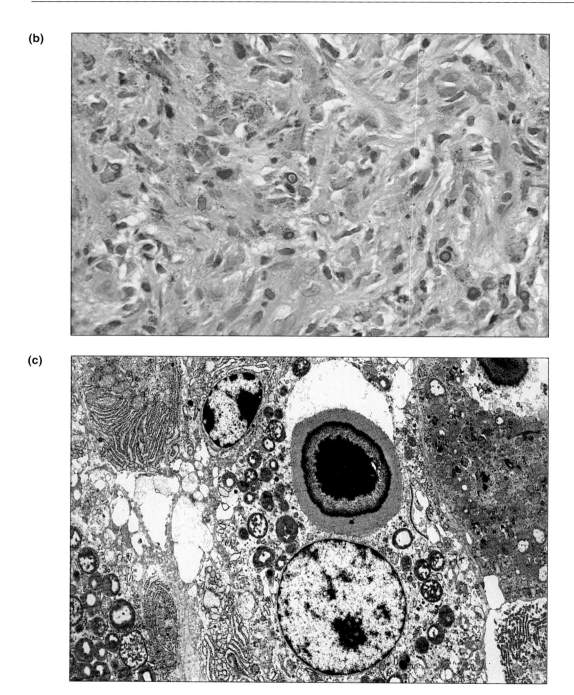

Figure 3.14 Malacoplakia. **(a):** Mucosal nodules in the ureter (arrows); **(b):** the submucosa contains a chronic inflammatory infiltrate with abundant Michaelis-Gutmann bodies. The periodic acid-Schiff stain highlights both mineralized and nonmineralized targetoid bodies; **(c):** ultrastructure, with large round laminated mineralized cytoplasmic body.

may coexist with encrusted cystitis (Berney et al, 1996).

3.2.6 Tuberculosis

Tuberculous cystitis is usually caused by *Mycobacterium tuberculosis*, although *M. bovis* accounts for up to 3% of cases (Cos & Cockett, 1980). Bladder involvement is a secondary event, occurring in 1% of patients with genitourinary tuberculosis and in about 65% of patients who undergo nephrectomy for renal involvement. Patients characteristically have frequency, dysuria, hematuria, and urgency.

The organisms implant in the vesical mucosa, often around the ureteral orifices via infected urine from the upper urinary tract. The initial microscopic changes occur around the ureteral orifices, and the earliest mucosal abnormality is marked hyperemia, sometimes with edema. The lesions progress to form discrete tubercles measuring up to 3 mm in diameter that may ulcerate and become covered with friable necrotic debris. Occasionally, there is abundant granulation tissue forming polypoid excrescences that macroscopically may be mistaken for carcinoma. The tubercles are sharply circumscribed and initially firm and solid; as they enlarge, they often coalesce and undergo central ulceration.

Microscopically, the tuberculous granuloma consists of an aggregate of epithelioid histiocytes with central caseous necrosis and variable numbers of multinucleated giant cells, plasma cells, lymphocytes, and circumferential fibrosis. Occasionally, caseating necrosis is absent, and the granulomas are not well formed; despite this, tuberculosis should still be strongly suspected with granulomatous inflammation, and efforts made to demonstrate mycobacteria (McClure & Young, 1989).

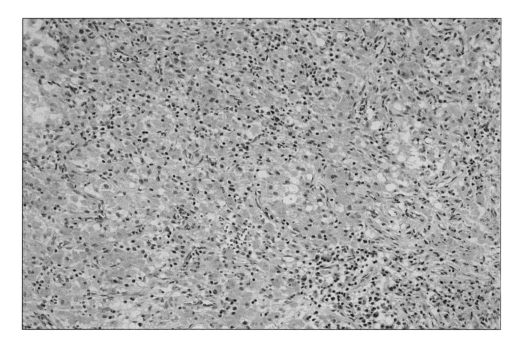

Figure 3.15 Idiopathic xanthogranulomatous cystitis in a transurethral resection specimen.

3.2.7 Xanthoma and Xanthogranulomatous Cystitis

Idiopathic cystitis consisting chiefly of sheets of vacuolated or foamy histiocytes is referred to as *xanthoma* or *xanthogranulomatous cystitis*, depending on the amount of associated inflammation (Fig 3.15). This lesion is rare and may occur in patients with recurrent urinary tract infections. Transmural involvement was described in one case (Walters et al, 1985).

Xanthogranulomatous cystitis may represent an early phase of malacoplakia. It should be noted that large numbers of xanthoma cells may rarely be seen in association with bladder cancer (Ash, 1940). Foamy histiocytes often accumulate within the fibrovascular cores of papilloma and low-grade papillary carcinoma of the bladder. Xanthoma can be identified by cold-cup biopsy (Nishimura et al, 1995), and stromal aggregates of xanthoma cells have also rarely been described in a fibroepithelial polyp of the ureter (Elson & McLaughlin, 1974).

3.2.8 Other Forms of Granulomatous Cystitis

Chronic granulomatous disease of childhood rarely affects the bladder, consisting of sheets of histiocytes, foreign-body giant cells, and neutrophils (Cyr et al, 1973).

The bladder is occasionally involved in autoimmune diseases such as systemic lupus erythematosus, Stevens-Johnson syndrome, pemphigus vulgaris, lichen planus, and rheumatoid arthritis (Orth et al, 1983). Patients with BCG instillation after bladder cancer have florid granulomatous inflammation in bladder biopsies (Bassi et al, 1992; Belmatough et al, 1993; Betz et al, 1993; Jufe et al, 1984). Granulomas may be seen in the bladder wall fistula in patients with Crohn's disease. One case of suture granuloma of the bladder has been described (Pearl &

Someren, 1980). Sarcoidosis may involve the urinary bladder (Tamella et al, 1989). Periurethral and submucosal bladder neck injections of polytetrafluoroethylene (Teflon) paste, used to treat urinary incontinence, sometimes result in an abundant foreign-body giant cell reaction with granulomas and stromal fibrosis (Kaczmarek, 1985). Histologically, refractile aggregates of Teflon are readily identified, particularly with polarization (McKinney et al, 1994).

3.3 OTHER INFECTIOUS CYSTITIDES

3.3.1 Fungal Cystitis

C. albicans is the most common fungal cause of cystitis, but it is relatively uncommon (Goldberg et al, 1979). Bladder involvement may occur from urethral spread or as part of hematogenous spread. Infection is usually restricted to the trigone. *Candida* infection usually occurs in debilitated or immunocompromised patients more than those on antibiotic therapy. Also, it is frequent in patients with diabetes mellitus, particularly women.

Symptoms of *Candida* cystitis include nocturia, unremitting pain and discomfort, and frequency. The urine is often turbid or bloody. Macroscopically, the mucosa is irregular and slightly elevated, with sharply demarcated adherent white plaques that bleed when removed. Diffuse erythema is occasionally present. Large lumenal fungus balls are rarely observed (Patel et al, 1996).

Microscopically, the urothelium is ulcerated, and the submucosa is inflamed. Some patients have emphysematous or gangrenous cystitis. Typical fungal spores and hyphae are present within fibrinoprurulent debris, often in large numbers.

Other rare forms of fungal cystitis are caused by *Torulopsis glabrata*, aspergillosis (Sakamoto, 1978), and *Coccidioides immitis*.

3.3.2 Actinomycosis

Actinomycosis of the bladder is rare. The bladder is usually secondarily involved by extension from adjacent organs such as the fallopian tube and ovary. Infection can also descend from the upper urinary tract or spread hematogenously (King & Lam, 1978).

Macroscopically, the bladder wall is usually focally or diffusely thickened. A localized mass simulating a bladder or urachal tumor may be present (Guermazi et al, 1996; Ozyurt et al, 1995). The mucosa is often ulcerated and edematous. Transmural necrosis often creates fistulae. Microscopically, the submucosa and muscularis propria contain abundant granulation tissue and numerous abscesses of variable size. "Sulfur granules" are present, consisting of masses of filamentous mycelia with a peripheral array of swollen eosinophilic "clubs." Periodic acid-Schiff and silver stains are helpful in recognizing these distinctive organisms.

3.3.3 Miscellaneous Infectious Cystitides

Uncommon infections of the bladder include trichomonal cystitis, hydatid cystitis, syphilis, and amebiasis. Trichomonal cystitis, as a result of *Trichomonas vaginalis* infection, is usually limited to the trigone and results from retrograde extension from the posterior urethra in women. In hydatid disease, the upper urinary tract becomes infected with the ova of *Echinococcus granulosus* during hematogenous spread, and typical cysts form. Rupture of these cysts leads to discharge of their contents into the lower urinary tract and subsequent infection of the bladder.

Syphilis of the urinary bladder is extremely rare and may occur in secondary or tertiary syphilis. The gummas are usually located near the urethral orifice and are typically single.

Infection of the bladder by *Entamoeba histolytica* (amebic cystitis) is rare, usually following colonic involvement in which the trophozoites perforate through the colonic wall and invade contiguous structures. Hematogenous spread typically involves the liver and rarely includes the urinary bladder, where lesions are concentrated in the trigone. Microscopically, there are varying degrees of chronic inflammation. The diagnosis is based on recognition of trophozoites in tissue sections, and this is facilitated by using the periodic acid–Schiff stain.

Early experimental studies in mice suggested that *Helicobacter pylori* may be a pathogen in the urinary bladder and renal pelvis, but this has not been confirmed in human studies (Isogai et al, 1994).

Pseudomembranous trigonitis, a curious disease that presents in women with the urethral syndrome, consists of vaginal-type glycogenated squamous metaplasia of the trigone associated with edema and vascular dilatation, but no significant inflammation (Henry & Fox, 1971).

Extremely uncommon lesions of the bladder may be caused by microfilariae (*Wuchereria bancrofti*), myasis (infestation with fly larvae), and Candirú (a tiny catfish living in the Amazon river) (Herman, 1973).

REFERENCES

Aabeck HS, Lien EN. Cystitis cystica in childhood: clinical findings and treatment procedures. *Acta Paediatr Scand*. 1982;71:247–252.

Abdou NI, NaPombejara C, Sagawa A, et al. Malakoplakia: evidence for monocyte lysosomal abnormality correctable by cholinergic agonist in vitro and in vivo. *N Engl J Med*. 1977;297:1413–1419.

Aldenborg F, Fall M, Enerback L. Proliferation and transepithelial migration of mast cells in interstitial cystitis. *Immunology*. 1986;58:411–416.

Algaba F. Papillo-polypoid cystitis. Focal cystitis with pseudoneoplastic aspect. *Acta Urol Esp*. 1991;15:260–264.

Ambinder RF, Burns W, Forman M, et al. Hemorrhagic cystitis associated with adenovirus infection in bone marrow transplantation. *Arch Intern Med*. 1986;146:1400–1401.

Anderstrom C, Ekelund P, Hansson HA, Johansson L. Scanning electron microscopy of polypoid cystitis—a reversible lesion of the human bladder. *J Urol*. 1984;131:242–244.

Antonakopoulous GN, Newman J. Eosinophilic cystitis with giant cells. *Arch Pathol Lab Med*. 1984;108: 728–731.

Arthur RR, Shah KV, Baust SM, et al. Association of BK viruria with hemorrhagic cystitis in recipients of bone marrow transplants. *N Engl J Med*. 1986;315:230–234.

Ash JE. Epithelial tumors of the bladder. *J Urol*. 1940;44:135.

Asvesti C, Delmas V, Dauge-Geffroy MC, et al. Multiple candylomata of the urethra and bladder disclosing HIV infection. *Ann Urol*. 1991;25:146–149.

Bailey H. Cystitis emphysematosa. *Am J Roentgenol Radium Ther Nucl Med*. 1961;86:850–862.

Baniel J, Shmulei D, Shapira Z, et al. Malacoplakia presenting as a pseudotumor of the bladder in cadaveric renal transplantation. *J Urol*. 1987;137:281–282.

Barry KA, Jafri SZ. Eosinophilic cystitis: CT findings. *Abdom Imaging*. 1994;19:272–273.

Bartkowski DP, Lanesky JR. Emphysematous prostatitis and cystitis secondary to *Candida albicans*. *J Urol*. 1988;139:1063–1065.

Bassi P, Milani C, Meneghini A, et al. Clinical value of pathologic changes after intravesical BCG therapy of superficial bladder cancer. *Urology*. 1992;40:175–179.

Belmatough N, Levy-Djebbour S, Appelboom T, et al. Polyarthritis in four patients treated with intravesical BCG-therapy for carcinoma of the bladder. *Rev Rheumatism*. 1993;60:162–166.

Berney DM, Thompson I, Sheaff M, Baithun SI. Alkaline encrusted custitis associated with malakoplakia. *Histopathology*. 1996;28:253–256.

Betz SS, See WA, Cohen MB. Granulomatous inflammation in bladder wash specimens after intravesical bacillus Calmette-Guerin therapy for transitional cell carcinoma of the bladder. *Am J Clin Pathol*. 1993;99:244–248.

Biggar WD, Kenting A, Bear RA. Malakoplakia: evidence for an acquired disease secondary to immunosuppression. *Transplantation*. 1981;31:109–112.

Bohne AW, Hudson JM, Rebuck JW, et al. An abnormal leucocyte response in interstitial cystitis. *J Urol*. 1962;88:387–392.

Brown EW. Eosinophilic granuloma of the bladder. *J Urol*. 1960;83:665–667.

Bruske T, Loch T, Thiemann O, et al. Panurothelial condyloma acuminatum with development of squamous cell carcinoma of the bladder and renal pelvis. *J Urol*. 1997;157:620–621.

Buck EG. Polypoid cystitis mimicking transitional cell carinoma. *J Urol*. 1984;131:963–965.

Bushman W, Goolsby C, Grayhack JT, et al. Abnormal flow cytometry profiles in patients with interstitial cystitis. *J Urol*. 1994;152:2262–2266.

Callea F, Damme BV, Desmet VJ. Alpha-1-antitrypsin in malakoplakia. *Virchows Arch Pathol Anat*. 1982;395:1–6.

Cardoza L. Postmenopausal cystitis. *Br Med J*. 1996;313:129.

Castillo J, Cartagena R, Montes M. Eosinophilic cystitis: a therapeutic challenge. *Urology*. 1988;32:535–537.

Choe JM, Kirkermo AK, Sirls LT. Intravesical thiotepa-induced eosinophilic cystitis. *Urology*. 1995;46:729–731.

Christmas TJ, Rode J. Characteristics of mast cells in normal bladder, bacterial cystitis and interstitial cystitis. *Br J Urol*. 1991;68:473–478.

Constantinides C, Gavras P, Stinios J, et al. Eosinophilic cystitis: a rare case which presented as an invasive bladder tumor. *Acta Urol Belgica*. 1994; 62:71–73.

Cos LR, Cockett AT. Genitourinary tuberculosis revisited. *Urology*. 1980;20:111–117.

Cox PJ. Cyclophosphamide cystitis—identification of acrolein as the causative agent. *Biochem Phamacol*. 1979;28:2045–2049.

Cristol DS, Greene LF. Gangrenous cystitis. Etiologic classification and treatment. *Surgery*. 1945;18:343–346.

Cyr WL, Johnson H, Balfour J. Granulomatous cystitis as a manifestation of chronic granulomatous disease of childhood. *J Urol*. 1973;110:357–359.

Damjanov I, Katz SM. Malakoplakia. *Pathol Annu*. 1981;16:103–126.

Dao AH. Gangrenous cystitis in chronic alcohol abuse. *J Tenn Med Assoc*. 1994;87:51–52.

de la Serna AR, Alarcon-Segovia D. Chronic interstitial cystitis as an initial major manifestation of systemic lupus erythematosus. *J Rheumatol*. 1981;8: 808–810.

Devitt AT, Sethia KK. Gangrenous cystitis: case report and review of the literature. *J Urol*. 1993;149: 1544–1545.

deVries CR, Freiha FS. Hemorrhagic cystitis: a review. *J Urol.* 1990;143:1–9.

Dubey NK, Tavadia HB, Hehir M. Malacoplakia: a case involving epididymis and a case involving a bladder complicated by calculi. *J Urol.* 1988;139: 359–361.

Eble JN, Banks ER. Postsurgical necrobiotic granulomas of the urinary bladder. *Urology.* 1990;35:454–457.

Ekelund P, Anderstrom C, Johansson SL, et al. The reversibility of catheter-associated polypoid cystitis. *J Urol.* 1983;130:456–459.

Elbadawi A. Interstitial cystitis: A critique of current concepts with a new proposal for pathologic diagnosis and pathogenesis. *Urology.* 1997;49(Suppl 5A):14–40.

Elliot GB, Moloney PJ, Anderson GH. Denuding cystitis and in situ urothelial carcinoma. *Arch Pathol.* 1977;96:91–94.

Elson EC, McLaughlin AP III. Xanthomatous ureteral polyp. *Urology.* 1974;4:214–216.

Erickson DR, Simon LJ, Belchis DA. Relationships between bladder inflammation and other clinical features in interstitial cystitis. *Urology.* 1994;44:655–659.

Estorc JJ, de La Coussaye JE, Viel EJ, et al. Teicoplanin treatment of alkaline encrusted cystitis due to Corynebacterium group D2. *Eur J Med.* 1992;1:183–184.

Fall M, Johansson SL, Vahlne A. A clinicopathological and virological study of interstitial cystitis. *J Urol.* 1985;133:771–773.

Farrow GM. Significant nonmalignant proliferative and neoplastic lesions of the urinary bladder. *Monogr Pathol.* 1992;34:54–76.

Feldman S, Levy LB, Prinz LM. Malakoplakia of the bladder causing bilateral ureteral obstruction. *J Urol.* 1980;123:588–589.

Feltis JT, Perez-Marrero R, Emerson LE. Increased mast cells of the bladder in suspected cases of interstitial cystitis: a possible disease marker. *J Urol.* 1987;138:42–43.

Fukushi Y, Orikasa S, Kagayama M. An electron microscopic study of the interaction between vesical epithelium and E. coli. *Invest Urol.* 1979;17:61–68.

George P. Haemorrhagic cystitis and cyclophosphamide. *Lancet.* 1963;2:942–945.

Goldberg PK, Lozinn PJ, Wise GJ. Incidence and significance of candiduria. *JAMA.* 1979;241:582–584.

Goldman RL, Warner NE. Hemorrhagic cystitis and cytomegalic inclusions in the bladder associated with cyclophosphamide therapy. *Cancer.* 1970;25: 7–11.

Goldstein M. Eosinophilic cystitis. *J Urol.* 1971;106: 854–856.

Gowing NFC. Pathological changes in the bladder following irradiation. *Br J Radiol.* 1960;33:484–487.

Gregg JA, Utz DC. Eosinophilic cystitis associated with eosinophilic gastroenteritis. *Mayo Clin Proc.* 1974;49:185–187.

Grignon, DJ, Sakr W. Inflammatory and other conditions that can mimic carcinoma in the urinary bladder. *Pathol Annu.* 1995;30:95–122.

Guermazi A, Kerviler E, Welker Y, et al. Pseudotumoral vesical actinomycosis. *J Urol.* 1996;156: 2002–2003.

Hanash KA, Pool TC. Interstitial and hemorrhagic cystitis: viral, bacterial and fungal studies. *J Urol.* 1970;104:705–706.

Hand JR. Instititial cystitis: report of 223 cases. *J Urol.* 1949;61:291–310.

Hansen MV, Kristensen PB. Eosinophilic cystitis simulating invasive bladder carcinoma. *Scand J Urol Nephrol.* 1993;27:275–277.

Hashida Y, Gaffney PC, Yunis EJ. Acute hemorrhagic cystitis of childhood and papovavirus-like particles. *J Pediatr.* 1976;89:85–87.

Hawtrey CE, Williams JJ, Schmidt JD. Cystitis emphysematosa. *Urology.* 1974;3:612–614.

Hellstrom HR, Davis BK, Shonnard JW. Eosinophilic cystitis: a study of 16 cases. *Am J Clin Pathol.* 1979;72:777–784.

Helms CA, Clark RE. Postherniorrhaphy granuloma simulating bladder neoplasm. *Radiology.* 1977; 124:56–59.

Henry L, Fox M. Histological findings in pseudomembranous trigonitis. *J Clin Pathol.* 1971;24:605–608.

Herman JR. Candiru: urinophilic catfish. Its gift to urology. *Urology.* 1973;1:265–267.

Hofmeister MA, Fang HE, Ratliff TL, et al. Mast cells and nerve fibers in interstitial cystitis (IC): An algorithm for histologic diagnosis via quantitative image analysis and morphometry (QIAM). *Urology.* 1997;49(Suppl 5A):41–47.

Holm-Bentzen M, Lose G. Pathology and pathogenesis of interstitial cystitis. *Urology.* 1987;29(suppl): 8–13.

Holm-Bentzen M, Jacobsen F, Nerstrom B, et al. Painful bladder disease: clinical and pathoanatomical differences in 115 patients. *J Urol.* 1987;138:500–502.

Hukanen V, Haarala M, Nurmi M, et al. Viruses and interstitial cystitis. Adenovirus genomes cannot be demonstrated in urinary bladder biopsies. *Urol Res.* 1996;24:235–238.

Hunner GL. A rare type of bladder ulcer in women: report of cases. *Trans South Surg Gynecol Assoc.* 1914;27:247–292.

Isogai H, Isogai E, Kimura K, et al. Helicobacter pylori induces inflammation in mouse urinary bladder and pelvis. *Microbiol Inmunol.* 1994;38:331–336.

Jimenez Lasanta JA, Mariscal A, Tenasa M, et al. Condyloma acuminatum of the bladder in a patient with AIDS: radiological findings. *J Clin Ultrasound.* 1997;25:338–340.

Johansson SL, Fall M. Pathology of interstitial cystitis. *Urol Clin N Am.* 1994;21:55–62.

Johnson DE, Lockatell CV, Hall-Craggs M, et al. Mouse models of short- and long-term foreign body in the urinary bladder: analogies to the bladder segment of urinary catheters. *Lab Anim Sci.* 1991;41:451–455.

Jufe RS, Molinolo AA, Fefer SA, et al. Plasma cell granuloma of the bladder: a case report. *J Urol.* 1984;131:1175–1176.

Kaczmarek A. Unusual complications of foreign body in the bladder. *Br J Urol.* 1985;57:106–107.

Keating MA, Young RH, Carr CP, et al. Condyloma acuminatum of the bladder and ureter: case report and review of the literature. *J Urol.* 1985;133:465–467.

Khafagy MM, El-Bolkainy MN, Mansour MA. Carcinoma of the bilharzial urinary bladder: a study of the associated mucosal lesions in 86 cases. *Cancer.* 1972;30:150–159.

King DT, Lam M. Actinomycosis of the urinary bladder. Association with an intrauterine contraceptive device. *JAMA.* 1978;240:1512–1513.

Koraitim MM, Metwalli NE, Atta MA, et al. Changing age incidence and pathological types of schistosoma-associated bladder carcinoma. *J Urol.* 1995;154:1714–1716.

Koziol JA. Epidemiology of interstitial cystitis. *Urol Clin N Am.* 1994;21:7–20.

Ladocsi LT, Sullivan B, Hanna MK. Eosinophilic granulomatous cystitis in children. *Urology.* 1995;46:732–735.

Lamm DC, Gittes RF. Inflammatory carcinoma of the bladder and interstitial cystitis. *J Urol.* 1977;117:49–53.

Larsen S, Thompson SA, Hald T, et al. Mast cells in interstitial cystitis. *Br J Urol.* 1982;54:283–286.

Libby JM, Frankel J, Scardino TT. Condyloma acuminatum of the bladder and associated urothelial malignancy. *J Urol.* 1985;134:134–136.

Littleton RH, Farah RN, Cerny JC. Eosinophilic cystitis: an uncommon form of cystitis. *J Urol.* 1982;127:132–133.

Long JP, Althausen AF. Malacoplakia: a 25-year experience with a review of the literature. *J Urol.* 1989;141:1328–1331.

Lopez-Beltran A, Munoz E. Transitional cell carcinoma of the bladder: low incidence of human papillomavirus DNA detected by the polymerase chain reaction and in situ hybridization. *Histopathology.* 1995;26:565–569.

Lund HG, Zingale FG, O'Dowd JA. Cystitis emphysematosa. *J Urol.* 1939;42:684–692.

Lynes WL, Flynn SD, Shortliffe LD, et al. Mast cell involvement in interstitial cystitis. *J Urol.* 1987;138:746–752.

MacDermott JP, Charpied GC, Tesluk H, Stone AR. Can histological assessment predict the outcome in interstitial cystitis? *Br J Urol.* 1981;67:44–47.

Maliwan N. Emphysematous cystitis associated with Clostridium perfringens bacteremia. *J Urol.* 1979;121:819–820.

Maloney PJ, Elliot GB, McLaughlin M, et al. In situ transitional carcinoma and the non-specifically inflamed contracting bladder. *J Urol.* 1974;111:162.

Marsh FP, Banerjee R, Panchamia P. The relationship between urinary infection, cystoscopic appearances, and pathology of the bladder in man. *J Clin Pathol.* 1974;27:297–307.

Marshall FF, Klinefelter HF. Late hemorrhagic cystitis following low-dose cyclophosphamide therapy. *Urology.* 1979;6:573–575.

Masukawa T, Garancis JC, Rytel MW, et al. Herpes genitalis virus isolation from human bladder urine. *Acta Cytol.* 1972;16:416–428.

McClurb FV, D'Agostino AN, Martin JH, et al. Ultrastructural demonstration of intercellular bacteria in three cases of malakoplakia of the bladder. *Am J Clin Pathol.* 1973;60:780–788.

McClure J, Young RH. Infectious disease of the urinary bladder, including malakoplakia. In: *Pathology of the urinary bladder* (1st ed.) New York: Churchill Livingstone;1989:351–376.

McKinney CD, Gaffey MJ, Gillenwater JY. Bladder outlet obstruction after multiple periurethral polytetrafluoroethylene injections. *J Urol.* 1994;153:149–151.

Menon EB, Tan ES. Urinary tract infection in acute spinal cord injury. *Singapore Med J.* 1992;33:359–361.

Messing EM, Stamey TA. Interstitial cystitis: early diagnosis, pathology, and treatment. *Urology.* 1978;12:381–392.

Milles G. Catheter induced hemorrhagic pseudopolyps of the urinary bladder. *JAMA.* 1965;193:968–969.

Mininberg DT, Watson C, Desquitado M. Viral cystitis with transient secondary vesicoureteral reflux. *J Urol.* 1982;127:983–985.

Mitas JA, Thompson T. Ureteral involvement complicating eosinophilic cystitis. *Urology.* 1985;26:67–69.

Moncada I, Lledo E, Verdu F, et al. Re: gangrenous cystitis: case report and review of the literature (Letter). *J Urol.* 1994;152:492.

Murphy WM. Diseases of urinary bladder, urethra, ureters, and renal pelves. In: *Urological pathology* (1st ed.). Philadelphia, PA: WB Saunders;1989:34–146.

Nash TE, Cheever AW, Ottesen EA, et al. Schistosome infections in humans: perspectives and recent findings. *Ann Intern Med.* 1982;97:740–746.

Neal DE Jr, Dilworth JP, Kaack MB. Tamm-Horsfall autoantibodies in interstitial cystitis. *J Urol.* 1991;145:37–39.

Nishimura K, Nozawa M, Hara T, et al. Xanthoma of the bladder. *J Urol.* 1995;153:1912–1913.

Numazaki Y, Shigeta S, Kumasaka T, et al. Acute hemorrhagic cystitis in children. Isolation of adenovirus type II. *N Engl J Med.* 1968;278:700–704.

O'Neill GF. Tiaprofenic acid as a cause of non-bacterial cystitis. *Med J Aust.* 1994;160:123–125.

Orth RW, Weisman MH, Cohen AH, et al. Lupus cystitis: primary bladder manifestations of systemic lupus erythematosus. *Ann Intern Med.* 1983;98:323–326.

Ozyurt C, Yurtseven O, Kocak I, et al. Actinomycosis simulating bladder tumor. *Br J Urol.* 1995;76:263–264.

Pang X, Cotreau-Bibbo MM, Sant GR, et al. Bladder mast cell expression of high affinity oestrogen receptors in patients with interstitial cystitis. *Br J Urol.* 1995;75:154–161.

Parsons CL, Mulholland SG. Bladder surface mucin. Its antibacterial effect against various bacterial species. *Am J Pathol.* 1978;93:423–432.

Patel B, Hhosla A, Chenoweth JL. Bilateral fungal bezoars in the renal pelvis. *Br J Urol.* 1996;78:651–652.

Pearl GS, Someron A. Suture granuloma simulating bladder neoplasm. *Urology.* 1980;15:304–308.

Peterson NE. Eosinophilic cystitis. *Urology.* 1985;26:167–171.

Ratliff TL, Klutke CG, MacDougall EM. The etiology of interstitial cystitis. *Urol Clin N Am.* 1994;21:21–30.

Ratliff TL, Klutke CG, Hofmeister M, et al. Role of the immune response in interstitial cystitis. *Clin Immunol Immunopathol.* 1995;74:209–216.

Raziuddin S, Masihuzzaman M, Shetty S, et al. Tumor necrosis factor alpha production in schistosomiasis with carcinoma of urinary bladder. *J Clin Immunol.* 1993;13:23–29.

Rosenberg HK, Eggli KD, Zerin JM, et al. Benign cystitis in children mimicking rhabdomyosarcoma. *J Ultrasound Med.* 1994;13:921–932.

Rosin MP, Anwar WA, Ward AJ. Inflammation, chromosomal instability, and cancer: the schistosomiasis model. *Cancer Res.* 1994a;54:1929–1933.

Rosin MP, Saad el Din Zaki S, Ward AJ, et al. Involvement of inflammatory reactions and elevated cell proliferation in the development of bladder cancer in schistosomiasis patients. *Mutation Res.* 1994b;305:283–292.

Rubin L, Pincus MB. Eosinophilic cystitis: the relationship of allergy in the urinay tract to eosinophilic cystitis and the pathophysiology of eosinophilia. *J Urol.* 1974;112:457–460.

Sakamoto S. Fungus ball formation of Aspergillus in the bladder. *Eur Urol.* 1978;4:388–391.

Sant GR, Theoharides TC. The role of the mast cell in interstitial cystitis. *Urol Clin N Am.* 1994;21:41–53.

Santamaria M, Molina I, Lopez-Beltran A, et al. Identification and characterization of a human cell line with dentritic cell features. *Virchows Archiv B Cell Pathol.* 1988;56:77–83.

Sarma KP. On the nature of cystitis follicularis. *J Urol.* 1970;104:709–714.

Schlomovitz BH. Cystitis follicularis. *J Urol.* 1942;47:168–174.

Seftel AD, Matthews LA, Smith MC, et al. Polyomavirus mimicking high grade transitional cell carcinoma. *J Urol.* 1996;156:1764–1765.

Shibutani YF, Schoenberg MP, Carpiniello VL. Human papillomavirus associated with bladder cancer. *Urology.* 1992;40:15–17.

Shindo K, Kitayama T, Ura T, et al. Acute hemorrhagic cystitis caused by adenovirus type II after renal transplantation. *Urol Int.* 1986;41:152–155.

Skudowitz RB, Weintraub CM. Malakoplakia association with transitional cell carcinoma of bladder. *J Urol.* 1977;118:482–484.

Smith JH, Christie JD. The pathology of Schistosoma haematobium infection in humans. *Hum Pathol.* 1986;17:333–345.

Smith BH, Dehner LP. Chronic ulcerating interstitial cystitis. *Arch Pathol.* 1972;93:76–81.

Spagnolo DV, Waring PM. Bladder granulomata after surgery. *Am J Clin Pathol.* 1986;86:430–437.

Speights VO, Edwards E, Jones KA, et al. In situ hybridization for viral detection in interstitial cystitis. *J Urol Pathol*. 1995;3:129–134.

Stillwell TJ, Benson RC Jr. Cyclophosphamide-induced hemorrhagic cystitis: a review of 100 patients. *Cancer*. 1988;61:451–457.

Stirling WC, Hopkins GA. Gangrene of the bladder. *J Urol*. 1934;31:517–525.

Tamella T, Kallioinen M, Kontturi M, et al. Sarcoidosis of the bladder: a case report and review of the literature. *J Urol*. 1989;141:608–609.

Ulker V, Apaydin E, Gursan A, et al. Eosinophilic cystitis induced by mitomycin-C. *Int Urol Nephrol*. 1996;28:755–759.

Utz DC, Zincke H. The masquerade of bladder cancer in situ as interstitial cystitis. *J Urol*. 1974;11:160–161.

Van de Merwe J, Kamerling R, Arendsen E, et al. Sjogren's syndrome in patients with interstitial cystitis. *J Rheumatol*. 1993;20:962–966.

Von Lichtenberg F, Edington GM, Nwabuebo I, et al. Pathologic effects of schistosomiasis in Ibadan, Western State of Nigeria: II. Pathogenesis of lesions of the bladder and ureters. *Am J Trop Med Hyg*. 1971;20:244–254.

Walters M, Glenn JF, Vellios F. Xanthogranulomatous cystitis. *J Urol*. 1985;134:745–746.

Warren JW. Interstitial cystitis as an infectious disease. *Urol Clin N Am*. 1994;21:31–39.

Wells HG. Giant cells in cystitis. *Arch Pathol*. 1938;26:32–38.

Wilson CB, Leopard J, Nakamura RM, et al. Selective type IV collagen defects in urothelial basement membrane in interstitial cystitis. *J Urol*. 1995;154:1222–1226.

Young RH. Papillary and polypoid cystitis: a report of eight cases. *Am J Surg Pathol*. 1988;12:542–546.

Young RH. Non-neoplastic epithelial abnormalities and tumor-like lesions. In: *Pathology of the urinary bladder*. New York: Churchill Livingstone;1989:1–63.

4
CHEMOTHERAPY- AND RADIATION-RELATED AND METABOLIC CHANGES

4.1 CHEMOTHERAPY-RELATED CHANGES

A handful of chemotherapeutic agents significantly alter the urothelium and may produce metabolic or toxic effects. The pathologist must be able to separate nonspecific toxicity and drug-specific alterations from tumor-related changes (Table 4.1). The clinical history is invaluable in this assessment. Bacillus Calmette-Guérin (BCG) granulomatous cystitis, the most common therapy-associated change, is discussed in Chapter 3.

4.1.1 Cyclophosphamide

This alkylating agent is used in the treatment of nonurothelial malignancies and diseases such as systemic lupus erythematosus (Plotz et al, 1979), rheumatoid arthritis, nephrotic syndrome, and lymphoproliferative disorders (Lawrence et al, 1975). Cyclophosphamide therapy may induce stromal fibrosis, vascular changes (intimal thickening, mural fibrin deposition, and ectasia), urothelial atypia, hemorrhagic cystitis, mural and mucosal fibrosis, and bladder cancer (Fig 4.1) (Berkson et al, 1973; Johnson & Meadows, 1971).

Table 4.1 Intravesical therapy–associated atypia and low-grade urothelial carcinoma

Feature	Therapy-associated atypia (thiotepa, mitomycin C)	Low-grade carcinoma
Cellularity	Early: high, late: low	Usually high
Cell size	Enlarged	Normal to minimal enlargement
Nucleus-to-cytoplasm ratio	Normal	Increased
Staining	Hyperchromatic	Hyperchromatic
Nuclear borders	Irregular	Irregular
Chromatin	Fine, regular	Fine, regular
Nucleoli	Variable	Variable
Architecture	Loose, dyscohesive	Papillary, loose clusters
Ploidy	Diploid	Usually diploid

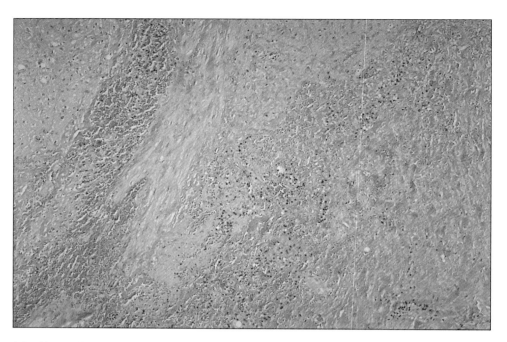

Figure 4.1 Hemorrhagic cystitis after cyclophosphamide therapy.

Cyclophosphamide induces epithelial necrosis, followed by rapid regeneration with hyperplasia and formation of papillary tumors. Bladder cancer associated with cyclophosphamide is uncommon but not rare (Wall & Clausen, 1975). The risk of neoplasm is apparently increased in patients with a history of cystitis (Rowland & Eble, 1983). Bladder cancer occurs most commonly in patients receiving cyclophosphamide for immunosuppression after organ transplantation or treatment of lymphoproliferative or myeloproliferative disorders, particularly multiple myeloma and Hodgkin's disease. Urothelial carcinoma is the most common cancer, although squamous cell carcinoma, adenocarcinoma, undifferentiated carcinoma, fibrosarcoma, leiomyosarcoma, and sarcomatoid carcinoma have also been reported (Fernandes et al, 1997; Kanno et al, 1985; Siddiqui et al, 1996; Talar-Williams et al, 1996). This occurs in a minority of patients following prolonged administration. The mean interval from primary tumor to bladder cancer is variable, although usually lengthy, and may be as long as 11 years.

The metabolic effects of cyclophosphamide, including arrest of cell and nuclear division, produce bi- and multinucleated cells, often with large bizarre nuclei resembling changes of radiation injury (Fig 4.2) (Forni et al, 1964; Heling & Okmian, 1973). This radiomimetic effect creates cellular changes that can be mistaken for malignancy. There is marked but variable cellular and nuclear enlargement. Nuclei are often eccentric, slightly irregular in outline, and usually markedly hyperchromatic (Goldman & Warner, 1970). Chromatin may be coarse but is usually evenly distributed. Nuclear pyknosis is a common late effect that results in loss of chromatin texture. Nucleoli are single or double and are occasionally large and distorted with irregular and sharp edges.

Cyclophosphamide may induce hemorrhagic cystitis. This spectrum of changes is described in Chapter 3.

4.1.2 Mitomycin C and Thiotepa

Mitomycin C, an antitumor antibiotic, and triethylenethiophosphoramide (thiotepa), a polyfunctional alkylating agent, are intravesical chemotherapeutic agents that reduce the likelihood of recurrence and thus prolong survival in patients with bladder cancer. Although these agents suppress tumor growth and progression, they do not eradicate cancer (Murphy et al, 1978). These topical chemotherapeutic agents produce identical histologic and cytologic changes, including an increase in exfoliation and denudation, multinucleation, cytoplasmic vacuolation, and the appearance of bizarre, nonmalignant nuclei in the superficial layer of the urothelium (Fig 4.3). Exfoliation of preserved cells is followed within 48 hours by the appearance of degenerated cells. The toxic effects do not become more severe with continued exposure and tend to subside after removal of the drug. Urothelial denudation makes recurrence of cancer difficult to detect cystoscopically and to document histologically; urine cytology is important for follow-up (Choe et al, 1995). A marked necroinflammatory process follows administration of topical mitomycin C. There is often a histiocytic response that extends deep into the bladder wall, and isolated single and clustered macrophages suggest an inflammatory neoplasm. Mitomycin C may also initiate eosinophilic cystitis (Choe et al, 1995; Ulker et al, 1996). These agents are not metabolic inhibitors of DNA replication and thus do not produce full-thickness atypical cells such as those seen after cyclophosphamide.

Thiotepa appears to affect only normal and not neoplastic urothelium. Superficial cells are large and often fused, with vacuolated cytoplasm and enlarged, hyperchromatic nuclei indicative of degeneration and regeneration. Typically, the cells have slightly or moderately enlarged nuclei, but there is no significant increase in chromatin density. When mild to moderate hyperchromasia occurs, it usually consists of smudged chromatin that lacks a sharply detailed pattern. Nuclei are round or oval, with smooth, thin chromatic rims or wrinkled rims because of degeneration. Large multinucleated superficial cells frequently contain multiple small nucleoli and display cytoplasmic

vacuolization with frayed borders (Murphy et al, 1980). These changes occur almost exclusively in superficial cells, recognized by their abundant cytoplasm and convex outer borders. The cytologic changes produced by thiotepa are not specific for topical chemotherapy and can be produced by chronic inflammation, catheterization, and instillation of saline. Morphologic features of malignancy, whether low or high grade, are not altered by these forms of therapy.

4.1.3 Other Chemotherapeutic Agents

Doxorubicin hydrochloride (adriamycin) causes chemical cystitis. Danazol (a synthetic anabolic steroid) and ortho-toluidine (a skin-absorbed chemical) may produce severe vesical hemorrhage (Scharf et al, 1977). Analgesic abuse with phenacetin, a drug with a chemical structure similar to that of aniline dyes, is associated with an increased risk of urothelial carcinoma of the renal pelvis and bladder (Piper et al, 1985). Busulfan-induced hemorrhagic cystitis rarely occurs but can be clinically significant (Pode et al, 1983).

4.1.4 Chemical Cystitis

Ether cystitis is uncommon and occurs when ether is introduced into the bladder to dissolve a catheter balloon that resists mechanical deflation. Formalin, instilled vesically to control bleeding, and turpentine, excreted by the kidney after ingestion, create an ether-type injury, including hemorrhagic urothelial necrosis, edema, and leukocytic infiltration. Bonney's blue may be instilled in the bladder during gynecologic surgery, but failure to dilute the concentrate to a 0.5% solution causes severe chemical cystitis.

4.2 RADIATION AND LASER-INDUCED CHANGES

Radiation therapy produces a variety of bladder lesions associated with diverse symptoms and pathologic findings (Figs 4.4–4.7) (Antona-

(a)

(b)

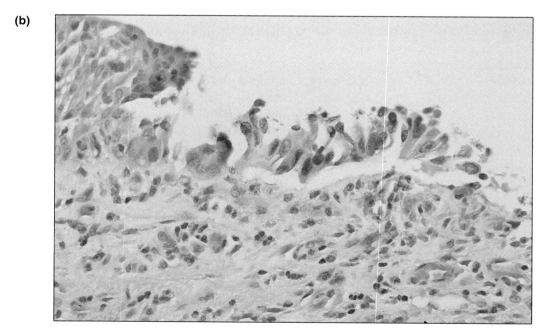

Figure 4.2   (a,b): The urothelium is distorted, hyperchromatic, and separated from the underlying inflamed submucosa after cyclophosphamide therapy.

(a)

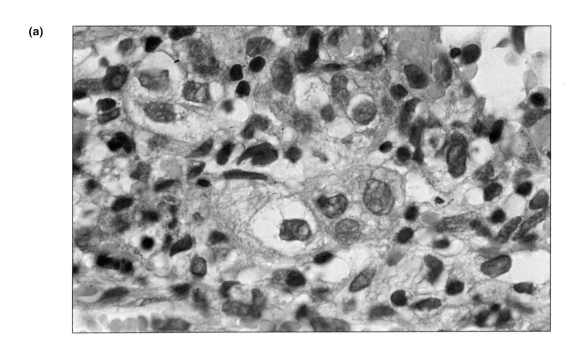

(b)

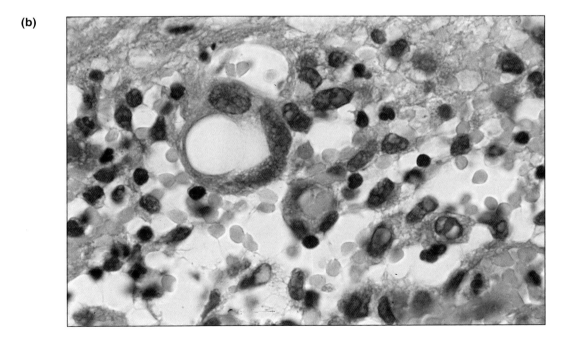

(c)

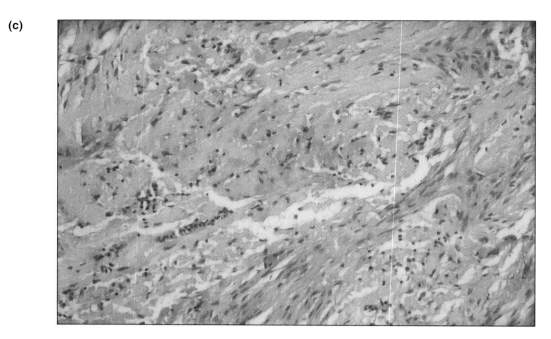

Figure 4.3 **(a,b):** Mitomycin C–induced changes, including stromal atypia, acute and chronic inflammation, and hemorrhage; **(c):** necrosis of the muscularis propria.

kopoulous et al, 1984). The clinical course has three phases according to the time of onset of symptoms: (1) acute (<6 months), (2) subacute (6 months to 2 years), and (3) chronic (2–5 years) (Fajardo et al, 1978; Marks et al, 1995; Pazzaglia et al, 1994). Bladder lesions are caused by mucosal, stromal, and vascular damage, and include acute and chronic radiation cystitis, with mucosal ulceration and bladder contracture as a late complication. Depending on the duration and the severity of vesical injury, the urine sediment contains cellular debris and degenerated or necrotic urothelial cells, variable hemorrhage, and other inflammatory cells, including histiocytes. Urothelial cells are enlarged and may show striking gigantism with or without bi- or multinucleation. Nuclear enlargement is also present, but the nucleus-to-cytoplasm ratio is low. Enlarged nuclei may contain macronucleoli but frequently show degenerative changes, including vacuolization, chromatin clearing, and loss of chromatin texture. Nuclear

irregularities and hyperchromasia reflect varying degrees of pyknosis. Cytoplasmic vacuolation and polychromasia are characteristic findings, and frayed borders indicate cellular degeneration. Cytologic changes may persist in the urine sediment for years.

4.2.1 Radiation Cystitis

A variety of abnormalities may be seen in the bladder as a result of radiation. The earliest change, usually seen after 3–6 weeks, consists of acute cystitis with desquamation of urothelial cells and hyperemia and edema of the lamina propria (Marks et al, 1995). The urothelial cells show varying degrees of atypicality, including cytoplasmic and nuclear vacuolization, karyorrhexis, normal nucleus-to-cytoplasm ratio, edema, prominent telangiectatic vessels, hyalinization, thrombosis of blood vessels, and atypical mesenchymal cells similar to those seen in giant cell cystitis (Fajardo et al, 1978; Hietala et

(a)

(b)

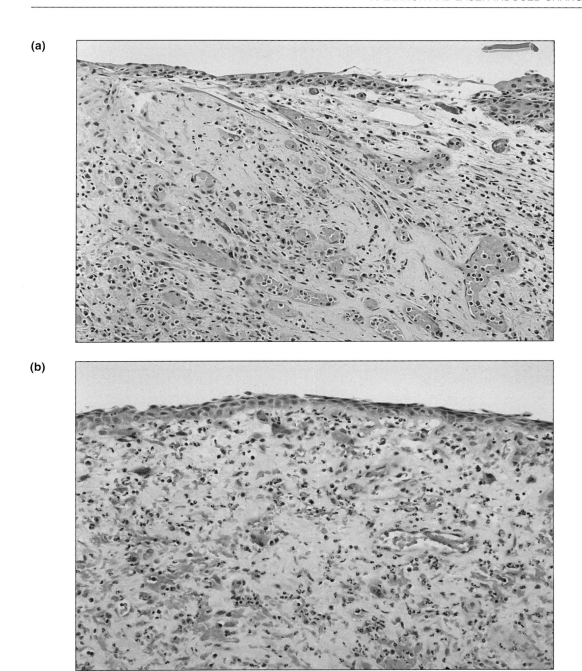

Figure 4.4 **(a,b):** Radiation-induced changes, including mucosal atrophy, inflammation of the lamina propria, and marked vascular congestion.

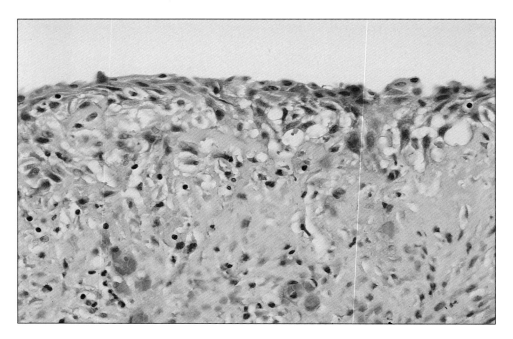

Figure 4.5 Radiation-induced change of the urothelium, including cytologic abnormalities, chronic inflammation, and submucosal fibrosis.

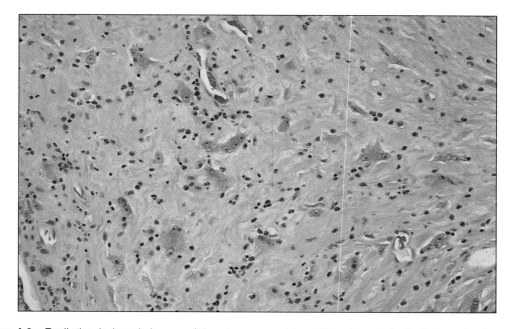

Figure 4.6 Radiation-induced change of the stroma consists of fibrosis and atypical stromal cells.

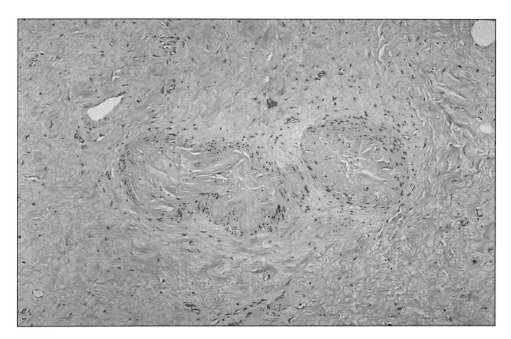

Figure 4.7 Radiation induces prominent accelerated arteriolosclerotic changes.

al, 1975; Marks et al, 1995). Late complications of radiation injury include ulcers, marked contraction of the bladder as a result of fibrosis, and ureteral stricture (Fajardo et al, 1978).

4.2.2 Photodynamic and Laser Therapy

Photodynamic and laser therapy for bladder cancer produces acute mucosal inflammation with sloughing and edema (Keane et al, 1994; Prout et al, 1987; Shanberg et al, 1987; Smith, 1985; Vicente et al, 1991). Other findings include dystrophic calcification and spindle cell artifact of urothelial cells (Fanning et al, 1993; Pisharodi & Bhan, 1995; Wong et al, 1996).

4.3 METABOLIC DEPOSITS

4.3.1 Amyloidosis

Amyloidosis is a disorder in which abnormal proteinaceous deposits occupy the parenchyma, interstitium, and blood vessel walls in multiple organs (Fig 4.8) (Fujiyara & Glenner, 1981). The condition is classified as primary or secondary. Most patients with bladder involvement present with primary amyloidosis that includes monoclonal immunoglobulin G abnormalities of serum, urine, or both, as well as amyloid deposits in the skin, tongue, heart, gastrointestinal tract, and carpal ligaments. Secondary amyloidosis accompanies chronic inflammation or infectious process such as rheumatoid arthritis, osteomyelitis, tuberculosis, syphilis, bronchiectasias, and ankylosing spondylitis. Amyloidosis is considered a generic term that refers to the deposition of various proteins that share a β-pleated sheet conformation. Different clinical types of amyloidosis are now more specifically associated with identifiable proteins usually derived from circulating serum precursors. The abnormal protein of the amyloid fibril in patients with nonhereditary primary systemic amyloidosis, or those with plasma cell dyscrasia, is either an intact immunoglobulin light chain (L) or a fragment of its variable region (amyloid L or AL).

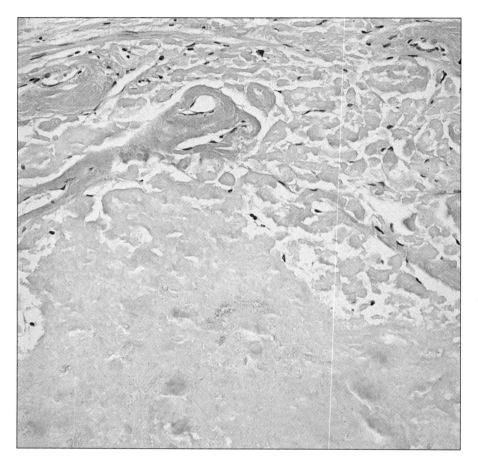

Figure 4.8 Amyloid deposit in the bladder.

In localized amyloidosis of the genitourinary tract, the amyloid fibrils appear to have kappa and lambda determinants, indicating immunocytic derivation. The abnormal protein associated with secondary amyloidosis is not immunoglobulin derived but appears to follow cleavage in the liver of the serum protein known as SAA, with the formation of amyloid A or AA. Anti-AA monoclonal antibodies may be used to identify this type of amyloid. AA also constitutes the abnormal protein in patients with hereditary amyloidosis (familial Mediterranean fever). Other types of inherited amyloidosis (autosomal dominant) are associated with other β-pleated proteins such as the variant of normal thyroxine-binding prealbumin, in the amyloidotic polyneuropathies, cardiomyopathies, or nephropathies. Fibrillar protein deposition of monomers and dimers of β_2-microglobulin occurs in patients on long-term dialysis, and this fibrillar protein has the same staining properties as amyloid. Most, but not all, cases of vesical amyloid are not associated with a systemic disorder and present with localized tumefactions in the bladder.

Primary vesical amyloidosis occurs with equal frequency in men and women and typically causes gross painless hematuria. Men appear to be affected at a younger age than women. The disorder may be associated with suprapubic pain, frequency, nocturia, dysuria, recurrent urinary tract infection, and ureteral obstruction. Primary vesical amyloidosis may clinically mimic interstitial cystitis. At cystoscopy, primary amyloidotic lesions are usually localized, appearing as hemorrhagic ulcers, erythematous and inflammatory excrescences, yellow tumefactions (ulcerated or necrotic), smooth round masses that are occasionally calcified, or as polyps (Malek et al, 1971). Localized deposits frequently resemble infiltrating neoplasms.

Microscopically, there is eosinophilic acellular, amorphous material in primary amyloidosis that thickens and distorts arteries and veins in the suburothelial stroma and inner layers of the muscularis propria. Connective tissue in these layers also becomes involved. There is usually no inflammatory response, although a lymphoplasmocytic and giant cell reaction may occasionally occur. Smooth muscle amyloid deposition apparently commences at the periphery of muscle bundles and progresses centrally (Fujiyara & Glenner, 1981).

Vesical amyloidosis associated with systemic disorders is similar to the primary type. The secondary type is uncommon and, rather than forming a localized mass, presents with diffuse erythema and petechiae or focal necrosis. There is more prominent vascular than stromal involvement, presumably accounting for the propensity for massive spontaneous hemorrhage or torrential bleeding after biopsy (Hinsch et al, 1996).

A distinctive subtype of AA amyloidosis shows massive vascular infiltration with protein AA fibrils. Amyloid stained by hematoxylin and eosin may be difficult to distinguish from hyalinized collagen, which usually is found in hyalinized blood vessel walls in the papillae of some urothelial carcinomas. Amyloid may be missed if there are few deposits and the pathologist is not considering this possibility. Unlike collagen, amyloid is not birefringent in polarized light. Its tinctorial qualities do not distinguish between primary and secondary types. However, β-pleated protein fibrils are metachromatic (red) with crystal or methyl violet; they fluoresce after thioflavin T staining and appear as bright apple green deposits after staining with alkaline Congo red and viewed with polarized light. Monoclonal antibodies may be used to further analyze these deposits.

4.3.2 Tamm-Horsfall Protein

Tamm-Horsfall protein (THP) is a high–molecular-weight glycoprotein synthesized exclusively by the ascending loop of Henle and the distal tubule of normal kidney. In pathologic conditions, THP may accumulate in the renal parenchyma, perirenal soft tissue, or renal hilar lymph nodes. Deposits of THP have been described in the bladder and ureter and are more frequent in men (male-to-female ratio: 8:1) between the ages of 45 and 78 years (mean: 68 years). Two morphologic patterns of presentation have been described (Truong et al, 1994). The most common pattern presents with THP appearing as large waxy pale or weakly eosinophilic masses (Fig 4.9). In such cases, THP is strongly positive by period acid-Schiff stain, pale on Masson's trichrome stain, and ultrastructurally composed of nonbranching 4-nm-wide fibrils arranged in a parallel fashion. In the second pattern, THP appears as inconspicuous flecks of interconnecting strands of eosinophilic material obscured by a large amount of adjacent fibrinous exudate or necrotic tissue. In these cases, Masson's trichrome and periodic acid-Schiff stains are not always helpful in making the diagnosis. Immunohistochemical studies using anti-THP antibody allow identification of even small amounts of THP. Also, staining is helpful in differentiating THP from amyloidosis or hyalinized collagen. Typically, the areas where THP is deposited invariably show necrosis, inflammation, fibrinous exudate, ulcer, or crystalline material. THP is frequently seen in bladder tissue and probably

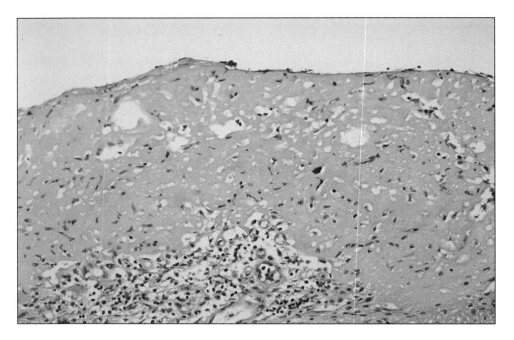

Figure 4.9 Tamm-Horsfall protein deposit in the bladder.

represents an incidental finding of morphologic interest but of no clinical significance (Truong et al, 1994). Recently, we observed two tumors of the renal pelvis that were associated with THP deposits, including an inflammatory myofibroblastic tumor and an invasive urothelial carcinoma.

REFERENCES

Antonakopoulous GN, Hicks RM, Berry RJ. The subcellular basis of damage to the urinary bladder induced by irradiation. *J Pathol.* 1984;143:103–116.

Berkson BM, Lome LG, Shapiro I. Severe cystitis induced by cyclophosphamide. Role of surgical management. *JAMA.* 1973;225:605–608.

Choe JM, Kirkemo AK, Sirls LT. Intravesical thiotepa-induced eosinophilic cystitis. *Urology.* 1995;46:729–731.

Fajardo LF, Berthrong M. Radiation injury in surgical pathology: I. *Am J Surg Pathol.* 1978;2:159–199.

Fanning CV, Staerkel GA, Sneige N, et al. Spindling artefact of urothelial cells in post-laser treatment urinary cytology. *Diagn Cytopathol.* 1993;9:279–281.

Fernandes ET, Manivel JC, Reddy PK, et al. Cyclophosphamide associated bladder cancer. A highly aggressive disease: analysis of 12 cases. *J Urol.* 1997;156:1931–1933.

Forni AM, Koss LG, Geller W. Cytological study of the effect of cyclophosphamide on the epithelium of the urinary bladder in man. *Cancer.* 1964;17:1348–1355.

Fujiyara S, Glenner GC. Primary localized amyloidosis of the genitourinary tract: immunohistochemical study of 11 cases. *Lab Invest.* 1981;44:55–60.

Goldman RL, Warner EN. Hemorrhagic cystitis and cytomegalic inclusion in the bladder associated with cyclophosphamide therapy. *Cancer.* 1970;25:7–16.

Heling I, Okmian L. Haemorrhagic cystitis complicating cyclophosphamide treatment in children. *Acta Pediatr Scand.* 1973;62:497–499.

Hietala SO, Winblad B, Hassler O. Vascular and morphological changes in the urinary bladder wall after irradiation. *Int Urol Nephrol.* 1975;7:119–125.

Hinsch R, Thompson L, Conrad R. Secondary amyloidosis of the urinary bladder. A rare cause of massive hematuria. *Aust NZ J Surg.* 1996;66:127–128.

Johnson WW, Meadows DC. Urinary-bladder fibrosis and telangiectasia associated with long-term cyclophosphamide therapy. *N Engl J Med.* 1971;284:290–292.

Kanno J, Sakamoto A, Washizuka M, et al. Malignant mixed mesodermal tumor of bladder occurring after radiotherapy for cervical cancer: report of a case. *J Urol.* 1985;133:854–855.

Keane TE, Petros JA, Velimirovich B, et al. Methoxypsoralen phototherapy of transitional cell carcinoma. *Urology.* 1994;44:842–846.

Lawrence HJ, Simone J, Aur RJA. Cyclophosphamide-induced hemorrhagic cystitis in children with leukemia. *Cancer.* 1975;36:1572–1579.

Malek RS, Greene LF, Farrow GM. Amyloidosis of the urinary bladder. *Br J Urol.* 1971;43:189–200.

Marks LB, Carrol PR, Dugan TC, et al. The response of the urinary bladder, urethra and ureter to radiation and chemotherapy. *Int J Radiat Oncol Biol Phys.* 1995;31:1257–1280.

Murphy WM, Soloway MS, Lin CJ. Morphological effects of thio-TEPA on mammalian urothelium: changes in abnormal cells. *Acta Cytol.* 1978;22:550–558.

Murphy WM, Soloway MS, Finebaum PJ. Pathologic changes associated with topical chemotherapy for superficial bladder cancer. *J Urol.* 1980;126:461–466.

Pazzaglia S, Chen XR, Aamodt CB, et al. In vitro radiation-induced neoplastic progression of low-grade uroepithelial tumors. *Radiation Res.* 1994;138:86–92.

Piper JM, Tonascia J, Matanowski GM. Heavy phenacetin use and bladder cancer in women aged 20 to 49 years. *N Engl J Med.* 1985;313:292–293.

Pisharodi LR, Bhan R. Spindling artefact of urothelial cells. *Diagn Cytopathol.* 1995;12:195–196.

Plotz PH, Klippel JH, Decker JL, et al. Bladder complications in patients receiving cyclophosphamide for systemic lupus erythematosus or rheumatoid arthritis. *Ann Intern Med.* 1979;91:221–225.

Pode D, Perlberg S, Steiner D. Busulfan-induced hemorrhagic cystitis. *J Urol.* 1983;130:347–348.

Prout GR Jr, Lin CW, Benson R Jr, et al. Photodynamic therapy with hematoporphyrin derivate in the treatment of superficial transitional cell carcinoma of the bladder. *N Engl J Med.* 1987;317:1251–1255.

Rowland RG, Eble JN. Bladder leiomyosarcoma and pelvic fibroblastic tumor following cyclophosphamide therapy. *J Urol.* 1983;130:344–346.

Scharf J, Nahir M, Eidelman S, et al. Carcinoma of the bladder with azathioprine therapy. *JAMA.* 1977;237:152–154.

Shanberg AM, Baghdassarian R, Tansey LA. Use of Nd:YAG laser in treatment of bladder cancer. *Urology.* 1987;29:26–30.

Siddiqui A, Melamed MR, Abbi R, et al. Mucinous (colloid) carcinoma of urinary bladder following long term cyclophosphamide therapy for Waldenström's macroglobulinemia. *Am J Surg Pathol.* 1996;20:500–504.

Smith JA Jr. Laser treatment of bladder cancer. *Semin Urol.* 1985;3:2–18.

Talar-Williams C, Hijazi YM, Walther MM, et al. Cyclophosphamide-induced cystitis and bladder cancer in patients with Wegener granulomatosis. *Ann Intern Med.* 1996;124:477–484.

Truong LD, Ostrowski ML, Wheeler TM. Tamm-Horsfall protein in bladder tissue. Morphologic spectrum and clinical significance. *Am J Surg Pathol.* 1994;18:615–622.

Ulker V, Apaydin E, Gursan A, et al. Eosinophilic cystitis induced by mitomycin-C. *Int Urol Nephrol.* 1996;28:755–759.

Vicente J, Salvador J, Laguna P, et al. Histological evaluation of superficial bladder tumors treated by Nd-YAG laser and transurethral resection. *Eur Urol.* 1991;20:192–196.

Wall RL, Clausen KP. Carcinoma of the urinary bladder in patients receiving cyclophosphamide. *N Engl J Med.* 1975;293:271–272.

Wong AK, Lupu AN, Shanberg AM. Laser ablation of renal pelvic transitional cell carcinoma in a solitary kidney. A 9 year follow up. *Urology.* 1996;48:298–300.

5

MISCELLANEOUS NON-NEOPLASTIC LESIONS

5.1 DIVERTICULOSIS

Diverticuli are saccular evaginations of the urinary bladder. They are most common in men (90% of cases) and occur in ages ranging from 21 to 90 years. Patients usually have bladder outlet obstruction at the bladder base (Peterson et al, 1973). Bladder diverticuli vary from a few millimeters to several centimeters in diameter, and about half are multiple. At surgery, most are inflamed with thinning of the sac wall, fibrosis, and loss of muscle fibers in the wall. Neutrophils often infiltrate the lamina propria, and focal squamous or glandular metaplasia of the mucosa may be present. Neoplasms are more common in diverticula than in the normal bladder, and a variety of mesenchymal and epithelial benign and malignant tumors may coexist (Peterson et al, 1973; Rajan et al, 1996). Survival with diverticular carcinoma is poor. Diverticular cancer is usually high-grade urothelial carcinoma, squamous cell carcinoma, or sarcoma.

5.2 ENDOCERVICOSIS

Endocervicosis is an uncommon glandular tumor-like condition occurring in the bladder of women between 31 and 44 years of age (Fig 5.1).

All reported lesions are diagnostically challenging, and some are misinterpreted as adenocarcinoma. Symptoms include suprapubic pain, dysuria, frequency, and hematuria (Nazeer et al, 1996).

Macroscopically, endocervicosis typically arises in the posterior wall and posterior dome of the bladder. Microscopically, there is extensive involvement of the wall by irregular benign-appearing or mildly atypical endocervical-type glands, some of which are typically cystically dilated. Clement and Young (1992) concluded that these lesions were müllerian and represented examples of endocervicosis, the mucinous counterpart of endometriosis. Occasionaly, tubules and cysts lined by tubal-type epithelium are observed that represent endosalpingiosis, including ciliated, intercalated, and peg cells (Young & Clement, 1996). In cases in which endosalpingiosis is associated with endocervicosis, endometriosis, or both, the term *müllerianosis* is proposed (Young & Clement, 1996). Curative treatment includes partial cystectomy and transurethral resection of the bladder (Bladamura et al, 1995; Parivar et al, 1995; Seman & Stewart, 1994).

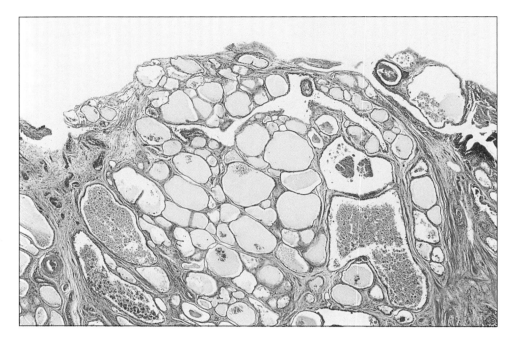

Figure 5.1 Endocervicosis of the bladder.

5.3 ENDOMETRIOSIS

The bladder is the most common organ in the urinary tract to harbor foci of ectopic endometrial tissue (Fig 5.2) (Vercellini et al, 1996). Most cases occur in women during the reproductive years, and many follow pelvic surgery. Endometriosis of the bladder has been rarely reported in men (Neto et al, 1984; Schrodt et al, 1980). Cystoscopically, the involved areas may be ulcerated, resulting in hematuria. If the implants are deep within the muscularis propria, they may elicit a prominent fibrous response, resulting in a mass lesion with wall distortion. The histologic appearance is similar to implants of endometriosis in other organs, consisting of a variable mixture of endometrial glands, stroma, and hemosiderin-laden macrophages. Rare cases of cancer arising in foci of endometriosis in the urinary bladder have been described, including cases of endometrioid ad-

enocarcinoma and adenosarcoma (Al-Izzi et al, 1989; Vara et al, 1990).

5.4 MELANOSIS (LIPOFUSCINOSIS VESICALIS)

Excess lipofuscin deposition is a normal process of aging but is rarely found in the bladder (Alroy et al, 1986; Henderson, 1991; Herrera et al, 1990). The cystoscopic or macroscopic appearance of multifocal dark pigmented spots or patches may create concern for melanoma, and coexistent melanosis and melanoma may occur (Kerley et al, 1991). Melanocytes are apparently not present in the normal urothelium; however, anti–S-100 protein-immunoreactive dendritic cells are present in inflamed urothelium, urothelial carcinoma, and cystitis follicularis (Anichkov & Nikonov, 1982). Adriamycin toxicity may be associated with vesicular melanosis (Rothberg et al, 1974).

(a)

(b)

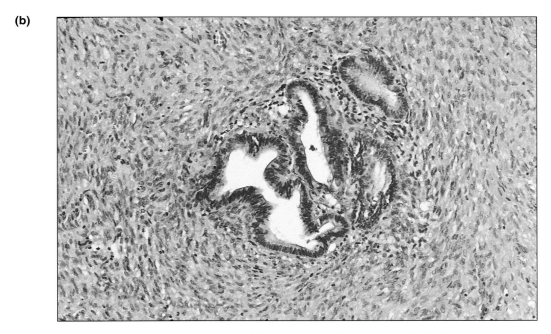

Figure 5.2 Endometriosis of the bladder. **(a):** Disabling diffuse endometriosis in a young woman, which required a cystectomy; **(b):** typical glands and stroma of endometriosis, with chronic inflammation.

5.5 OTHER NON-NEOPLASTIC TUMOR-LIKE CONDITIONS

5.5.1 Submucosal Calcification and Ossification

Massive calcification rarely occurs in the bladder, similar to its counterpart in the renal pelvis (Firstater & Farkas, 1981). Patients have a long history of chronic cystitis, often with nephrogenic metaplasia or urachal carcinoma (Lopez-Beltran et al, 1984). A case of massive submucosal bone metaplasia was reported in association with encrusted cystitis (Collins & Welebir, 1941).

5.5.2 Hemorrhage and Bladder Rupture

Subepithelial hemorrhage similar to the Antopol-Goldman lesion of the renal pelvis rarely occurs in the bladder (Fig 5.3) (Antopol & Goldman, 1948; Iczkowski et al, in press; Levitt et al, 1984). Pseudoneoplastic healing reactions may occur after traumatic bladder rupture. Spontaneous rupture of the urinary bladder is a late complication of radiotherapy (Addar et al, 1996). A unique case of prolapse of the fallopian tube into the bladder was misinterpreted as carcinoma (Anastasiades & Majmudar, 1983).

REFERENCES

Addar MH, Stuart GCE, Nation JG, et al. Spontaneous rupture of the urinary bladder. A late complication of radiotherapy. A case report and review of the literature. *Gynecol Oncol.* 1996;62:314–316.

Al-Izzi MS, Horton LW, Kelleher J, et al. Malignant transformation of endometriosis of the bladder. *Histopathology.* 1989;14:191–198.

Alroy J, Ucci AA, Heaney JA, et al. Multifocal pigmentation of prostatic and bladder urothelium. *J Urol.* 1986;136:96–97.

Anastasiades KD, Majmudar B. Prolapse of fallopian tube into urinary bladder mimicking bladder carcinoma. *Arch Pathol Lab Med.* 1983;107:613–615.

Antopol W, Goldman L. Subepithelial hemorrhage of renal pelvis simulating neoplasm. *Urol Cutan Rev.* 1948;52:189–192.

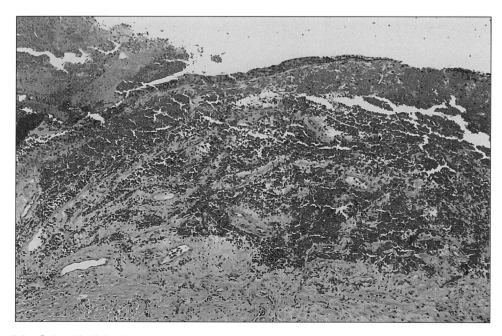

Figure 5.3 Subepithelial pelvic hematoma of the renal pelvis that clinically mimicked cancer in a 56-year-old man.

Bladamura S, Palma PD, Meneghini A. Paramesonephric remnants with prominent mucinous secretion, so-called endocervicosis of the urinary bladder. *J Urol Pathol.* 1995;3:165–172.

Clement PB, Young RH. Endocervicosis of the urinary bladder. A report of 6 cases of a benign mullerian lesion that may mimic adenocarcinoma. *Am J Surg Pathol.* 1992;16:533–540.

Collins CW, Welebir F. Osteoma of the bladder. *J Urol.* 1941;46:494–498.

Firstater M, Farkas A. Submucosal renal pelvic calcification simulating a pelvic stone. *J Urol.* 1981;126:802–803.

Henderson DW. Unusual pigmented vesical lesion in a middle-aged woman. *Ultrastruct Pathol.* 1991;15:311–314.

Herrera GA, Turbat-Herrera EA, Lockard VG. Unusual pigmented vesical lesion in a middle-aged woman. *Ultrastruct Pathol.* 1990;14:529–535.

Iczkowski KA, Sweat SD, Bostwick DG. Subepithelial pelvic hematoma of the kidney clinically mimicking cancer: Report of six cases and review of the literature. *Urology.* In press.

Kerley SW, Blute ML, Keeney GL. Multifocal malignant melanoma arising in vesicovaginal melanosis. *Arch Pathol Lab Med.* 1991;115:950–952.

Levitt S, Waisman J, de Kernion J. Subepithelial hematoma of the renal pelvis (Antopol-Goldman lesion): a case report and review of the literature. *J Urol.* 1984;131:939–940.

Lopez-Beltran A, Nogales F, Donne CH, Sayag JL. Adenocarcinoma of the urachus showing extensive calcification and stromal osseous metaplasia. *Urol Int.* 1984;53:110–113.

Nazeer T, Ro JY, Tornos C, et al. Endocervical type glands in urinary bladder. A clinicopathological study of 6 cases. *Hum Pathol.* 1996;27:816–820.

Neto WA, Lopes RN, Cury M, et al. Vesical endometriosis. *Urology.* 1984;24:271–273.

Parivar F, Bolton DM, Stoller ML. Endocervicosis of the bladder. *J Urol.* 1995;153:1218–1220.

Peterson LJ, Paulson DF, Glenn JF. The histopathology of vesical diverticula. *J Urol.* 1973;110:62–64.

Rajan N, Makhuli ZN, Humphrey DM, et al. Metastatic umbilical transitional cell carcinoma from a bladder diverticulum. *J Urol.* 1996;155:1700–1701.

Rothberg H, Place CH, Shteir O. Adriamycin (NSC-123127) toxicity: unusual melanotic reaction. *Cancer Chemother Rep.* 1974;58(5, pt 1):749–751.

Schrodt GR, Alcorn MO, Ibanez J. Endometriosis of the male urinary system: a case report. *J Urol.* 1980;124:722–723.

Seman EI, Stewart CJ. Endocervicosis of the urinary bladder. *Aust N Z J Obstet Gynaecol.* 1994;34:496–497.

Vara AR, Ruzics EP, Moussabeck O, et al. Endometrioid adenosarcoma of the bladder arising from endometriosis. *J Urol.* 1990;143:813–815.

Vercellini P, Meschia M, Giorgi O, et al. Bladder detrusor endometriosis: clinical and pathogenetic implications. *J Urol.* 1996;155:84–86.

Young RH, Clement PB. Mullerianosis of the urinary bladder. *Mod Pathol.* 1996;9:731–737.

6

Urothelial Metaplasia
and Hyperplasia

6.1 BRUNN'S NESTS

Brunn's nests (von Brunn's nests) are round to oval aggregates of benign urothelial cells in the superficial lamina propria that arise by invagination of the overlying urothelium (Fig 6.1). The term *Brunn's buds* is sometimes used when attachment to the urothelium is still apparent (Wiener et al, 1979). Brunn's nests are a common finding, present in virtually all serially sectioned bladders at autopsy, present in all age groups, and frequently associated with cystitis cystica and glandularis. They occur most commonly in the trigone. The etiology is uncertain, and the link with inflammation is disputed by some authors. Early reports suggested that Brunn's nests are precancerous, but this view is no longer accepted.

Brunn's nests are typically round, circumscribed nests of urothelial cells devoid of atypia located immediately beneath the urothelium. Squamous metaplasia is uncommon. Occasionally, urothelial carcinoma may extend into Brunn's nests, causing bulbous expansion that may be misinterpreted as lamina propria invasion (Wiener et al, 1979). Useful distinguishing features for invasive carcinoma include irregular infiltration of the stroma by

nests of cells and single cells with cytologic abnormalities, often accompanied by a stromal response (Wiener et al, 1979; Young, 1988). Diagnostic difficulty occurs when Brunn's nests are present deep within the lamina propria; this deep separation from the overlying epithelium may result in the overdiagnosis of carcinoma. The rare nested variant of urothelial carcinoma should also be considered (Chapter 10). The benign cytologic findings in Brunn's nests usually stand in contrast to the changes in urothelial cancer, but the epithelium in Brunn's nests, similar to the surface urothelium, may exhibit hyperplasia and reactive atypia, including the presence of occasional mitotic figures.

6.2 CYSTITIS CYSTICA

Cystitis cystica probably results from central cavitation of Brunn's nests (Fig 6.2). It is found in up to 60% of serially sectioned bladders (Ito et al, 1981) and is most common in adults but often occurs in children. Like cystitis glandularis, it occasionally simulates a neoplasm.

Grossly, cystitis cystica consists of one or more discrete translucent 2–5 mm diameter submucosal beads or cysts, varying from pearl-white to yellow-brown (Jost et al, 1993;

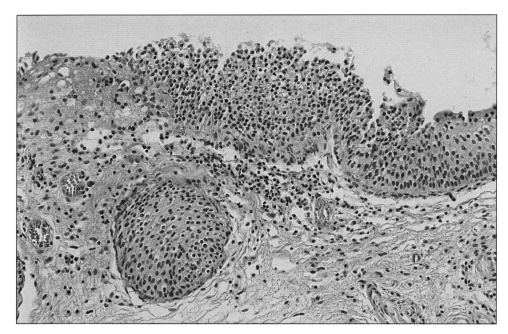

Figure 6.1 Brunn's nest beneath intact urothelium.

Parker, 1970). It contains clear or slightly yellow fluid, is lined by cuboidal or flattened urothelium (Wiener et al, 1979), and is often filled with eosinophilic fluid containing inflammatory cells. Cystitis cystica is not considered premalignant.

6.3 CYSTITIS GLANDULARIS AND INTESTINAL METAPLASIA

Cystitis glandularis is thought to arise from Brunn's nests, similar to cystitis cystica (Figs 6.3 and 6.4). It is present in 71% of serially sectioned bladders and, like Brunn's nests, is most common in the trigone (Ito et al, 1981). The cells in cystitis glandularis are considered mucinous but do not usually have a conspicuous mucinous appearance in hematoxylin- and eosin-stained sections. Special stains for mucin are often negative or weakly positive (Edwards et al, 1972).

Intestinal-type mucinous metaplasia is similar to the intestinal form of cystitis glandularis,

but the term *metaplasia* is restricted to cases in which the surface urothelium contains columnar cells with goblet cells (Gordon, 1963; Mostofi, 1954). Intestinal metaplasia and the intestinal form of cystitis glandularis are not strong risk factors for bladder adenocarcinoma (Bell & Wendel, 1968; Belman, 1978; Bullock et al, 1987; Corica et al, 1997; Susmano et al, 1971; Theuring, 1992; Willeman et al, 1992). Occasionally, the cystoscopic appearance of cystitis glandularis suggests malignancy, particularly with polypoid cystitis glandularis. Metaplastic bone and cartilage may appear in the stroma of polypoid cystitis glandularis (Quilter, 1956).

Two forms of cystitis glandularis may coexist: glandular and intestinal. The glandular form is most common, consisting of glands lined by cuboidal to columnar cells surrounded by a layer of urothelial cells. The intestinal form of cystitis glandularis consists of tall columnar and goblet cells with prominent mucin production resembling colonic epithelium (Davies & Castro, 1977; Davis et al, 1974; Lin et al, 1980;

(a)

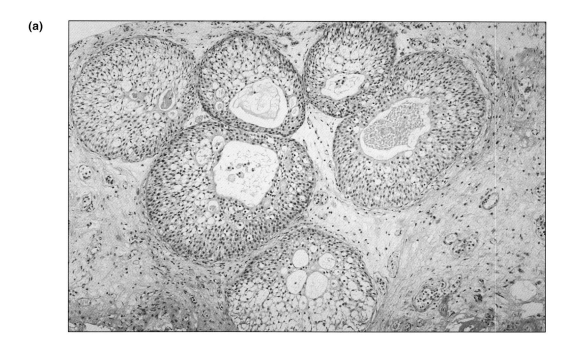

(b)

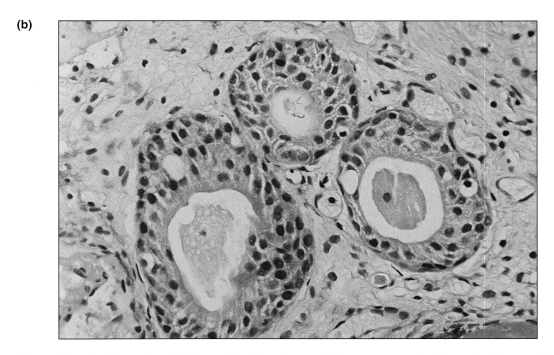

Figure 6.2 Cystitis cystica. **(a):** Nests of proliferative urothelium are punctuated by central lumens. **(b):** The urothelial cells display reactive features; pink proteinaceous secretions are present in the lumens.

(a)

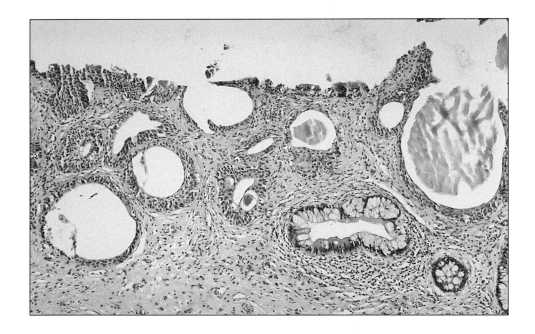

(b)

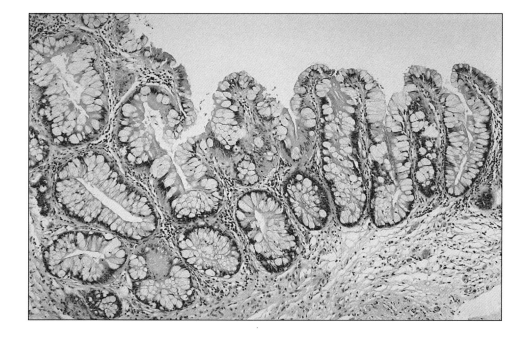

(c)

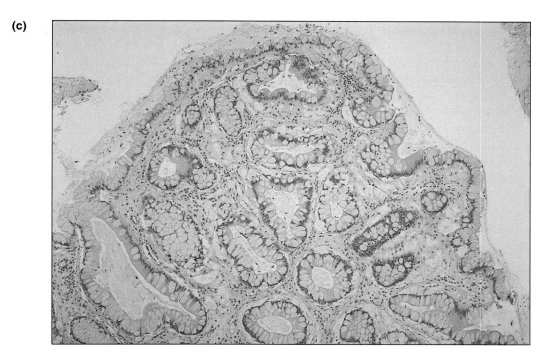

Figure 6.3 Cystitis glandularis. **(a):** Cystitis cystica with focal cystitis glandularis; **(b):** the normal urothelium is replaced by intestinal-type (colonic) metaplasia; **(c):** polypoid form of cystitis glandularis, intestinal type.

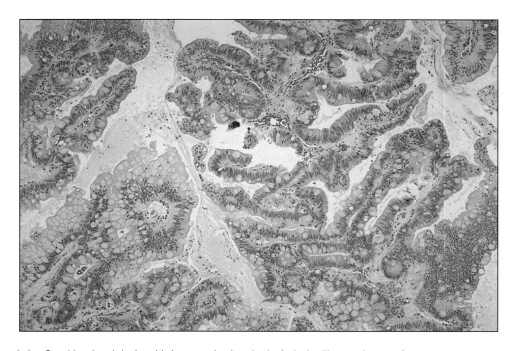

Figure 6.4 Cystitis glandularis with low-grade dysplasia (tubulovillous adenoma).

Theuring, 1992). Paneth cells, argentaffin cells, and argyrophilic cells are rarely present. The intestinal form of cystitis glandularis has the same histochemical profile as colonic epithelium.

Florid cystitis glandularis is uncommon and is distinguished from adenocarcinoma by the lack of stromal infiltration and marked cytologic abnormalities (Heynes et al, 1991; Ward, 1971). Cases in which there are distorted glands in the stroma or deep within the lamina propria, particularly with cytologic abnormalities (even if minor), should be evaluated carefully to exclude malignancy (O'Brien & Urbanski, 1985). A recent report highlighted the importance of recognizing intestinal metaplasia in the presence of superficial muscularis propria involvement, cytologic atypia, scattered mitotic figures, and, most remarkably, dissecting mucin in the lamina propria and muscularis propria (Fig 6.5) (Young & Bostwick, 1996).

Occasionally, a prolonged history of cystitis glandularis of intestinal form precedes adenocarcinoma (Ward, 1971; Wells & Anderson, 1985). In such cases, the bladder often contains a variety of abnormalities, including adenocarcinoma in situ.

6.4 SQUAMOUS METAPLASIA

Squamous metaplasia is a frequent finding in patients with *schistosomiasis haematobium* infection, nonfunctioning bladder, exstrophy, or severe chronic cystitis (Kaufman et al, 1977; Montgomerie et al, 1993; Stonehill et al, 1996; Widran et al, 1974). It is more common in women than men and often occurs on the anterior wall.

At cystoscopy, the mucosa is thickened and typically white or gray-white. The appearance may be striking, with irregular flaky keratinizing material (Morgan & Cameron, 1980). Mi-

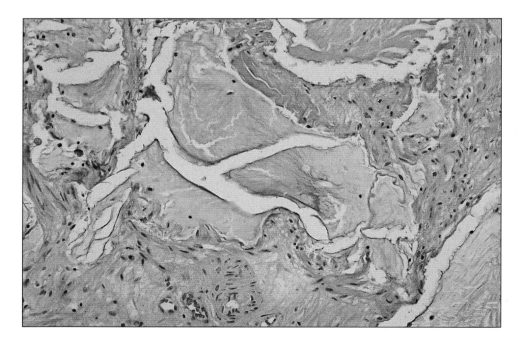

Figure 6.5 Acellular mucin within the bladder wall in association with intestinal metaplasia. This finding should not be confused with mucinous carcinoma.

(a)

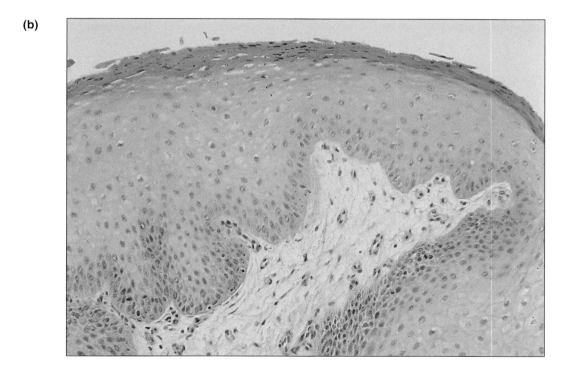

(b)

Figure 6.6 Squamous metaplasia of the bladder. **(a):** The mucosal surface is thickened, leathery, and grey-white; **(b):** the epithelium is typical mature keratinizing squamous mucosa without evidence of atypia.

croscopically, there is squamous mucosa of variable thickness that is often covered by a layer of keratin (Fig 6.6). Cytologic atypia is uncommon but may include carcinoma in situ, raising the possibility of invasive carcinoma elsewhere in the specimen (Locke et al, 1985; Young, 1988). The relationship of squamous metaplasia and squamous cell carcinoma is a matter of debate with contradictory findings (O'Flynn & Mullaney, 1974; Reece & Koontz, 1975; Stonehill et al, 1996; Walts & Sacks, 1977). In a series from the Mayo Clinic, 22% of patients with squamous metaplasia had synchronous carcinoma, and another 20% subsequently developed carcinoma when followed for as long as 30 years (Benson et al, 1984). The mean interval from the diagnosis of squamous metaplasia to the development of carcinoma was 11 years. The high frequency of squamous metaplasia and squamous cell carcinoma in patients with schistosomiasis supports this association (Khafagy et al, 1972).

Squamous metaplasia should be distinguished from nonkeratinizing glycogenated squamous epithelium, similar to that of the vaginal type, which is a normal finding in the trigone and bladder neck in up to 86% of women during reproductive and menopausal years (Fig 6.7) (Longe & Shepherd, 1983; Tyler, 1962). Epithelium of this type rarely occurs in men, except in those receiving estrogen therapy for prostatic carcinoma. Glycogenated squamous epithelium in the trigone may be very thick (Young, 1988).

6.5 NEPHROGENIC METAPLASIA (NEPHROGENIC ADENOMA)

Nephrogenic metaplasia is most common in the bladder (55% of cases) but may also involve the urethra (41%) and ureter (4%) (Bhagavan et al, 1981; Ford et al, 1985; Friedman & Kuhlenbeck, 1950; Molland et al, 1976; Oliva & Young, 1995).

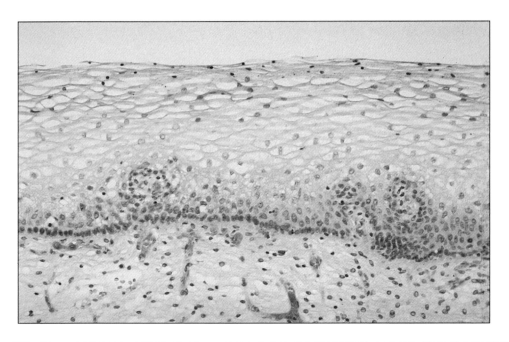

Figure 6.7 Normal trigonal urothelium of a woman during the reproductive years. Note the vaginal-type nonkeratinizing glycogenated squamous epithelium that may be mistaken for squamous metaplasia.

It usually occurs in adults (90% of cases) (Young & Scully, 1985), and men predominate (2:1 ratio). Most patients have a history of an operative procedure or one or more irritants, including calculi, trauma, cystitis, and tuberculosis (Davis, 1949; Muto et al, 1993); approximately 8% of patients have undergone kidney transplantation (Fournier et al, 1996). Symptoms include hematuria, frequency, and dysuria.

Typically, nephrogenic metaplasia is 1 cm or less in diameter and single, but exceptions occur (O'Shea et al, 1981). Microscopically, tubules are the most common histologic finding (Pierre-Louis et al, 1985), but the proliferation may also be cystic, polypoid, papillary, and rarely, diffuse (Figs 6.8 and 6.9). The tubules appear as small, round, hollow acini reminiscent of renal tubules (Devine et al, 1984). They are occasionally solid and surrounded by a prominent basement membrane that is highlighted by the periodic acid-Schiff stain (Emmett & MacDonald, 1942). The tubules frequently become dilated and cystic but may also appear as solid nests. The tubules and cysts often contain an eosinophilic or basophilic secretion that is weakly mucicarminophilic. Most of the cells lining the tubules, cysts, and papillae are cuboidal or low columnar with scant cytoplasm; occasionally, the cells have an abundant clear cytoplasm (McIntire et al, 1987). Hobnail cells line the tubules and cysts in up to 70% of cases, and large cysts may be lined by flattened cells. Small amounts of mucin may be present in the cells of nephrogenic metaplasia, but glycogen is scant or absent. Nuclear abnormalities are uncommon and, when present, appear reactive or degenerative. Mitotic figures are rare or absent. There is often marked chronic cystitis that may partially obscure the nephrogenic metaplasia; squamous and glandular metaplasia may coexist. Rare cases of nephrogenic metaplasia are associated with prominent stromal calcification or malacoplakia (Raghavaiah et al, 1980).

The most common differential diagnosis of nephrogenic metaplasia is adenocarcinoma. In some cases, the metaplasia is composed of minute mucin-containing tubules lined by single cells with compressed nuclei that simulate signet-ring cell carcinoma (Malpica et al, 1994). Hobnail cells suggest the possibility of clear cell carcinoma of the bladder, but such cells are focally present in 70% of cases of nephrogenic metaplasia. Solid tubules with cells containing clear cytoplasm also suggest clear cell carcinoma (Schultz et al, 1984), but this is an uncommon and focal finding in nephrogenic metaplasia (Alsanjari et al, 1995; Malpica et al, 1994). The greatest difficulty in distinguishing nephrogenic metaplasia from clear cell carcinoma arises in small specimens and biopsies of urethral diverticuli (Table 6.1).

6.6   UROTHELIAL HYPERPLASIA

6.6.1   Flat Urothelial Hyperplasia

Flat urothelial hyperplasia is associated with a wide variety of inflammatory disorders, lithiasis, and vesical neoplasms, particularly those with papillary growth (Ayala & Ro, 1989; Koss, 1975). It may represent an early stage in the development of papillary urothelial neoplasms, but current evidence is inconclusive.

Histologically, urothelial hyperplasia is usually focal, consisting of an increase in the number of cell layers, usually 10 or more (but at least >7). There are few or no significant cytologic abnormalities, although slight nuclear enlargement may be present (Fig 6.10). Hyperplasia may occasionally be associated with dysplasia or carcinoma in situ in the adjacent mucosa. Pseudopapillary growth is uncommon in flat hyperplasia and characteristically lacks well-formed vascular cores. Mimics of flat urothelial hyperplasia include urothelial compression, artifact, and tangential sectioning of the mucosa (Koss, 1975).

(a)

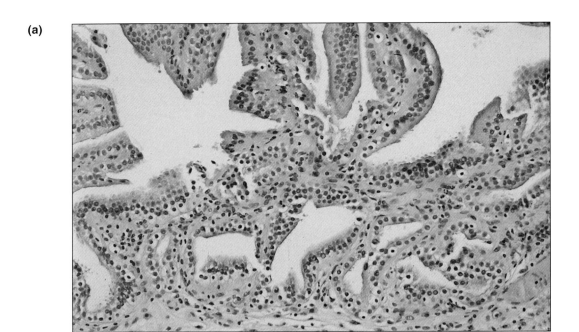

(b)

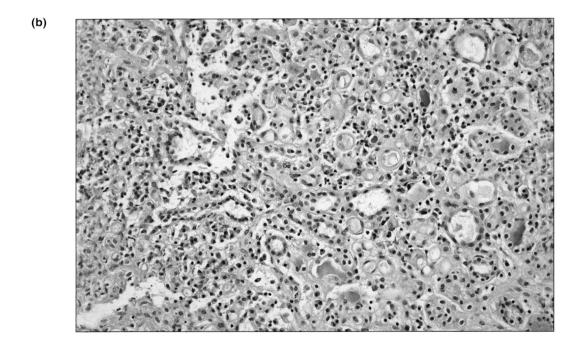

(c)

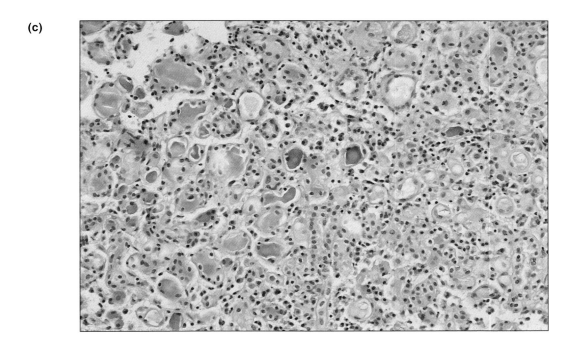

(d)

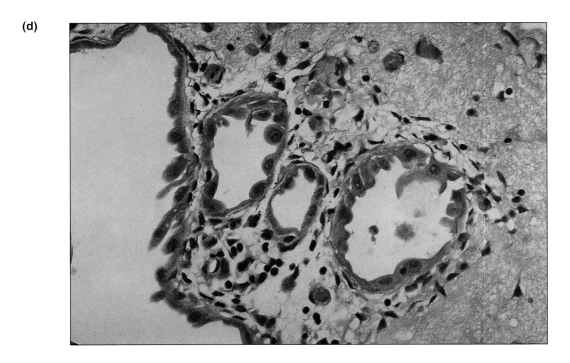

Figure 6.8 Nephrogenic metaplasia. **(a):** Polypoid pattern; **(b):** tubular pattern with abundant inflammation; **(c):** near-solid pattern; **(d):** dilated tubules lined by hobnail cells.

(a)

(b)

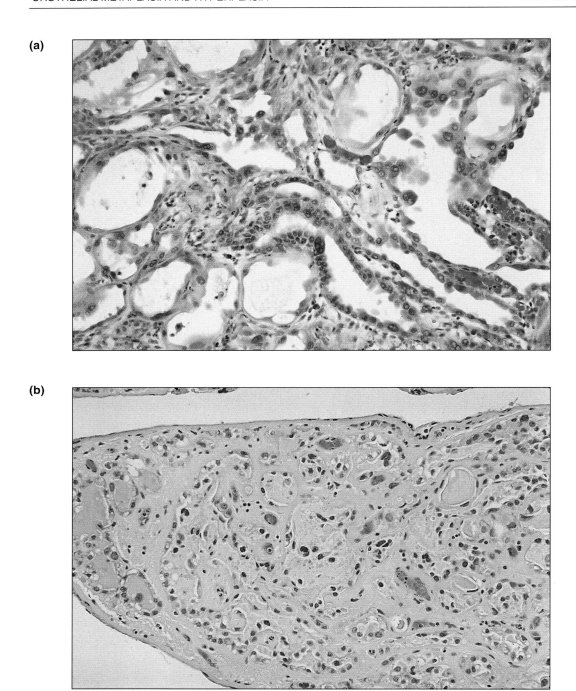

Figure 6.9 **(a):** Nephrogenic metaplasia with dilated tubules and mild to moderate cytologic atypia; **(b):** another case with smudged hyperchromatic nuclei.

Table 6.1 Comparison of nephrogenic adenoma and clear cell carcinoma of the bladder

Characteristic	Nephrogenic metaplasia	Clear cell carcinoma
Sex	Male predominance	Female predominance
Patient age	One-third <30 years old	Virtually none <43 years old
Predisposing factors (trauma, infection)	Common	Rare
Large size	Rare	Common
Diffuse growth	Uncommon (14%)	Common
Clear cells	Uncommon (15%)	Common
Hobnail cells	Usually rare and focal	Common
Cytologic atypia	Rare	Common
Mitotic figures	Rare	Common
Nucleoli	Absent, inconspicuous; focally prominent in 20%	Prominent
Cytoplasmic glycogen	Scant	Abundant
Keratin (CAM 5.2)	+	+ (focal)
Epithelial membrane antigen	+	+
Carcinoembryonic antigen	–	– (in biopsy) + (focal in partial cystectomy)
S-100 protein	–	–
MIB 1	+ (1.5%–10%)	+ (15%–30%)

– = Negative immunoreactivity; + = positive immunoreactivity.

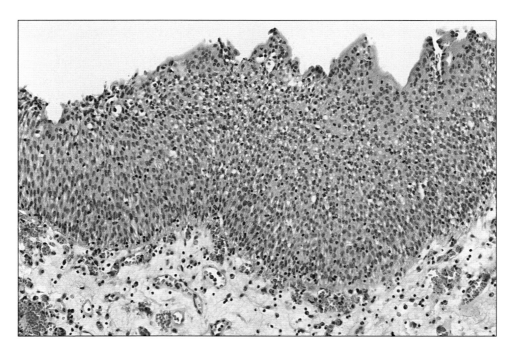

Fig 6.10 Flat urothelial hyperplasia. The urothelium displays normal maturation without papillae, uniform spacing, and no nuclear abnormalities; however, it is substantially thicker than normal.

6.6.2   Papillary Hyperplasia

The term *papillary hyperplasia* is appropriate for cases in which papillae are not usually seen macroscopically but are present microscopically (Taylor et al, 1996; Young, 1988). Papillary urothelial hyperplasia is a nonspecific reaction of the urothelium following irritation of the bladder by an inflammatory or neoplastic process (Figure 6.11). Occasionally, inflammatory papillary hyperplasia of the bladder may be confused with cancer at cystoscopy. Microscopically, there is characteristic granulation tissue with varying amounts of acute and chronic inflammation and occasionally denuded papillae. Cases of this type are referred to in the old literature as *cystitis granulosa*. It is possible that some cases represent early papilloma.

REFERENCES

Alsanjari N, Lynch MJ, Fisher C, et al. Vesical clear cell adenocarcinoma. V: nephrogenic adenoma: a diagnostic problem. *Histopathology.* 1995;27:43–49.

Ayala A, Ro J. Premalignant lesions of the urothelium and transitional cell tumors. In: Young RH, ed. *Pathology of the Urinary Bladder.* Philadelphia, PA: Churchill Livingstone; 1989:65–101.

Bell TE, Wendel RC. Cystitis glandularis: benign or malignant? *J Urol.* 1968;100:462–466.

Belman AB. The clinical significance of cystitis cystica in girls: results of a prospective study. *J Urol.* 1978;119:661–663.

Benson RC Jr, Swanson SK, Farrow GM. Relationship of leukoplakia to urothelial malignancy. *J Urol.* 1984;131:507–511.

Bhagavan BS, Tiamon EM, Wenk RE, et al. Nephrogenic adenoma of the urinary bladder and urethra. *Hum Pathol.* 1981;12:907–916.

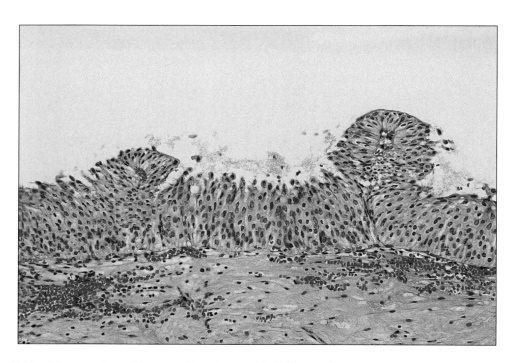

Figure 6.11 Microscopic papillary growth without urothelial hyperplasia or cytologic atypia. This represents early papilloma or papillary hyperplasia.

Bullock PS, Thoni DE, Murphy WM. The significance of colonic mucosa (intestinal metaplasia) involving the urinary tract. *Cancer.* 1987;59:2086–2090.

Corica FA, Husmann, DA, Churchill BM, Young RH, Pacelli A, Lopez-Beltran A, Bostwick DG. Intestinal metaplasia is not a strong risk factor for bladder cancer: study of 53 cases with long term follow-up. *Urology.* 1997;50:427–431.

Davies G, Castro JE. Cystitis glandularis. *Urology.* 1977;10:128–129.

Davis TA. Hamartoma of the urinary bladder. *Northwest Med.* 1949;48:182–185.

Davis EL, Goldstein AMB, Morrow JW. Unusual bladder mucosal metaplasia in a case of chronic prostatitis and cystitis. *J Urol.* 1974;111:767–769.

Devine P, Ucci AA, Krain H, et al. Nephrogenic adenoma and embryonic kidney tubules share PNA receptor sites. *Am J Clin Pathol.* 1984;81:728–732.

Edwards PD, Hurm R, Jaeschke WH. Conversion of cystitis glandularis to adenocarcinoma. *J Urol.* 1972;108:568–570.

Emmett JL, McDonald JR. Proliferation of glands of the urinary bladder simulating malignant neoplasm. *J Urol.* 1942;48:257–261.

Ford TF, Watson GM, Cameron KM. Adenomatous metaplasia (nephrogenic adenoma) of urothelium: an analysis of 70 cases. *Br J Urol.* 1985;57:427–433.

Fournier G, Menut P, Moal MC, et al. Nephrogenic adenoma of bladder in renal transplant recipients: report of 9 cases with assessment of deoxyribonucleic acid ploidy and long term follow-up. *J Urol.* 1996;156:41–44.

Friedman NB, Kuhlenbeck H. Adenomatoid tumors of the bladder reproducing renal structures (nephrogenic adenomas). *J Urol.* 1950;64:657–661.

Gordon A. Intestinal metaplasia of the urinary tract epithelium. *J Pathol Bacteriol.* 1963;85:441–444.

Heynes CF, De Kock ML, Kirsten PH, et al. Pelvic lipomatosis associated with cystitis glandularis and adenocarcinoma of the bladder. *J Urol.* 1991;145:364–366.

Ito N, Hirose M, Shirai T, et al. Lesions of the urinary bladder epithelium in 125 autopsy cases. *Acta Pathol Jpn.* 1981;31:545–557.

Jost SP, Dixon JS, Gosling JA. Ultrastructural observations on cystitis cystica in human bladder urothelium. *Br J Urol.* 1993;71:28–33.

Kaufman JM, Fam B, Jacobs SC, et al. Bladder cancer and squamous metaplasia in spinal cord injury patients. *J Urol.* 1977;118:967–971.

Khafagy MM, El-Bolkainy MN, Mansour MA. Carcinoma of the bilharzial urinary bladder: a study of the associated mucosal lesions in 86 cases. *Cancer.* 1972;30:150–159.

Koss L. Tumors of the urinary bladder. In: *Atlas of Tumor Pathology* (2nd series, fascicle 11). Washington, DC: AFIP; 1975.

Lin JI, Tseng CH, Choy C, et al. Diffuse cystitis glandularis. *Urology.* 1980;15:411–415.

Locke JR, Hill DE, Walzer Y. Incidence of squamous cell carcinoma in patients with long-term catheter drainage. *J Urol.* 1985;133:1034–1035.

Longe ED, Shepherd RT. The incidence and significance of vaginal metaplasia of the bladder trigone in adult women. *Br J Urol.* 1983;55:189–194.

Malpica A, Ro JY, Troncoso P, et al. Nephrogenic adenoma of the prostatic urethra involving the prostate gland: a clinicopathologic and immunohistochemical study of eight cases. *Hum Pathol.* 1994;25:390–395.

McIntire TL, Soloway MS, Murphy WM. Nephrogenic adenoma. *Urology.* 1987;29:237–241.

Molland EA, Trott PA, Paris AMI, et al. Nephrogenic adenoma: a form of adenomatous metaplasia of the bladder. A clinical and electron microscopical study. *Br J Urol.* 1976;48:453–462.

Montgomerie JZ, Holshuh HJ, Keyser AJ, et al. 28 K in squamous metaplasia of the bladder in patients with spinal cord injury. *Paraplegia.* 1993;31;105–110.

Morgan RJ, Cameron KM. Vesical leukoplakia. *Br J Urol.* 1980;52:96–100.

Mostofi FK. Potentialities of bladder epithelium. *J Urol.* 1954;71:705–714.

Muto G, Comi L, Baldini D. Nephrogenic adenoma of the bladder associated with urinary tuberculosis: case report. *Minerva Urol Nefrol.* 1993;45:77–81.

O'Brien AME, Urbanski SJ. Papillary adenocarcinoma in situ of the bladder. *J Urol.* 1985;134:544–546.

O'Flynn JD, Mullaney J. Vesical leukoplakia progressing to carcinoma. *Br J Urol.* 1974;46:31–37.

Oliva E, Young RH. Nephrogenic adenoma of the urinary tract: a review of the microscopic appearance of 80 cases with emphasis on unusual features. *Mod Pathol.* 1995;8:722–730.

O'Shea PA, Callaghan JF, Lawlor JB, et al. "Nephrogenic adenoma": an unusual metaplastic change of urothelium. *J Urol.* 1981;125:249–252.

Parker C. Cystitis cystica and glandularis: a study of 40 cases. *Proc R Soc Med.* 1970;63:239–242.

Pierre-Louis ML, Kovi J, Jackson A, et al. Nephrogenic adenoma: a light and electron microscopic and immunohistochemical study. *J Natl Med Assoc.* 1985;77:201–205.

Quilter TN. Embryoma of the urinary bladder. *J Urol.* 1956;76:392–395.

Raghavaiah NV, Noe HN, Parham DM, et al. Nephrogenic adenoma of the urinary bladder associated with malakoplakia. *Urology.* 1980;15:190–193.

Reece RW, Koontz WW Jr. Leukoplakia of the urinary tract: a review. *J Urol.* 1975;114:165–171.

Schultz RE, Bloch MJ, Tomaszewski JE, et al. Mesonephric adenocarcinoma of the bladder. *J Urol.* 1984;132:263–265.

Stonehill WH, Dmochowski RR, Patterson AL, et al. Risk factors for bladder tumors in spinal cord injury patients. *J Urol.* 1996;155:1248–1250.

Susmano D, Rubenstein AB, Dakin AR, et al. Cystitis glandularis and adenocarcinoma of the bladder. *J Urol.* 1971;105:671–674.

Taylor DC, Bhagavan BS, Larsen MP, et al. Papillary urothelial hyperplasia. A precursor to papillary neoplasms. *Am J Surg Pathol.* 1996;20:1481–1488.

Theuring F. Cystitis glandularis vom intestinalen Typ (intestinale Metaplasie) in der Harnblasenschleimhaut mit funktionell bedeutsamer Pseudotumorbildung [Glandular cystitis of intestinal type (inteniale metaplasia) of the urinary bladder mucosa with functionally relevant pseudotumor]. *Pathologe.* 1992;13:235–240.

Tyler DE. Stratified squamous epithelium in the vesical trigone and urethra: findings correlated with the menstrual cycle and age. *Am J Anat.* 1962; 111:319–335.

Walts AE, Sacks SA. Squamous metaplasia and invasive epidermoid carcinoma of bladder. *Urology.* 1977;9:317–320.

Ward AM. Glandular neoplasia within the urinary tract. The aetiology of adenocarcinoma of the urothelium with a review of the literature. I. Introduction: the origin of glandular epithelium in the renal pelvis, ureter, and bladder. *Virchows Arch A Pathol Anat Histopathol.* 1971;352:296–311.

Wells M, Anderson K. Mucin histochemistry of cystitis glandularis and primary adenocarcinoma of the urinary bladder. *Arch Pathol Lab Med.* 1985; 109:59–61.

Widran J, Sanchez R, Gruhn J. Squamous metaplasia of the bladder: a study of 450 patients. *J Urol.* 1974;112:479–482.

Wiener DP, Koss LG, Sablay B, et al. The prevalence and significance of Brunn's nests, cystitis cystica and squamous metaplasia in normal bladders. *J Urol.* 1979;122:317–321.

Willemen P, Van Poppel H, Baert L. Ectopic colonic epithelium of the bladder complicated by development of an adenocarcinoma. *Acta Urol Belg.* 1992;60:147–149.

Young RH. Pseudoneoplastic lesions of the urinary bladder. *Pathol Annu.* 1988;23:67–104.

Young RH, Scully R. Clear cell adenocarcinoma of the bladder and urethra: a report of three cases and review of the literature. *Am J Surg Pathol.* 1985; 9:816–826.

Young RH, Bostwick DG. Florid cystitis glandularis of intestinal type with mucin extravasation: a mimic of adenocarcinoma. *Am J Surg Pathol.* 1996;20:1462–1468.

7

POLYPS AND OTHER BENIGN EPITHELIAL NEOPLASMS

This chapter deals with predominantly benign epithelial and mixed epithelial-stromal polyps of the urothelium. Inflammatory polyps such as polypoid and papillary cystitis are discussed in Chapter 3.

7.1 POLYPS

7.1.1 Fibroepithelial Polyp

This rare lesion usually occurs in children (Wolgel et al, 1982). Histologically, it is similar to a fibroepithelial polyp seen elsewhere, appearing as a solitary polyp with a fibrous core usually devoid of significant inflammation (Fig 7.1). One unusual case contained stromal xanthoma cells (Elson & McLaughlin, 1974). Benign atypical stromal cells similar to those in giant cell cystitis are sometimes present, referred to as *pseudosarcomatous stroma*, and may be mistaken for sarcoma (see Fig 10.11) (Young, 1986). The epithelial lining is flat and metaplastic in some cases. One case was associated with the Beckwith-Wiedemann syndrome (Wolgel et al, 1982).

7.1.2 Ectopic Prostatic Tissue in the Bladder

Papillary, polypoid, and sessile masses of benign prostatic epithelium are rarely found in the male bladder, resembling similar findings in the urethra (Remick & Kumar, 1984). This lesion is more common at the trigone, arising in men between 20 and 80 years of age. Hematuria is the usual presenting symptom. Ectopic prostatic tissue consists of acini lined by columnar epithelium that displays prostate-specific antigen immunoreactivity (Yajima et al, 1993). Rarely, the acini of ectopic prostatic tissue are partially covered by urothelium.

7.1.3 Polypoid Hamartoma

Hamartoma of the bladder invariably arises in children between 10 and 15 years of age, often in association with hamartomatous polyps of the gastrointestinal tract. It consists of a mixture of tissues resembling Brunn's nests, cystitis cystica, and cystitis glandularis. The stroma may be muscular, fibrous, or edematous (McCallion et al, 1993). The intestinal form of

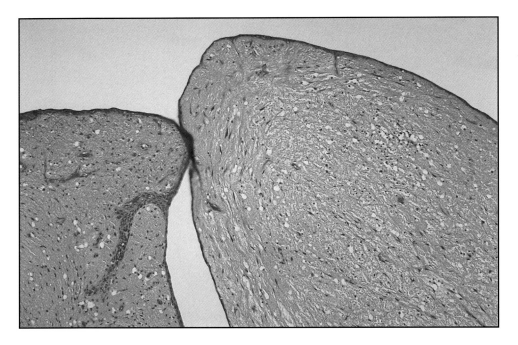

Figure 7.1   Fibroepithelial polyp, with a flat atrophic urothelial surface lining.

cystitis glandularis may be present, and some authors consider this an unusual and florid variant of cystitis glandularis.

7.1.4   Villous Adenoma and Tubular Adenoma

There are few documented examples of villous adenoma and tubular adenoma of the bladder, and these are histologically identical to their counterparts in the colon (Fig 7.2) (Cheng L, Montironi R, Bostwick DG, unpublished observations, 1998; Miller et al, 1983; Trotter et al, 1994); such a lesion is more common in the urachus. Pure forms of tubular adenoma have also been described (Rubin et al, 1981). Patients with these tumors may present with gross hematuria (Husain et al, 1996). Villous adenoma of the urinary bladder is more common in men than women (3:1 ratio), presenting in patients between 52 to 79 years of age (Billis et al, 1980). All tumors appear cystoscopically as exophytic

papillary masses. Histologically, papillary fronds are covered by columnar mucus-secreting epithelium with goblet cells. Nuclear crowding and pseudostratification of the epithelium characteristic of dysplasia are present. Argyrophilic neuroendocrine cells may be present, as well as loss of the normal ABH(O) blood isoantigens by immunohistochemistry. Tumor cells are invariably cytokeratin 20 immunoreactive (Cheng L, et al, unpublished observations, 1998). A confounding histologic feature is the uncommon finding of lakes of extravasated mucin in the stroma, raising the possibility of invasion (Grignon & Sakr, 1995). One case was associated with invasive urothelial carcinoma of the bladder (West et al, 1995). Transurethral resection of the bladder (TURB) is the treatment of choice, with no reported recurrences.

The differential diagnosis of villous adenoma includes florid intestinal-type cystitis glandularis (polypoid cystitis glandularis), well-differ-

(a)

(b)

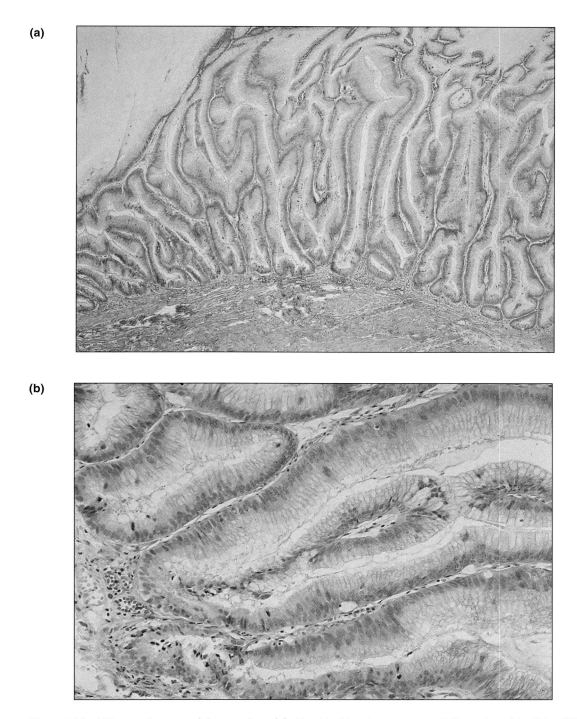

Figure 7.2 Villous adenoma of the urachus. **(a):** The bladder dome was partially replaced by this villiform growth that, on high magnification **(b)**, displayed typical features of villous adenoma with low-grade dysplasia. Resection revealed extension into the urachal canal.

entiated adenocarcinoma, and ectopic prostate tissue with cytologic abnormalities. Adenocarcinoma with villous architecture occurs in the urinary bladder, usually with severe anaplasia of the pseudoestratified epithelium and invasion of the underlying stroma.

7.2   UROTHELIAL PAPILLOMA

The proper diagnosis of a urothelial papilloma of the urinary bladder is controversial (Lerman et al, 1970; Nichols & Marshall, 1956). Much of the difficulty in diagnosis and acceptance of this lesion is based on varying diagnostic criteria. If one employs restrictive diagnostic criteria as recommended by the World Health Organization and the International Society of Urologic Pathologists, this lesion is uncommon, representing no more than about 3% of papillary urothelial tumors (Eble & Young, 1989). Several authors believe that papilloma should include all grade 1

urothelial carcinomas as defined by the World Health Organization (Murphy et al, 1994; Reuter & Melamed, 1994), but most others do not follow this recent suggestion (Epstein et al, 1998).

The restrictive criterion for papilloma as defined by the World Health Organization is a small, usually solitary, papillary lesion with a delicate fibrovascular core lined by cytologically and architecturally normal urothelium without mitotic figures (Figs 7.3–7.5 and Table 7.1) (Mostofi et al, 1973) (see Chapter 9). Such lesions usually occur in patients under 50 years of age. Mild cytologic atypia of the superficial cells does not exclude the diagnosis of papilloma, particularly when accompanied by an inflammatory infiltrate (Fig 7.6).

Papilloma by itself does not have the capacity to invade or metastasize, and most authors consequently consider it benign (Jordan et al, 1987). It is, however, considered neoplastic,

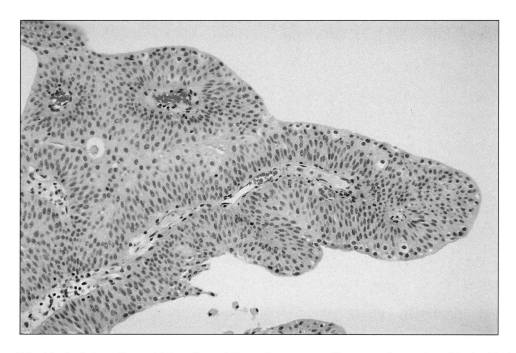

Figure 7.3   Urothelial papilloma. This solitary 1.5-cm diameter papillary growth was found in the bladder of a 45-year-old man. The urothelium is focally thickened but in most areas was of normal thickness.

(a)

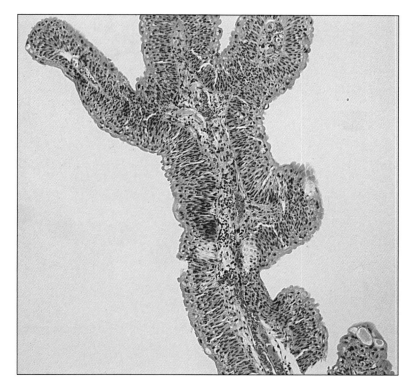

(b)

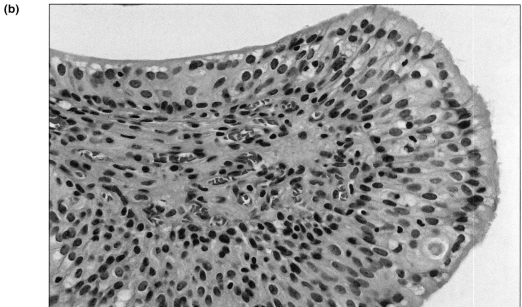

Figure 7.4 Urothelial papilloma. **(a):** A single delicate elongate 1.1-cm-long papillary growth was present in the posterior wall of the bladder of a 51-year-old woman. **(b):** The urothelium is of normal thickness, with no cytologic atypia and an intact superficial cell layer.

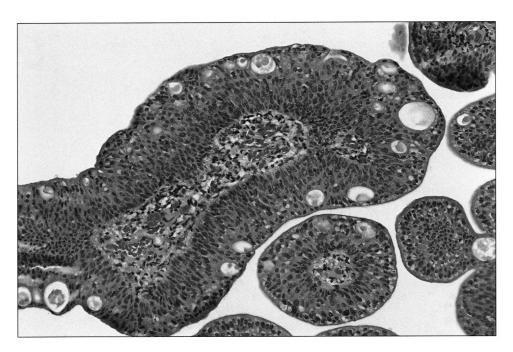

Figure 7.5 Urothelial papilloma. A 39-year-old woman was found to have a 2.1-cm diameter solitary papillary growth at the right ureteral orifice that consisted of a proliferation of urothelium without cytologic atypia.

Table 7.1 Papilloma versus papillary urothelial neoplasm of low malignant potential

	No. epithelial cell layers	Superficial (umbrella) cells	Nuclear enlargement	Nuclear hyperchromasia
Papilloma	7 or less	Present/small*	No†	Absent
Papillary urothelial neoplasm of low malignant potential	>7	Usually present/small	Slight to moderate	Slight; occasional cells

*In rare instances superficial cell may be conspicuous and enlarged.
†Some nuclear enlargement of superficial cells may be present.

(a)

(b)

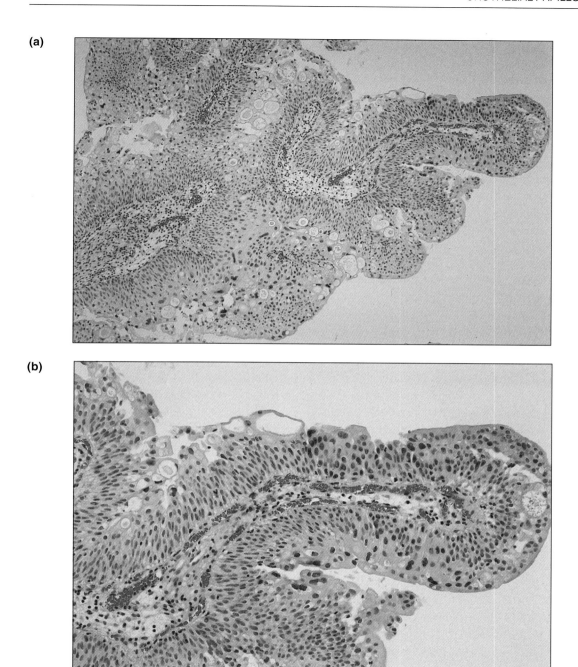

Figure 7.6 Urothelial papilloma with nuclear atypia of the superficial cells. **(a):** A 2.0-cm diameter papillary growth was removed from the left bladder wall of a 47-year-old man. **(b):** Cytologic atypia is present but restricted to the superficial cells.

based on the potential for recurrence and the occasional association with subsequent development of carcinoma. Additional papillary tumors arise in up to 73% of cases, according to the results of one study of 100 patients followed for a minimum of 15 years. Invasive carcinoma develops in up to 10% of patients (Greene et al, 1973; Prout et al, 1992). In one study, urothelial papilloma accounted for 25% of papillary neoplasms of the bladder; of these patients, 3.3% developed higher grade lesions, and 4.4% died of urothelial carcinoma (Jordan et al, 1987). In the National Bladder Cancer Study Group series, 61% of patients with noninvasive grade 1 tumors subsequently developed other papillary tumors, and 4.5% developed invasive carcinoma, 16% of whom had a higher histologic grade (Prout et al, 1992).

7.2.1 Inverted Papilloma (Urothelial Adenoma; Brunnian Adenoma)

Inverted papilloma occurs at all ages, although most patients are middle-aged, with a mean age of 55 years. It is more common in men than women (7:1 ratio) and usually presents with hematuria and irritative symptoms. The etiology is uncertain. Some consider this to be a neoplasm with malignant potential (Urakami et al, 1996), whereas others consider it a reactive process similar to proliferative urothelial lesions such as cystitis glandularis and cystitis cystica. Ultrastructural and immunohistochemical studies indicate a similarity to normal urothelium and low-grade urothelial carcinoma (Goertchen et al, 1994).

Most cases of inverted papilloma are located in the trigone. Macroscopically, it is characteristically sessile or pedunculated, smooth surfaced, small (<3 cm in diameter), and single, but large multifocal lesions may occur (Matz et al, 1974; Rozanski et al, 1996).

Microscopically, inverted papilloma consists of intramucosal and submucosal anastomosing islands and trabeculae of urothelium (Figs 7.7 and 7.8). The surface urothelium may be normal, attenuated, or elevated. There are two main patterns of inverted papilloma, including trabecular and glandular patterns (Kunze et al, 1983). The trabecular pattern is composed of anastomosing cords and sheets of urothelium that are arranged at various angles to the mucosal surface. In some cases, cystic spaces lined by attenuated urothelium are present within the epithelial islands. These spaces may contain eosinophilic secretions that stain with periodic acid-Schiff stain but not mucicarmine. The glandular pattern is composed of nests of urothelium with pseudoglandular or true glandular differentiation with goblet cells. Pseudoglandular spaces are lined by urothelium, whereas true glandular spaces contain mucous-secreting cells with mucicarminophilic secretions, sometimes with intestinal metaplasia with goblet cells (Kunze et al, 1983). In both patterns of inverted papilloma, the epithelial elements are surrounded by an intact basement membrane and delicate fibrovascular stroma.

Unusual growth patterns of inverted papilloma include basaloid, hyperplastic, spindle cell (medullary), and neuroendocrine patterns, often with mixed forms (Fig 7.9). Neuroendocrine differentiation in inverted papilloma is characterized by numerous granular eosinophilic cells that are immunoreactive for chromogranin. Such cells are present in 40% of cases of typical inverted papilloma. Nonkeratinizing squamous metaplasia is also common.

Mild cytologic atypia is often encountered in inverted papilloma, and the precise demarcation with carcinoma is unresolved; fortunately, this is an uncommon problem, but there are cases that are difficult to resolve (Fig 7.10). Mitotic figures are usually rare or absent in inverted papilloma, unlike carcinoma. It is possible that inverted papilloma and papillary urothelial carcinoma are related, but this possibility is controversial (Caro & Tessler, 1998;

(a)

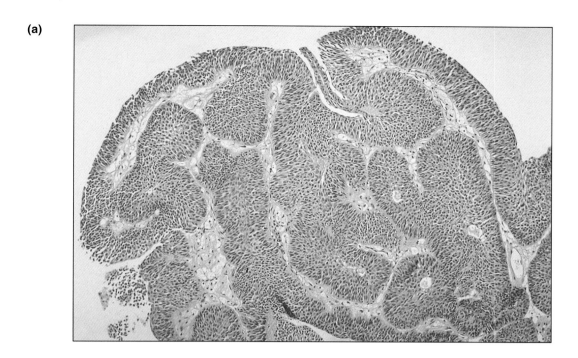

(b)

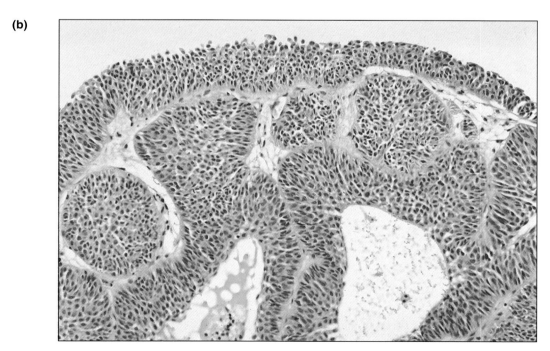

Figure 7.7 Inverted papilloma. **(a):** This solitary 3.0-cm diameter mass formed a protruberant nodule in the trigone of a 55-year-old woman. **(b):** The tumor contains typical anastomosing trabeculae of uniform urothelial cells.

(a)

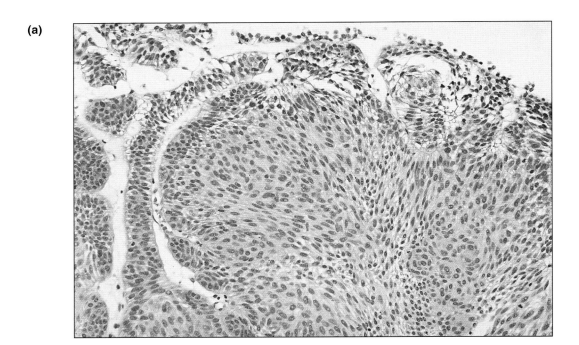

(b)

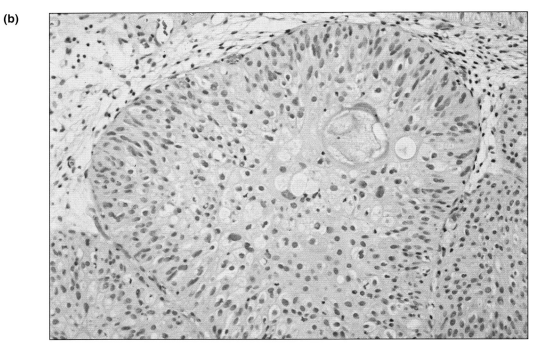

(c)

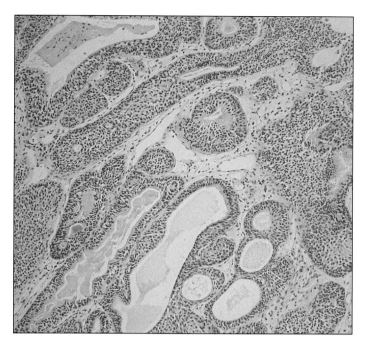

Figure 7.8 Inverted papilloma. The nests may be **(a)** solid with whorled masses of uniform spindle cells, **(b)** punctuated by small cysts filled with mucin, or **(c)** contain large cysts with variable amounts of proteinacous material.

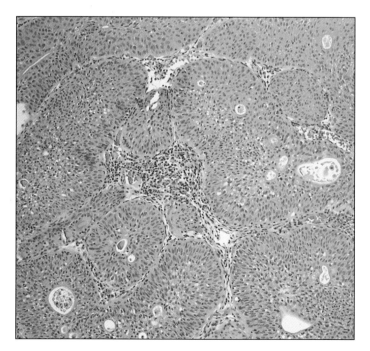

Figure 7.9 Inverted papilloma, hyperplastic pattern.

109

(a)

(b)

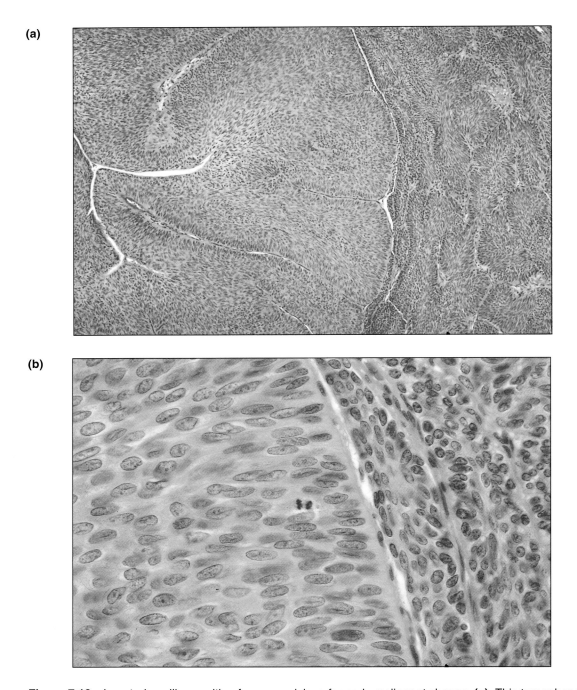

Figure 7.10   Inverted papilloma with a focus suspicious for early malignant change. **(a):** This tumor has the typical architectural features of inverted papilloma, but **(b)** focal increased cellularity and mitotic figures are worrisome for malignancy.

(a)

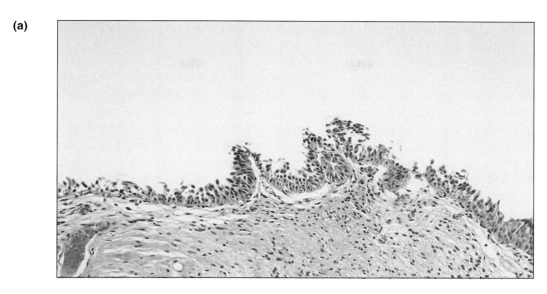

(b)

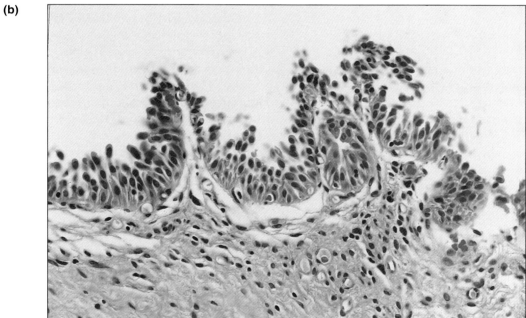

Figure 7.11 Diffuse papillomatosis. **(a):** Multiple minute papillary excrescences were identified in the posterior wall of the bladder of a 46-year-old man. **(b):** The urothelium was invariably <7 cells in thickness, with no cytologic atypia.

Chan et al, 1996; Lazarevic & Garret, 1978; Stein et al, 1983; Urakami et al, 1996). The number of cases with coexistent urothelial carcinoma in situ or carcinoma has increased recently (Altaffer et al, 1982). In some cases, foci of papillary urothelial carcinoma appear to arise from an otherwise typical inverted papilloma (Goertchen et al, 1994; Stosiek et al, 1993). Some cases of inverted papilloma probably represent urothelial carcinoma with an inverted growth pattern (Amin et al, 1997; Khoury et al, 1985). A unique case associated with leiomyoma has been reported (Urakami et al, 1996). Inverted papilloma is diploid (Urakami et al, 1996), although one of three cases with associated urothelial carcinoma was aneuploid (Kunimi et al, 1994).

7.2.2 Squamous Papilloma

Squamous papilloma, presumably the squamous counterpart of urothelial cell papilloma, is a rare benign neoplasm. It should be differentiated from papillary cystitis, a lesion in which the urothelium is occasionally replaced by metaplastic squamous epithelium.

7.2.3 Diffuse Papillomatosis

Diffuse papillomatosis is a rare lesion characterized by replacement of most or all of the bladder mucosa by delicate papillary processes, creating a velvety cystoscopic appearance (Mostofi, 1968). The papillae are covered by urothelium that is indistinguishable from normal mucosa or may have slight cytologic changes (Fig 7.11). Histologically, there is a proliferation of small papillae covered by cells with conspicuous eosinophilic cytoplasm, minimal or no architectural distortion, little or mild nuclear atypia, and no mitotic figures. These lesions are occasionally focal (Eble & Young, 1989). The malignant potential of this lesion is uncertain.

7.3 BENIGN NEOPLASMS OF THE URACHUS

Benign epithelial neoplasms of the urachus are rare (Eble et al, 1986, 1989). Adenoma most often occurs in the lower one-third of the urachus and involves the bladder wall (Fig 7.2) (Hamm, 1940). Macroscopically, adenoma is cystic and may be multilocular, varying in size from 1 cm to 8 cm in diameter. The cysts are often filled with mucus, and mucinuria is a characteristic finding (Eble, 1989). Microscopically, the epithelium consists of tall columnar cells and goblet cells, often with a striking resemblance to colonic glandular epithelium. Accordingly, these tumors are often referred to as *villous*, *tubulovillous*, or *tubular adenoma*. The epithelium may be papillary or flat, sometimes admixed with urothelium. The distinction between multilocular urachal cyst and adenoma may be difficult in some cases, particularly when the lesion is not complex and the surface epithelium is simple. Occasionally, dysplasia may be present, raising the possibility of adenocarcinoma in situ. Invasion may be difficult to evaluate in superficial specimens, and repeat biopsy or transurethral resection may be of value.

REFERENCES

Altaffer LF III, Wilkerson SY, Jordan GH, Lynch DF. Malignant inverted papilloma and carcinoma in situ of the bladder. *J Urol.* 1982;128:816–818.

Amin MB, Gomez JA, Young RH. Urothelial transitional cell carcinoma with endophytic growth patterns. A discussion of patterns of invasion and problems associated with assessment of invasion in 18 cases. *Am J Surg Pathol.* 1997;21:1057–1068.

Billis A, Queroz LS, Oliveira ER, et al. Adenoma of the bladder in siblings with renal displasia. *Urology.* 1980;16:299–301.

Caro DJ, Tessler A. Inverted papilloma of the bladder: a distinct urological lesion. *Cancer.* 1978;42:708–710.

Chan KW, Lam KY, Srivastava G. Accumulation of p53 protein in inverted transitional cell papilloma of the urinary bladder. *J Clin Pathol.* 1996;49:M43–M45.

Eble JN. Abnormalities of the urachus. In: Young, RH, ed. *Pathology of the Urinary Bladder.* New York: Churchill Livingstone; 1989: 213–243.

Eble JN, Young RH. Benign and low grade papillary lesions of the urinary bladder: a review of the papilloma-papillary carcinoma controversy and a report of five typical papillomas. *Sem Diagnost Pathol.* 1989;6:351–371.

Eble JN, Hull MT, Rowland RG, et al. Villous adenoma of the urachus with muscusuria: a light and electron microscopic study. *J Urol.* 1986;135:1240–1242.

Elson EC, McLaughlin AP. Xanthomatous ureteral polyp. *Urology.* 1974;4:214-216.

Epstein JI, Amin MB, Reuter VR, et al. WHO/ISP consensus classification of urothelial (transitional cell) neoplasms of the urinary bladder. Am *J Surg Pathol* 1998;22:1435-1448.

Goertchen R, Seidenschnur A, Stosiek P. Clinical pathology of inverted papillomas of the urinary bladder. A complex morphologic and catamnestic study. *Pathologe.* 1994;15:279–285.

Greene LF, Hanash KA, Farrow GM. Benign papilloma or papillary carcinoma of the bladder. *J Urol.* 1973;110:205–209.

Grignon DJ, Sakr W. Inflammatory and other conditions that can mimic carcinoma in the urinary bladder. *Pathol Annu.* 1995;30:95–122.

Hamm FC. Benign cystadenoma of the bladder probably of urachal origin. *J Urol.* 1940;44:227.

Husain AS, Papas P, Khatib G. Villous adenoma of the urinary bladder presenting as gross hematuria. *J Urol Pathol.* 1996;4:299–306.

Jordan AM, Weingarten J, Murphy WM. Transitional cell neoplasms of the urinary bladder: can biologic potential be predicted from histologic grading? *Cancer.* 1987;60:2766–2774.

Khoury JM, Stutzman RE, Sepulveda RA. Inverted papilloma of the bladder with focal transitional cell carcinoma: a case report. *Mil Med.* 1985;150:562–563.

Kunimi K, Uchibayashi T, Lee SW, et al. Nuclear desoxyribonucleic acid content in inverted papilloma of the urothelium. *Eur Urol.* 1994;26:149–152.

Kunze E, Schauer A, Schmitt M. Histology and histogenesis of two different types of inverted urothelial papillomas. *Cancer.* 1983;51:348–358.

Lazarevic B, Garret R. Inverted papilloma and papillary transitional cell carcinoma of urinary bladder. Report of four cases of inverted papilloma, one showing papillary malignant transformation and review of the literature. *Cancer.* 1978;42:1904–1911.

Lerman RI, Hutter RVP, Whitmore WF Jr. Papilloma of the urinary bladder. *Cancer.* 1970;25:333–338.

Matz LR, Wishart A, Goodman MA. Inverted urothelial papilloma. *Pathology.* 1974;6:37–44.

McCallion WA, Herron BM, Keane PF. Bladder hamartoma. *Br J Urol.* 1993;72:382–383.

Miller DC, Gang DL, Gavris V, et al. Villous adenoma of the urinary bladder: a morphologic or biologic entity? *Am J Clin Pathol.* 1983;79:728–731.

Mostofi FK. Pathological aspects and spread of carcinoma of the bladder. *JAMA.* 1968;206:1764–1769.

Mostofi FK, Sobin LH, Torloni H. Histological typing of urinary bladder tumours. In: *International Classification of Tumours* (19th ed). Geneva, Switzerland: WHO; 1973:25–26.

Murphy WM, Beckwith JB, Farrow GM. Tumors of the kidney, urinary bladder, and related structures. In: *Atlas of Tumor Pathology* (3rd series, fascicle 11). Washington, DC: AFIP; 1994:193–288.

Nichols JA, Marshall BF. Treatment of histologically benign papilloma of the urinary bladder by local excision and fulguration. *Cancer.* 1956;9:566–571.

Prout GR, Barton BA, Griffin PP. Treated history of noninvasive grade 1 transitional cell carcinoma. *J Urol.* 1992;148:1413–1419.

Remick DG, Kumar NB. Benign polyps with prostatic-type epithelium of the urethra and the urinary bladder. A suggestion of histogenesis based on histologic and immunohistochemical studies. *Am J Surg Pathol.* 1984;8:833–839.

Reuter VE, Melamed MR. The lower urinary tract. In: Sternberg SS, ed. *Diagnostic Surgical Pathology* (2nd ed). New York: Raven Press; 1994:1784–1785.

Rozanski TA. Inverted papilloma: an unusual recurrent, multiple, and multifocal lesion. *J Urol.* 1996;155:1391–1393.

Rubin J, Khanna OP, Damjanov I. Adenomatous polyp of the bladder: A rare case of hematuria in young men. *J Urol.* 1981;126:549–550.

Stein BS, Rosen S, Kendall R. The association of inverted papilloma and transitional cell carcinoma of the urothelium. *J Urol.* 1983;131:751–752.

Stosiek P, Kasper M, Seidenschnur A, et al. Cytokeratins in inverted papillomas of the urinary bladder. Part 1. *Pathologe.* 1993;14:330–333.

113

Trotter SE, Philp B, Luck R, et al. Villous adenoma of the bladder. *Histopathology.* 1994;24:491–493.

Urakami S, Igawa M, Shirikawa H, et al. Biological characteristics of inverted papilloma of the urinary bladder. *Br J Urol.* 1996;77:55–60.

West D, Orihuela E, Pow-sang M, et al. Villous adenoma-like lesions associated with invasive transitional cell carcinoma of the bladder. *J Urol Pathol.* 1995;3:263–268.

Wolgel CD, Parris AC, Mitty HA, et al. Fibroepithelial polyp of renal pelvis. *Urology.* 1982;19:436–439.

Yajima I, Ogawa H, Yamaguhi K, et al. Ectopic prostatic tissue in the bladder. *Acta Urol Jpn.* 1993;39:761–764.

Young RH. Fibroepithelial polyp of the bladder with atypical stromal cells. *Arch Pathol Lab Med.* 1986;110:241–242.

8

FLAT UROTHELIAL LESIONS INCLUDING CARCINOMA IN SITU

Intraepithelial neoplasia of the bladder is strongly linked with invasive carcinoma, including flat lesions (dysplasia and carcinoma in situ), discussed in this chapter, and papillary lesions (noninvasive papillary carcinoma), discussed in Chapter 9 (Fig 8.1). Related lesions such as papilloma, inverted papilloma, papillary hyperplasia, and a variety of metaplastic lesions may also be associated with carcinoma, but the evidence is inconclusive.

8.1 UROTHELIAL ATYPIA AND DYSPLASIA

Epithelial changes that have some but not all of the features of carcinoma in situ are variously referred to as *atypia, atypical hyperplasia,* or *dysplasia* (Figs 8.2–8.5). The synonymous terms *intraepithelial neoplasia, grades 1, 2, and 3* and *intraurothelial neoplasia* (IUN) were proposed more than a decade ago but were not widely adopted (Mostofi & Sesterhenn, 1984).

The difficulty in standardizing nomenclature for urothelial cytologic abnormalities is compounded by the lack of reproducibility in classification and grading. Carcinoma in situ (CIS) and high-grade dysplasia are considered synonymous by most but not all investigators (Adsay et al, 1997), because there are no apparent distinguishing histologic features and there is a rela-

tively high level of agreement for classification of these lesions (see below). However, separation of epithelial changes with fewer cytologic and architectural abnormalities than CIS such as intermediate (moderate)-grade dysplasia and low-grade dysplasia is difficult, and the morphologic continuum does not provide any absolute features that allow unequivocal separation. Some authors propose categories of reactive atypia and dysplasia, culminating in the final preinvasive stage of CIS (Murphy & Soloway, 1982; Nagy et al, 1982); others (Amin et al, 1996; Nagy & Friedell, 1993; Reuter & Melamed, 1994) suggest a two- or four-tiered system. One group (Reuter & Melamed, 1994) lumps all neoplastic epithelial lesions into the category of CIS, apparently in response to the clinical and biologic uncertainty of these changes, whereas others (Nagy & Friedell, 1993) grade CIS as 1, 2, or 3. Recently, a concensus classification on flat urothelial lesion terminology was proposed by the World Health Organization (WHO) and the International Society of Urologic Pathologists (ISUP) (Table 8.1) (Epstein et al, in press).

The WHO/ISUP recommends a three-tier system (Table 8.1) and restricts the diagnosis of CIS (the third and final tier) to lesions considered severe or high-grade dysplasia or CIS by others (Epstein et al, in press). Lesions with fewer changes that are still classified as dysplas-

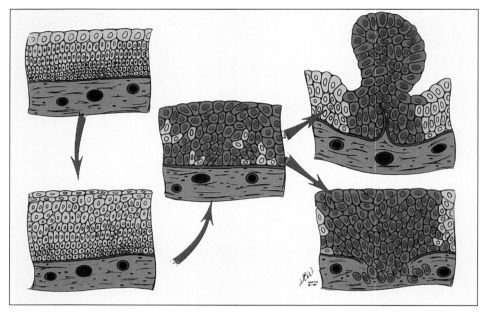

Figure 8.1 Diagrammatic representation of the evolution of invasive bladder cancer through a flat in situ phase. Formation of a papillary neoplasm may also occur, although this is unproven. Reprinted with permisison from Farrow & Utz (1982).

(a)

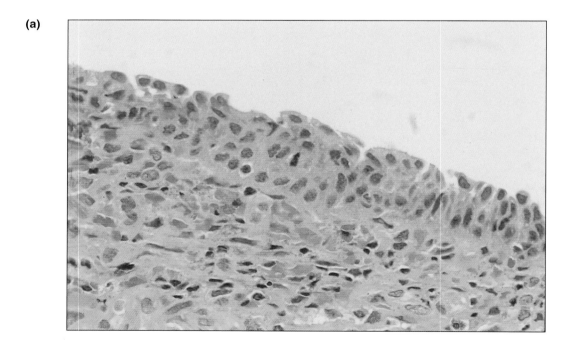

(b)

(c)

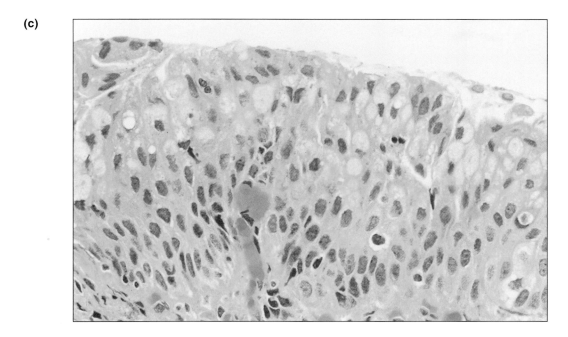

Figure 8.2 Reactive urothelial atypia. **(a):** There is some thickening and loss of polarity and crowding of the mucosal cells, but they are relatively uniform in size and show maturation at the surface. **(b):** The mucosa is thickened, with enlargement of the nuclei of the basal epithelium. Note the presence of eosinophils. **(c):** In the superficial urothelium, many of the cells show mucinous metaplasia.

(a)

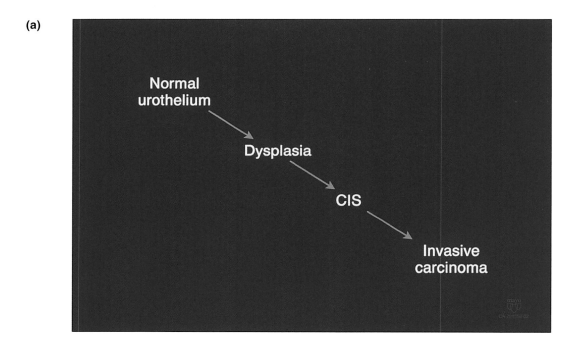

(b)

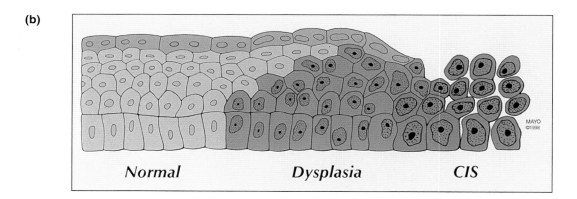

Figure 8.3 Continuum from normal urothelium through dysplasia to carcinoma in situ according to the disease-continuum concept. **(a):** Progression schema; **(b):** morphologic continuum.

tic and not reactive are considered dysplasia; most of these would be considered moderate dysplasia or moderate intraepithelial neoplasia (intraurothelial neoplasia grade 2). The greatest difficulty is encountered in separating the lowest grade of dysplasia (so-called intraurothelial neoplasia grade 1) and reactive atypia, and the WHO/ISUP recommends classifying this lesion as atypia of unknown clini-cal significance, recognizing that the biologic significance of this lesion is probably very low (Adsay et al, 1997) (Tables 8.1 and 8.2). Many pathologists prefer to use the term *atypia* to encompass reactive atypia and dysplasia falling short of CIS, but this is now discouraged by international consensus (Epstein et al, in press).

The cytologic abnormalities in dysplasia are less severe than in CIS and are usually restricted

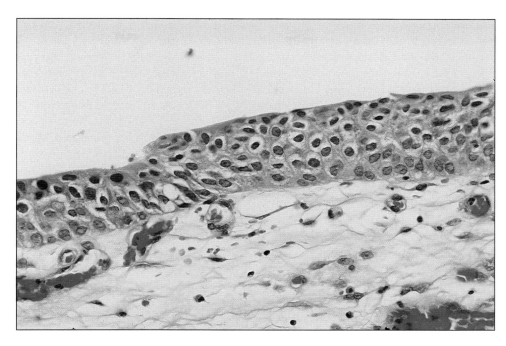

Figure 8.4 Dysplasia. Despite cytologic changes, including nuclear enlargement and hyperchromasia, the urothelium maintains cellular polarity and maturation. Multiple observers felt this focus was dysplastic and not reactive due largely to the lack of coexistent inflammation.

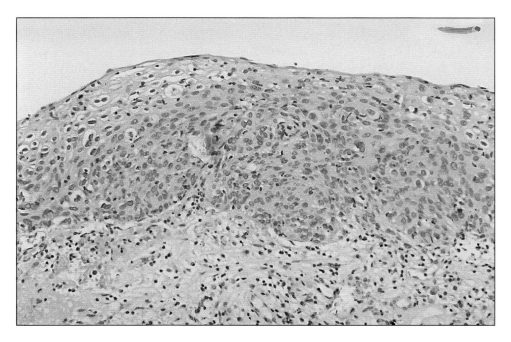

Figure 8.5 Dysplasia. There is partial thickness involvement by cytologic abnormalities of the urothelium. Although considered dysplastic by multiple observers, this focus has many features of partial thickness involvement by immature squamous metaplasia as described in other organs.

to the basal and intermediate layers (Fig 8.6). The abnormalities include nuclear enlargement, coarse chromatin, variation in nuclear shape, and notching of the chromatinic rim. Nucleoli may be small and inconspicuous or rarely enlarged. Mitotic figures are usually absent. The superficial cell layer is intact. Nuclear and architectural features are considered most useful in distinguishing atypia and dysplasia (Murphy & Soloway, 1982). It should be noted that nuclear and nucleolar enlargement and crowding may be seen in reactive conditions (atypia of unknown clinical significance), and we rarely if ever diagnose dysplasia in the setting of cystitis resulting from infection, calculus, instrumentation, or therapy.

The incidence of isolated (primary) dysplasia is unknown because there is a lack of screening studies and an inability to identify most cases cystoscopically. A retrospective study of 15 cases of primary dysplasia revealed subsequent CIS in only two patients (13%) (Zuk et al, 1988). Similarly, only 1 of 19 cases (5%) of primary dyspalsia diagnosed cytologically developed carcinoma (Murphy & Miller, 1984). Dysplasia in the mucosa adjacent to papillary urothelial carcinoma is associated with an increased risk of recurrence and progression; in one study, 73% of patients with dysplasia relapsed, whereas only 43% of those without dysplasia recurred (Friedell et al, 1986; Heney, 1992; Kiemeney et al, 1994; Smith et al, 1983; Wolf & Hojgaard, 1983).

Isolated urothelial dysplasia is rare (Cheng L, Cheville JC, Neumann RM, Bostwick DG, unpublished data, 1998; Zuk et al, 1988). Zuk et al studied 15 patients with dysplasia without con-comitant cancer and found that 15% developed CIS (mean follow-up: 4.8 years). Similarly, we studied 36 patients with isolated urothelial dysplasia at the Mayo Clinic (Cheng L, Cheville JC, Neumann RM, Bostwick DG, unpublished data, 1998). Patients ranged in age from 25 to 79 years (mean: 60 years), and the male-to-female ratio was 2.6:1. Patients presented with urinary tract obstructive symptoms (11 of 36), hematuria (10), both (3), and incidentally (12). Dysplasia had a predilection for the posterior wall. Nineteen percent of patients developed biopsy-proven progression, including 11% with CIS and 8% with invasive cancer (mean follow-up: 8.2 years). Mean time to progression was 2.5 years (range: 0.5 to 8 years). We concluded that isolated urothelial dysplasia was a significant risk factor for urothelial carcinoma.

Cytokeratin 20 immunoreactivity may be an objective marker of dysplasia, and its routine use in equivocal cases has been recommended (Harnden et al, 1996). Expression of cytokeratin 20 in benign urothelium is limited to the superficial cells, whereas dysplasia and CIS show more extensive or full-thickness immunoreactivity.

Studies of blood group isoantigen expression, nuclear morphometry, and DNA ploidy indicate that the findings in dysplasia are, as expected, intermediate between benign urothelium and CIS.

8.2 UROTHELIAL CARCINOMA IN SITU

CIS is defined as a flat noninvasive neoplastic mucosal change of the urothelium with substantial cytologic and architectural abnormali-

Table 8.1 Classification of flat urothelial lesions (WHO/ISUP)

Lesion	Description
Atypia of unknown clinical significance	Minimal architectural and cytologic changes in flat urothelium; uncertain whether it is neoplastic or merely reactive
Dysplasia	Appreciable architectural and cytologic changes in flat urothelium that fall short of the diagnostic threshold of carcinoma in situ
Carcinoma in situ	High-grade (malignant-appearing) nuclei in flat urothelium. Cells may be large or small; full thickness involvement is not necessary for diagnosis.

Table 8.2 Histologic comparison of atypical urothelium, hyperplasia, dysplasia, and carcinoma in situ

	Atypia of unknown clinical significance	Hyperplasia*	Dysplasia	Carcinoma in situ
Cell layers	Variable	>7 cells	Variable	Variable
Polarization	Slightly abnormal	Normal	Slightly abnormal	Abnormal
Cytoplasm	Vacuolated	Homogeneous	Homogeneous	Homogeneous
N:C ratio	Normal or slightly increased	Normal or slightly increased	Slightly increased	Increased
Nuclei				
Position	Normal	Normal	Eccentric	Eccentric
Borders	Regular/smooth	Regular/smooth	Notches/creases	Pleomorphic
Chromatin	Fine/dusty	Fine	Fine	Coarse
Distribution	Even	Even	Even	Uneven
Nucleoli	Large	Small/absent	Small/absent	Large
Mitotic figures	Variable	Absent	Variable	Variable
Denudation	Variable	No	No	Variable

N:C =nucleus-to-cytoplasm ratio.
*Very rare.

ties that lacks papillary changes (Figs 8.7–8.9). In most cases, CIS is multifocal, appearing cystoscopically as erythematous, velvety, or granular patches, although it may be visually undetectable (Wolf et al, 1994; Zincke et al, 1985).

CIS exists in two settings: primary or isolated CIS and secondary CIS associated with noninvasive or invasive papillary urothelial carcinoma. There is strong indirect evidence that this lesion is a precursor of invasive carcinoma, but direct evidence in humans is lacking.

8.2.1 Primary CIS

Primary (de novo or isolated) CIS is uncommon, accounting for <10% of cases of CIS and 1% of bladder tumors (Cifuentes et al, 1970; Farrow, 1992; Okaneya et al, 1991; Orozco et al, 1994). It occurs in the absence of other urothelial tumors, almost exclusively in men over 50 years of age. Symptoms typically include dysuria, pain, frequency, hematuria, nocturia, and sterile pyuria. The clinical presentation may closely mimic interstitial cystitis. Primary CIS is asymptomatic in about 25% of patients. It may be present throughout the bladder but usually involves the trigone, floor, and neck.

8.2.2 Secondary CIS

Secondary CIS is more common than primary CIS, accounting for about 90% of cases of CIS. Secondary CIS is the association of CIS with a prior or synchronous urothelial tumor, including noninvasive or invasive urothelial carcinoma (Altaffer et al, 1982; Althausen et al, 1976; Batista et al, 1994; Brawn, 1982; Prout et al, 1983).

The frequency of CIS increases with increasing grade and stage of the associated urothelial neoplasm. Up to 24% of random biopsies from patients with Ta and T1 carcinoma show epithelial abnormalities that include dysplasia and CIS. Mapping studies of cystectomy specimens show extensive CIS with involvement of the prostatic urethra in up to 67% of cases and involvement of the ureter in up to 57% of cases (Batista et al, 1994; Khan et al, 1979; Mahadevia et al, 1986; Vicente et al, 1991).

8.2.3 Diagnostic Criteria for CIS

The cells of CIS may form a layer that is only one cell layer thick, of normal thickness (up to 7 cells) , or the thickness of hyperplasia (greater than 7 cells). The diagnosis of CIS requires the

(a)

(b)

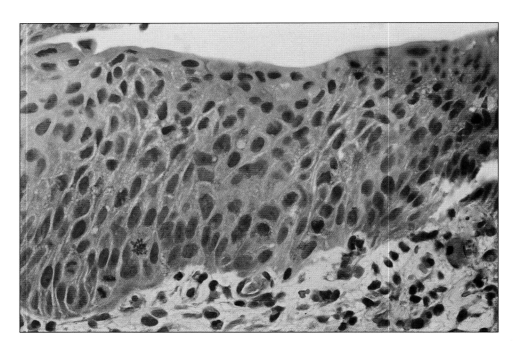

Figure 8.6 **(a):** Dysplasia bordering on carcinoma in situ. **(b):** Thickened urothelium with dysplastic changes, including marked nuclear hyperchromasia.

(a)

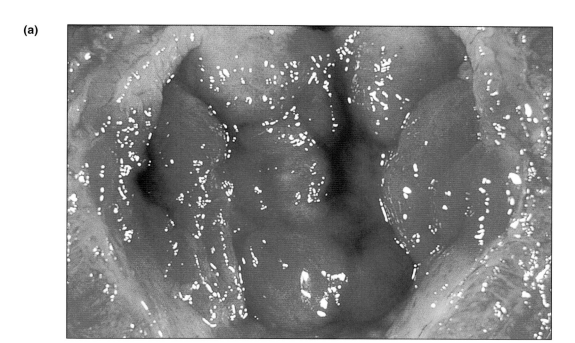

(b)

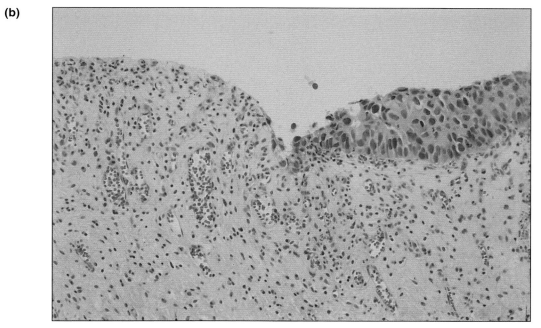

(c)

(d)

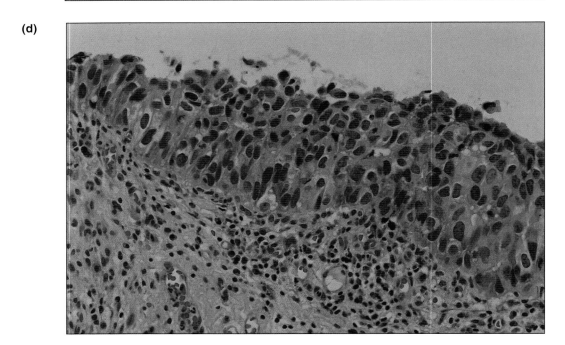

Figure 8.7 Carcinoma in situ (CIS). **(a):** Partially denuded urothelium; the remainder is lined by cells with marked cytologic abnormalities. **(b):** Bizarre hyperchromatic cells of CIS separating from the basement membrane; note the underlying chronic cystitis. **(c):** CIS involving a thickened urothelium. **(d):** Another focus of CIS.

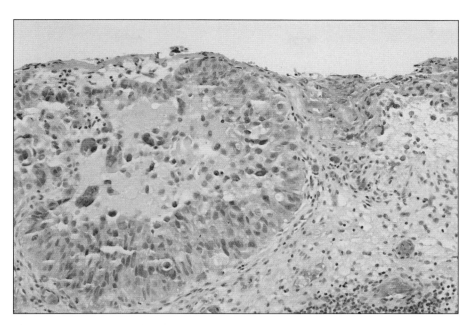

Figure 8.8 Carcinoma in situ involving Brunn's nests.

presence of severe cytologic atypia (nuclear anaplasia); full-thickness change is not essential, although it is usually present. Interobserver agreement with CIS is high (Sharkey & Sarosdy, 1997).

Prominent disorganization of cells is characteristic, with loss of polarity and cohesiveness. Superficial (umbrella) cells may be present except in areas of full-thickness abnormality. The tumor cells tend to be large and pleomorphic, with moderate to abundant cytoplasm, although they are sometimes small with a high nucleus-to-cytoplasmic ratio. The chromatin tends to be coarse and clumped. Morphometrically, the cells display increased nuclear area, nuclear perimeter, and maximum nuclear diameter. Nucleoli are usually large and prominent in at least some of the cells and may be multiple. Mitotic figures are often seen in the uppermost urothelium and may be atypical. The adjacent mucosa often contains lesser degrees of cytologic abnormality.

The small cell pattern of CIS is usually associated with an increased number of cell layers. In such cases, the cytoplasm is scant and the nuclei are enlarged and hyperchromatic, with coarse unevenly distributed chromatin; scattered prominent nucleoli are distorted and angulated. Mitotic

figures are frequently present, often with abnormal forms. The cells are randomly oriented and disorganized, often with striking cellular dyscohesion that, in some cases, results in few or no recognizable epithelial cells on the surface, a condition referred to as *denuding cystitis* (Elliot et al, 1973). In rare instances, there is an undermining (lepidic) growth pattern of CIS (Amin & Young, 1997). Careful search of all residual mucosa is important in biopsies that have little or no mucosa to exclude the denuding cystitis of CIS.

CIS is often associated with focal discontinuity of the basement membrane. There may be intense chronic inflammation in the superficial lamina propria in some cases, and vascular ectasia and proliferation of small capillaries are frequent. In denuded areas, residual CIS may involve Brunn's nests. Rarely, CIS exhibits pagetoid growth, characterized by large single cells or small clusters of cells within otherwise normal urothelium, in squamous metaplasia, or within prostatic ducts (Begin et al, 1991; Farrow, 1992; Jendresen et al, 1994; Orozco et al, 1993). Individual cells showing pagetoid spread have enlarged nuclei with coarse chromatin, single or multiple nucleoli, and abundant pale to eosino-

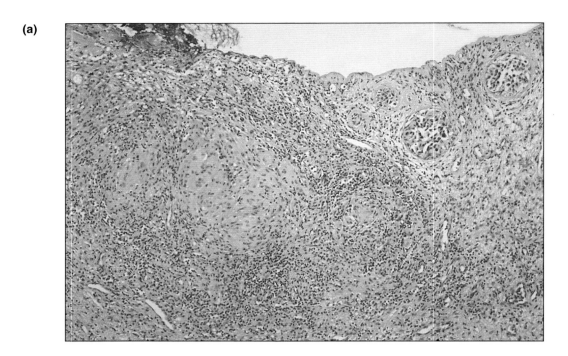

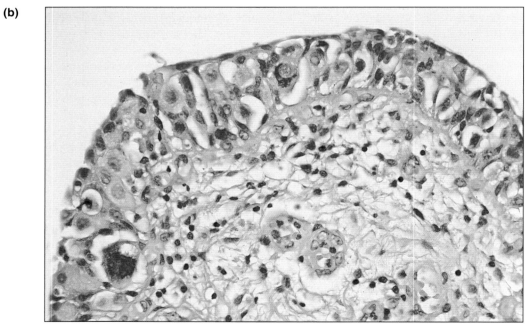

Figure 8.9 Recurrent carcinoma in situ. **(a):** There is prominent granulomatous inflammation resulting from therapy with bacillus Calmette-Guérin, but **(b):** carcinoma in situ persists.

philic cytoplasm that is negative for mucin . Careful search should be made for subepithelial invasion (microinvasion), often appearing as single cells or small nests of cells with retraction artifact. Microinvasion may be masked by chronic inflammation, denuded mucosa, or stromal fibrosis.

CIS typically does not express normal A, B, and O (H) blood group isoantigens (Coon et al, 1985). Conversely, carcinoembryonic antigen, usually absent in normal urothelium, is frequently found in the cells of CIS. DNA ploidy studies by flow cytometry and image analysis reveal a high frequency of aneuploidy (Norming et al, 1992a, 1992b; Sanchez-Fernandez de Sevilla et al, 1992; Tyrkus et al, 1992).

8.2.4   Clinical Course of CIS

Urothelial CIS has a high likelihood of progressing to invasive carcinoma if untreated, occurring in up to 83% of cases (Daly, 1976; Dean & Murphy, 1987; Hudson & Herr, 1995; Utz & Farrow, 1980, 1984; Utz et al, 1980). Cystectomy reveals foci of microinvasion in 34% of bladders with CIS and muscle-invasive cancer in up to 9% (Farrow & Utz, 1982). Patients with CIS treated by radical cystectomy have up to 100% 5-year survival rates (Amling et al, 1994). Intravesical therapy is also commonly employed, including treatment with thiotepa, mitomycin C, and bacillus Calmette-Guérin.

Primary CIS has a lower risk of progression (28% vs. 59%) and death (7% vs. 45%) than secondary CIS (Orozco et al, 1994). Factors predictive of high risk of progression include multifocality, a coexistent bladder neoplasm, prostatic urethral involvement, and recurrence after treatment (Table 8.3).

Table 8.3   Clinical and anatomic predictive factors of progression in CIS

Multifocal and extensive CIS (versus focal CIS)
Involvement of prostatic urethra
Coexistent urothelial neoplasm
Recurrence after treatment

REFERENCES

Adsay NV, Sakr WA, Grignon DJ. Flat-type transitional cell carcinoma in situ. *Pathol Case Rev.* 1997;2:115–121.

Altaffer LF III, Wilkerson SY, Jordan GH, et al. Malignant inverted papilloma and carcinoma in situ of the bladder. *J Urol.* 1982;128:816–820.

Althausen AF, Prout GR Jr, Daly JJ. Non-invasive papillary carcinoma of the bladder associated with carcinoma in situ. *J Urol.* 1976;116:575–580.

Amin MB, Young RH. Intraepithelial lesions of the urinary bladder with a discussion of the histogenesis of urothelial neoplasm. *Sem Diagn Pathol.* 1997;14:84–97.

Amin MB, Murphy WM, Reuter VE, et al. Controversies in the pathology of transitional cell carcinoma of the urinary bladder. In: Rosen PP, Flechner RE, eds. *Reviews in pathology.* Chicago, IL: ASCP Press; 1996:1–38.

Amling CL, Thrasher JB, Dodge KR, et al. Radical cystectomy for stages TA, TIS, and T1 transitional cell carcinoma of the bladder. *J Urol.* 1994;151:31–36.

Batista JE, Palou J, Iglesias J, et al. Significance of ureteral carcinoma in situ in specimens of cystectomy. *Eur Urol.* 1994;25:313–315.

Begin LR, Deschenes J, Mitmaker B. Pagetoid carcinomatous involvement of the penile urethra in association with high-grade transitional cell carcinoma of the urinary bladder. *Arch Pathol Lab Med.* 1991;115:632–635.

Brawn PN. The origin of invasive carcinoma of the bladder. *Cancer.* 1982;50:515–520.

Cifuentes L, Oliva H, Navarro V. Intraepithelial carcinoma of the bladder. *Urol Int.* 1970;25:169–186.

Coon JS, McCall C, Miller AW III, et al. Expression of blood-group-related antigens in carcinoma in situ of the urinary bladder. *Cancer.* 1985;56:797–802.

Daly JJ. Carcinoma in situ of the urothelium. *Urol Clin North Am.* 1976;3:87–95.

Dean PJ, Murphy WM. Carcinoma in situ and dysplasia of the bladder urothelium. *World J Urol.* 1987;5:103–107.

Elliot GB, Moloney PJ, Anderson GH. Denuding cystitis and in situ urothelial carcinoma. *Arch Pathol.* 1973;96:91–94.

Epstein JI, Amin MB, Reuter V, et al. WHO/ISUP consensus classification of urothelial (transitional cell) lesions. *J Urol Pathol.* In press.

Farrow GM. Pathology of carcinoma in situ of the urinary bladder and related lesions. *J Cell Biochem.* 1992;161:39–43.

Farrow GM, Utz DC. Observations on microinvasive transitional cell carcinoma of the urinary bladder. *Clin Oncol.* 1982;1:609–615.

Friedell GH, Soloway MS, Hilgar AG, et al. Summary of the workshop on carcinoma in situ of the bladder. *J Urol.* 1986;136:1047–1048.

Harnden P, Eardley I, Joyce AD, Southgate J. Cytokeratin 20 as an objective marker of urothelial dysplasia. *Br J Urol.* 1996;78:870–875.

Heney NM. Natural history of superficial bladder cancer. Prognostic features and long-term disease course. *Urol Clin North Am.* 1992;19:429–433.

Hudson MA, Herr HA. Carcinoma in situ of the bladder. *J Urol.* 1995;153:564–572.

Jendresen M, Kvist E, Beck B. Paget's disease in a squamous metaplasia of the urinary bladder. *Scand J Urol Nephrol.* 1994;28:327–329.

Khan AU, Farrow GM, Zincke H, et al. Primary carcinoma in situ of the ureter and renal pelvis. *J Urol.* 1979;121:681–686.

Kiemeney LA, Witjes JA, Heijbroek RP, et al. Dysplasia in normal-looking urothelium increases the risk of tumor progression in primary superficial bladder cancer. *Eur J Cancer.* 1994;30A:1621–1625.

Mahadevia PS, Koss LG, Tar IJ. Prostatic involvement in bladder cancer: prostate mapping in 20 cystoprostatectomy specimens. *Cancer.* 1986;58: 2096–2102.

Mostofi FK, Sesterhenn IA. Pathology of epithelial tumors and carcinoma in situ of the bladder. *Prog Clin Biol Res.* 1984;162A:55–74.

Murphy WM, Miller AW. In: Javadpour NE, ed. *Bladder cancer.* Baltimore, MD: Williams & Wilkins; 1984:100–122.

Murphy WM, Soloway MS. Developing carcinoma/dysplasia of the urinary bladder. *Pathol Ann.* 1982;17:197–212.

Nagy GK, Friedell GHY. Urinary bladder. In: Henson DE, Albores-Saavedra J, eds. *Pathology of incipient neoplasia* (2nd ed). Philadelphia, PA: WB Saunders; 1993:334–356.

Nagy GK, Frable WJ, Murphy WM. The classification of premalignant urothelial abnormalities. A Delphi Study of the National Bladder Clinical Collaborative Group A. *Pathol Ann.* 1982;17:219–229.

Norming U, Tribukait B, Gustafson H, et al. Deoxyribonucleic acid profile and tumor progression in primary carcinoma in situ of the bladder: a study of 63 patients with grade 3 lesions. *J Urol.* 1992a;147:11–15.

Norming U, Tribukait B, Nyman CR, et al. Prognostic significance of mucosal aneuploidy in stage Ta/T1 grade 3 carcinoma of the bladder. *J Urol.* 1992b;148:1420–1426.

Okaneya T, Ikado S, Ogawa A. The progress pattern of carcinoma in situ of the urinary bladder. *Jpn J Urol.* 1991;82:1227–1231.

Orozco RE, Vander Zwaag R, Murphy WM. The pagetoid variant of urothelial carcinoma in situ. *Hum Pathol.* 1993;24:1199–1206.

Orozco RE, Martin AA, Murphy WM. Carcinoma in situ of the urinary bladder. Clues to host involvement in human carcinogenesis. *Cancer.* 1994;74: 115–122.

Prout GR Jr, Griffin PP, Daly JJ, et al. Carcinoma in situ of the urinary bladder with and without associated vesical neoplasms. *Cancer.* 1983;52:524–531.

Reuter V, Melamed M. The lower urinary tract. In: Sternberg S, ed. *Diagnostic surgical pathology* (vol 2). New York: Raven Press; 1994:1784–1785.

Sanchez-Fernandez de Sevilla MC, Morell-Quadreny L, Gil-Salom M, et al. Morphometric and immunohistochemical characterization of bladder carcinoma in situ and its preneoplastic lesions. *Eur Urol.* 1992;21:5–9.

Sharkey FE, Sarosdy MF. The significance of central pathology review in clinical studies of transitional cell carcinoma in situ. *J Urol.* 1997;157:68–70.

Smith G, Elton RA, Beynon LL. Prognostic significance of biopsy results of normal looking mucosa in cases of superficial bladder cancer. *Br J Urol.* 1983;55:665–669.

Tyrkus M, Powell I, Fakr W. Cytogenetic studies of carcinoma in situ of the bladder: prognostic implications. *J Urol.* 1992;148:44–46.

Utz DC, Farrow GM. Management of carcinoma in situ of the bladder: the case for surgical management. *Urol Clin North Am.* 1980;7:533–542.

Utz DC, Farrow GM. Carcinoma in situ of the urinary tract. *Urol Clin North Am.* 1984;11:735–748.

Utz DC, Farrow GM, Rife CC, et al. Carcinoma in situ of the bladder. *Cancer.* 1980;45:1842–1850.

Vicente J, Laguna MP, Duarte D, et al. Carcinoma in situ as a prognostic factor for G3pT1 bladder tumours. *Br J Urol.* 1991;68:380–382.

Wolf H, Hojgaard K. Urothelial dysplasia concomitant with bladder tumours as a determinant factor for future new occurrences. *Lancet.* 1983;2:134–136.

Wolf H, Melsen F, Pedersen SE, et al. Natural history of carcinoma in situ of the urinary bladder. *Scand J Urol Nephrol.* 1994;157:147–151.

Zincke H, Utz DC, Farrow GM. Review of Mayo Clinic experience with carcinoma in situ. *Urology.* 1985;26:39–46.

Zuk RJ, Rogers HS, Martin JE, Baithun SI. Clinicopathological importance of primary dysplasia of bladder. *J Clin Pathol.* 1988;41:1277–1280.

9

PAPILLARY UROTHELIAL LESIONS, INCLUDING UROTHELIAL CARCINOMA

This chapter describes the spectrum of papillary urothelial tumors and invasive urothelial cancer (Fig 9.1) (Table 9.1). Papilloma is described in Chapter 7.

9.1   PAPILLARY NEOPLASM OF LOW MALIGNANT POTENTIAL AND UROTHELIAL CARCINOMA

Most noninvasive urothelial carcinomas are papillary neoplasm of low malignant potential (formerly World Health Organization grade 1) or low-grade carcinoma (formerly WHO grade 2) (Figs 9.2 and 9.3) (Briggs et al, 1992; Soto et al, 1977). Approximately 70% of these tumors are noninvasive (stage 0; pTa), and 30% invade the lamina propria (stage A; pT1) (El Ouakdi et al, 1991).

Noninvasive papillary carcinoma may be single or multiple (70% vs. 30% of cases, respectively). The majority of stage pTa tumors are papillary neoplasm of low malignant potential, whereas up to 70% of stage pT1 are low-grade carcinoma. More than 60% of noninvasive tumors recur locally, and the remainder progress to invasion (Friedell et al, 1982; Holmäng et al, 1995; Itoku & Stein, 1992; Kiemeney et al, 1993; Mostofi, 1956; Sanchez de la Muela et al, 1993). Papillary tumors frequently have a pushing border with no desmoplastic stromal reaction and may abut the muscularis propria (Abou Farha et al, 1993; Bostwick, 1992; Koch et al, 1986). Some authors have combined pTa and pT1 cancer as "superficial" cancer, but the World Health Organization and International Society of Urologic Pathologists (ISUP) recommends elimination of this imprecise term; stratification by TNM stage is more appropriate and avoids misinterpretation (Epstein et al, 1998).

Papillary neoplasm of low malignant potential and low-grade papillary urothelial carcinoma are occasionally associated with infiltrating cancer at the base (Heney et al, 1983). Sometimes, the invasive component is higher grade than the noninvasive component.

Patients at risk for recurrence or progression can be identified by a variety of prognostic factors, including tumor grade, depth of invasion, presence of vascular or lymphatic invasion, the number and size of tumors, associated mucosal abnormalities, and numerous biologic markers (Chen et al, 1996; Deen & Ball, 1994; Esrig et al, 1994; Hemstreet et al, 1991; Holmäng et al, 1995; Torti & Lum, 1987). Koilocytosis is uncommon in urothelial carcinoma by light microscopy or molecular techniques (Hartveit et al, 1992; Lopez-Beltran et al, 1992).

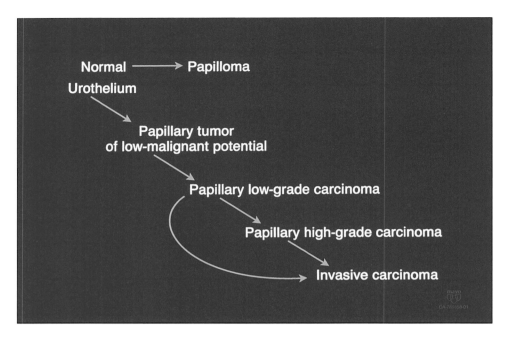

Figure 9.1 Continuum of papillary urothelial lesions and evolution to invasive carcinoma (terminology of the World Health Organization and the International Society of Urologic Pathologists).

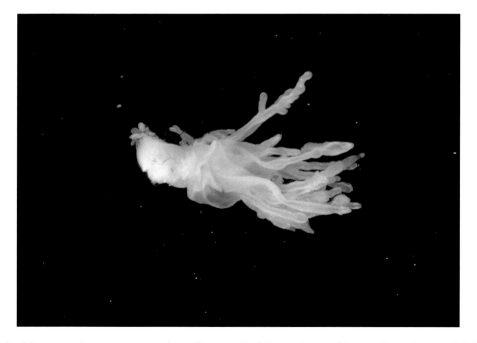

Figure 9.2 Macroscopic appearance of papillary urothelial neoplasm of low malignant potential. Courtesy of Dr. Paul Dundore, Mayo Clinic, Jacksonville, FL.

Table 9.1 Classification of papillary urothelial neoplasms (WHO/ISUP)

Lesion	Description
Papilloma	Uncommon, benign lesion with papillary growth and a delicate fibrovascular core; lined by a normal urothelium; usually small, usually solitary, usually in patients under 50 years of age
Papillary neoplasm of low malignant potential	Analogous to WHO grade 1 carcinoma; papillary growth with minimal architectural and cytologic abnormalities; almost never invades but is a risk factor
Low-grade papillary urothelial carcinoma	Analogous to WHO grade 2 carcinoma (all but the highest end of the spectrum); papillary growth with architectural and cytologic abnormalities; can progress
High-grade papillary urothelial carcinoma	Analogous to WHO grades 2 (highest end of the spectrum) and 3 carcinoma; papillary growth with marked architectural and cytologic abnormalities that are apparent at medium magnification; usually associated with invasion

In this new classification, the term *papilloma* is retained as in the 1973 WHO classification (see Chapter 7). The category *papillary neoplasm of low malignant potential* describes a papillary urothelial lesion with minimal cytological and architectural abnormalities, irrespective of the cell thickness, in contrast to papilloma that has no cytological or architectural atypia. It is analogous to what has been called grade 1 urothelial carcinoma in the 1973 WHO classification. It is understood that this lesion, given its cytologic and growth pattern characteristics, is incapable of invasion or metastases in the overwhelming majority of cases. Nevertheless, it is a clinically important lesion given that these patients have increased risk of developing recurrent or new papillary lesions. These new lesions are occasionally of higher grade and, thus, may progress. Pathologists are encouraged to include the following note in cases diagnosed as papillary neoplasm of low malignant potential: "Note: Patient with these tumors are at risk of developing new bladder tumors, usually of similar histology. However, occasionally, these subsequent lesions manifest as urothelial carcinoma, such that follow-up is warranted." If one encounters a lesion with the cytologic and growth pattern characteristics of papillary urothelial neoplasm of low malignant potential with evidence of invasion, the diagnosis of low-grade papillary urothelial carcinoma should be rendered. The category "papillary urothelial carcinoma, low grade" describes a papillary urothlial lesion with cytologic and architectural abnormalities, both of which may be observed at medium magnification. The abnormalities include what has been called WHO grade 2 cancer (1973). These tumors can and do progress and may be associated with invasion at the time of presentation. The last category "papillary urothelial carcinoma, high grade" describes a papillary urothelial lesion with moderate to marked cytologic and growth pattern abnormalities, which may be observed at medium and sometimes low magnification. The abnormalities include the spectrum of 1973 WHO grade 3 carcinoma (in other words, high grade). These tumors do progress and are more often than not associated with invasion at the time of presentation.

9.2 MICROINVASIVE CARCINOMA

Microinvasive carcinoma of the urinary bladder is defined as invasion into the lamina propria to a depth of no more than 5 mm from the basement membrane (Farrow & Utz, 1982). In the original study, cystectomy specimens with urothelial carcinoma in situ were totally embedded, with extensive CIS involving at least 25% of the bladder (Farrow et al, 1976, 1977). Of 70 cases, 24 contained microinvasion, and 2 patients died of cancer.

9.3 INVASIVE UROTHELIAL CARCINOMA

The term *urothelial carcinoma* usually refers to invasive cancer of the urinary bladder and should be distinguished from carcinoma in situ and noninvasive papillary carcinoma (Friedell et al, 1986; Holmäng et al, 1995; Melamed, 1992). Urothelial carcinoma is rare in patients under age 40 years (Bostwick, 1992; Njeh et al, 1994) and is more common in men than women. Frequently, there is coexistent urothelial carcinoma

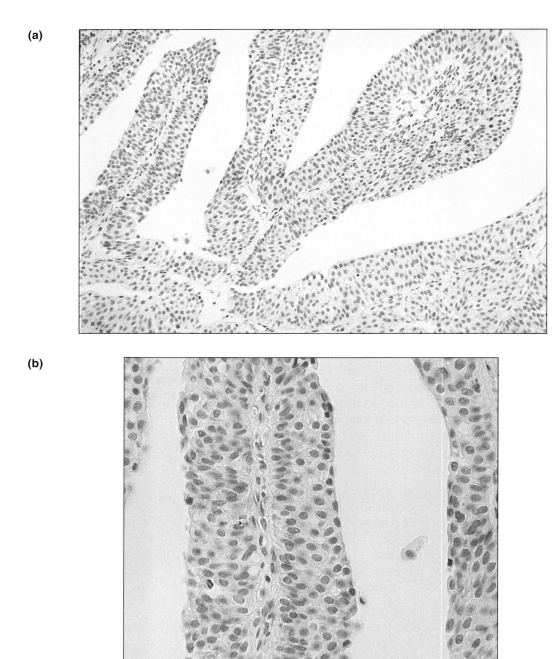

Figure 9.3 Papillary neoplasm of low malignant potential. Although sharing some features with papilloma, this tumor was large (4 cm diameter) and multifocal, occurring in a 75-year-old man.

of the upper urinary tract (Mukamel et al, 1994); rarely, urachal carcinoma is associated with primary urothelial carcinoma of the bladder. Urothelial carcinoma may occur or recur after placement of an ileal neobladder (Shokeir, 1995). Rare cases of urothelial carcinoma present with hypercalcemia.

9.3.1. Gross and Microscopic Features

The single most important element in biopsy interpretation of bladder cancer is recognition of the presence and extent of invasion (Montie, 1994). Foci of invasion are often single and solid but may be mixed with papillary carcinoma and other growth patterns (Figs 9.4 and 9.5). Commonly, there are nests and small clusters of cells that irregularly infiltrate the bladder wall and elicit a stromal fibrous response. Conversely, there may be solid diffuse growth with little intervening stroma. The pattern of growth is clinically important; a broad front of invasion has a more favorable prognosis than tentacular invasion (Farrow & Utz, 1982). In small, fragmented, and cauterized specimens, it may be particularly difficult to determine the presence or extent of subepithelial invasion. In such cases, we sometimes employ broad-spectrum antikeratin immunostaining (AE1/AE3) to identify epithelial differentiation in suspicious cells.

Invasive cancer tends to be high grade and is often deeply invasive (pT2 or higher), although rare cases have deceptively benign-appearing cytologic features (see section 9.3.2). In most cases, the stroma contains a lymphocytic infiltrate with a variable number of plasma cells. The inflammation is usually mild to moderate and focal, although it may be severe, dense, and widespread. Neutrophils and eosinophils are rarely prominent unless there is coexistent cystitis. Urothelial carcinoma without inflammation may be more aggressive than inflamed cancer (Lipponen et al, 1992; Lopez-Beltran et al, 1989). Occasionally, mucoid cyto-plasmic inclusions may be present, particularly in low-grade carcinoma (Lopez-Beltran et al, 1986; Yang and Campbell, 1996).

9.3.2 Differential Diagnosis

Low-grade urothelial carcinoma may be mistaken for urothelial papilloma, inverted papilloma, benign hyperplasia, and papillary cystitis, although the identification of unequivocal invasion is diagnostic of malignancy. With some small and fragmented specimens, it is essential that the pathologist consider the clinical and cystoscopic findings in attemping this separation, particularly in cases with questionable foci of invasion.

The differential diagnosis of high-grade urothelial carcinoma includes high-grade prostatic adenocarcinoma, sarcoma, and high-grade malignant lymphoma. Rare considerations include lymphoepithelioma-like carcinoma of the urinary bladder, particularly in cases with extensive inflammation (Amin et al, 1994).

9.3.3 Grading Urothelial Carcinoma

Grading of urothelial carcinoma is based on the worst grade present. The 1973 World Health Organization (WHO) grading system and equivalent 1973 WHO/ISUP system are the most commonly used internationally (Epstein et al, 1998; Mostofi et al, 1973) (Tables 9.1–9.3), but others have been proposed in recent years. WHO/ISUP papillary neoplasm of low malignant potential (formerly WHO grade 1 carcinoma) consists of a urothelium more than seven cell layers thick containing cells that display minimal to slight nuclear enlargement, normal or slightly distorted architecture, and rare or absent mitotic figures (Figs 9.2 and 9.3). ISUP low-grade carcinoma (formerly WHO grade 2 carcinoma) displays greater nuclear pleomorphism, coarsely clumped chromatin,

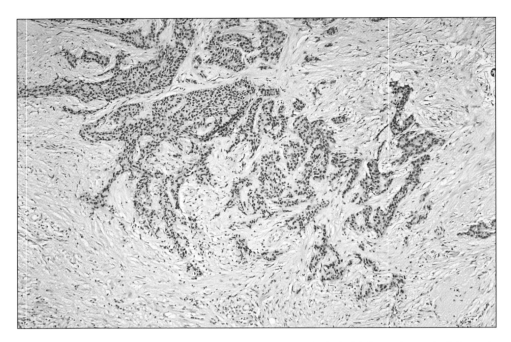

Figure 9.4 Tentacular pattern of stromal invasion with desmoplasia in high-grade urothelial carcinoma.

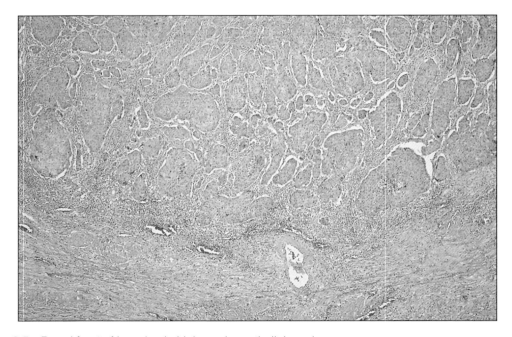

Figure 9.5 Broad front of invasion in high-grade urothelial carcinoma.

Table 9.2 WHO/ISUP grading of papillary urothelial neoplams of the bladder

Features	Grade		
	Papillary neoplasm of low malignant potential (formerly WHO grade 1)	Low-grade (formerly WHO grade 2)	High-grade (formerly WHO grade 2)
Increased cell layer	Yes	Variable	Variable
Superficial cells	Usually present	Absent	Absent
Clear cytoplasm	Often absent	Often absent	Absent
Nuclear size	Increased	Increased	Greatly increased
Pleomorphism	Slight	Moderate	Marked
Nuclear polarization	Slightly abnormal	Abnormal	Absent
Hyperchromatism	Slight	Moderate (<50%)	Marked (>50%)
Mitotic figures	None/rare	Present	Prominent
Nuclear grooves	Present	Present	Absent

Table 9.3 Histologic grading of papillary urothelial neoplasms

ISUP (Epstein et al, 1998)	Mostofi et al (1973)	Murphy (1987)	Carbin et al (1991)	Pauwels et al (1988)
Papilloma	Papilloma	Papilloma	Papilloma	Papilloma
Papillary neoplasm of low malignant potential	Grade 1		Grade 1	Low grade
Low-grade carcinoma	Grade 2	Low grade	Grade 2a-A	Grade 2a low grade
High-grade carcinoma	Grade 3	High grade	Grade 2b-B	Grade 2b high grade
			Grade 3 -B	Grade 3 high grade

and some disruption of the normal architecture (Figs 9.6 and 9.7). WHO/ISUP high-grade carcinoma (formerly WHO grade 3 carcinoma) displays the most extreme nuclear abnormalities, similar to those seen in carcinoma in situ, including loss of normal architecture and cell polarity, noncohesive cells, and frequent mitotic figures (Figs 9.8 and 9.9). Cellular anaplasia, characteristic of high-grade carcinoma, is defined as increased cellularity, nuclear crowding, disturbance of cellular polarity, absence of differentiation from the base to the mucosal surface, nuclear pleomorphism, irregularity in the size of the cells, variation in nuclear shape and chromatin pattern, increased number of mitotic figures, and the occasional presence of neoplastic giant cells (Mostofi et al, 1973).

Most cases of urothelial carcinoma are WHO/ISUP low-grade carcinoma (formerly WHO grade 2 carcinoma). However, difficulty in precisely defining the cut point between WHO/ISUP papillary neoplasm of low malignant potential (formerly WHO grade 1 carcinoma) and WHO/ISUP low-grade carcinoma (formerly WHO grade 2) and between WHO/ISUP low-grade carcinoma and WHO/ISUP high-grade carcinoma (formerly WHO grade 3) has resulted in a wide variety of incidences for WHO/ISUP low-grade carcinoma, ranging from 13% (Jordan et al, 1987) to 58% (Lipponen et al, 1993a) and 69% (Pauwels et al, 1988). A study of 103 invasive nodular urothelial carcinomas revealed that 14% were WHO/ISUP papillary neoplasms of low malignant potential (formerly WHO grade 1 carcinoma); 58%, WHO/ISUP low-grade carcinoma; and 28%, WHO/ISUP high-grade carcinoma (Lipponen et al, 1993b). Despite this variation in histologic grading, virtually all studies have concluded that tumor grade is one of the most powerful predictive factors for all patient outcome variables (Carbin et al, 1991; Jordan et al, 1987;

(a)

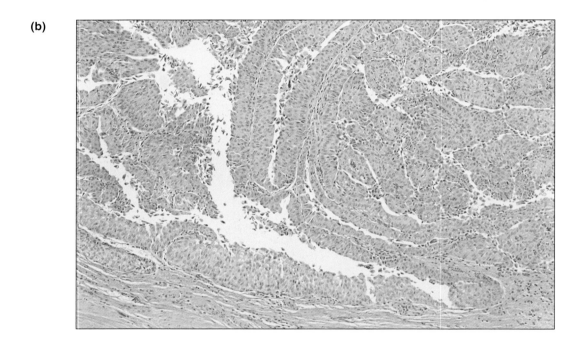

(b)

(c)

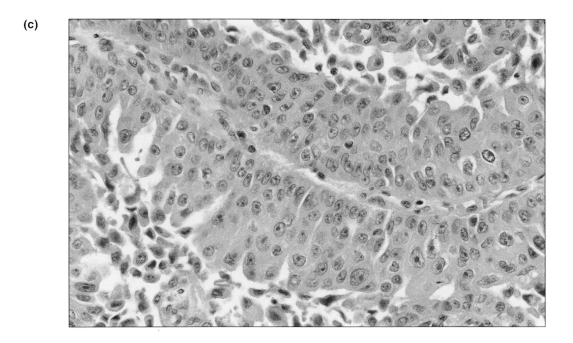

(d)

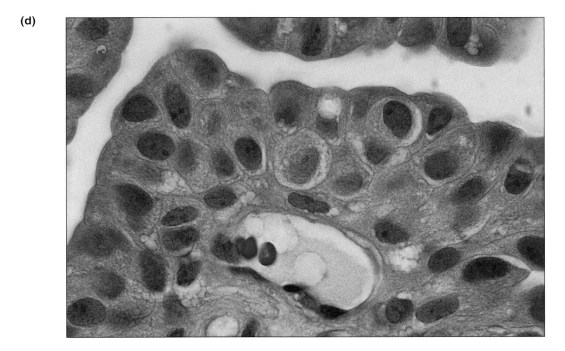

Figure 9.6   Noninvasive low-grade papillary urothelial carcinoma. **(a):** The bladder is partially filled by a soft velvety mass. **(b):** Closely packed papillae are characteristic. **(c, d):** There are mild to moderate cytologic abnormalities, including nucleomegaly and anisonucleosis. Multiple observers considered this diagnostic of low-grade carcinoma rather than papillary urothelial neoplasm of low malignant potential.

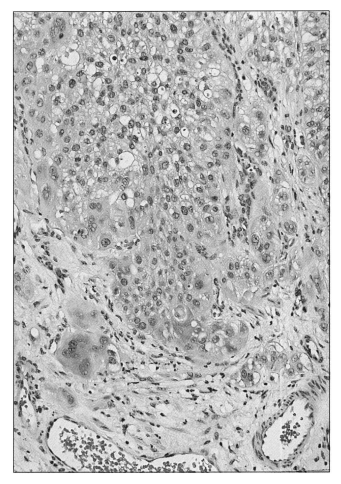

Figure 9.7 Lamina propria invasion in low-grade urothelial carcinoma.

Lipponen et al, 1993a; Lopez-Beltran et al, 1992, 1994; Pauwels et al, 1988).

To improve stratification of the large WHO/ISUP low-grade carcinoma group, some investigators subdivide these cases into two smaller groups (A and B) based on the degree of nuclear deviation and polarity of cells. In one study, low-grade A carcinoma (formerly WHO grade 2A) consisted of urothelial cancer with slight cellular deviation, some variation in nuclear size, and normal polarity of cells, whereas low-grade B carcinoma (formerly WHO grade 2B) had obvious variability in nuclear size and shape, with some loss of normal polarity (Pauwels et al,

1988). Using this modification, the authors identified tumor progression in 4% of low-grade A carcinomas (formerly WHO grade 2A) (pTA and pT1) and 33% of low-grade B carcinomas (formerly WHO grade 2B) (pTA and pT1) (Pauwels et al, 1988). This subdivision of WHO/ISUP low-grade carcinoma was also of prognostic significance for muscle-invasive cancer (Pauwels et al, 1988; Shapers et al, 1994).

Other investigators considered both nuclear pleomorphism and mitotic counts as criteria for subdividing WHO/ISUP low-grade carcinoma and were successful in identifying groups of cancers with different outcomes (Carbin et al,

(a)

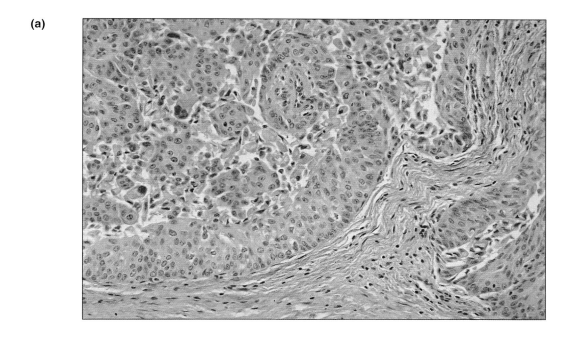

(b)

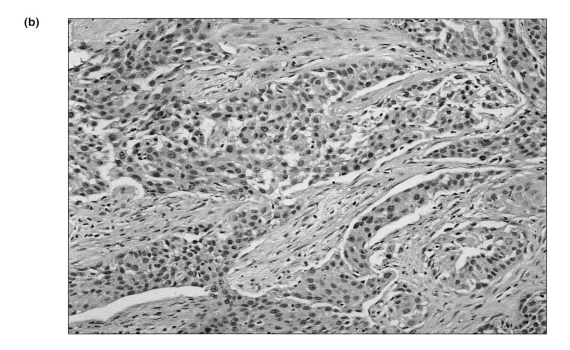

Figure 9.8 **(a):** High-grade papillary urothelial carcinoma; **(b):** desmoplastic response to tumor.

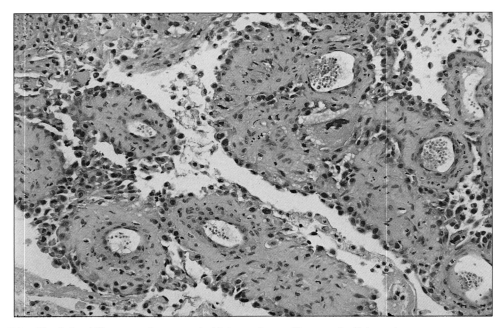

Figure 9.9   Hyalinized fibrovascular cores in high-grade papillary urothelial carcinoma.

1991). Low-grade A carcinoma (formerly WHO grade 2A) had a 5-year survival rate of 92%, similar to papillary neoplasm of low malignant potential, whereas low-grade B carcinoma (formerly WHO grade 2B) was comparable to WHO/ISUP high-grade carcinoma, with a 5-year survival rate of 43% (Jakse et al, 1987; Kakizoe et al, 1992; Takashi et al, 1991). This grading system is reproducible, with interobserver agreement of more than 90% (Carbin et al, 1991). The authors' final classification based on these data was to include papillary neoplasm of low malignant potential and low-grade A carcinoma (formerly WHO grade 2A) in one category (A), low-grade B carcinoma (formerly WHO grade 2B) and WHO/ISUP high-grade carcinoma together in a second category (B), and to introduce a third category (C), which included anaplastic carcinoma. Others found that mitotic index was the single most useful criterion for bladder cancer grading (Lipponen & Eskelinen, 1991; Lipponen et al, 1993a).

Recent efforts to grade urothelial carcinoma using image analysis based on nuclear morphometry, silver-staining nucleolar organizer regions, and other markers have also been successful but are not routinely used (Choi et al, 1994; Cohen et al, 1993; Helpap et al, 1994; Jarkrans et al, 1995; Kruger & Muller, 1995; Portillo et al, 1992a, 1992b; Tachibana et al, 1994; van Velthoven et al, 1995).

Urothelial carcinoma grade correlates with cancer stage, including the probability of muscle invasion and metastases as well as survival (Kaubisch et al, 1991; Thrasher et al, 1994; Torti et al, 1987). The actuarial 20-year survival rate for patients with papillary neoplasm of low malignant potential is more than 90%, and most patients have a normal life expectancy, regardless of the number of recurrences; only 4% of these patients die of cancer, and 3% of papillary neoplasm of low malignant potential progress to WHO/ISUP high-grade carcinoma (Jordan et al, 1987). The 20-year survival rate for treated WHO/ISUP low-grade carcinoma is more than 80%.

9.3.4 Staging

Pathologic staging of bladder cancer remains the single most important determinant of prognosis. The pathologist plays a central role in this determination and therefore must have an understanding of the staging systems and terminology (Table 9.4). Currently, the Marshall modification of the Jewett-Strong system and the American Joint Committee on Cancer/ Union International Contre le Cancer (AJCC-UICC) classifications are the two main systems in practice, and the pathology report should indicate the specific AJCC-UICC stage as far as possible in bladder biopsy or transurethral resection specimens (Witjes et al, 1994).

Pathologic staging of bladder cancer is critical in stratifying patients for therapy (Fig 9.10) (Gospodarowitz, 1994; Lopez-Beltran et al, 1992, 1994; Mazzucchelli et al, 1994). There is a sig-

Table 9.4 Pathologic staging of bladder carcinoma (TNM 1997)

Depth of invasion	AJCC/ UICC	Jewett/ Marshall
Noninvasive, papillary	Ta	0
Noninvasive, flat	TIS	0
Lamina propria	T1	A
Superficial muscularis propria	T2a	B1
Deep muscularis propria	T2b	B2
Perivesicle fat	T3	C
Adjacent structures	T4	D1
Lymph node metastases	N1–3*	D1
Distant metastases	M1	D2

*N1 = regional lymph node, <2 cm; N2 = regional lymph nodes, 2–5 cm; N3 = regional lymph nodes, >5 cm, or other lymph nodes.

nificant difference in outcome between urothelial carcinoma that does not penetrate beyond the basement membrane (pTa) and that which invades the lamina propria (pT1). Up to 46% of patients with pT1 cancers progress to muscle invasion (Angulo et al, 1995; Jewett,

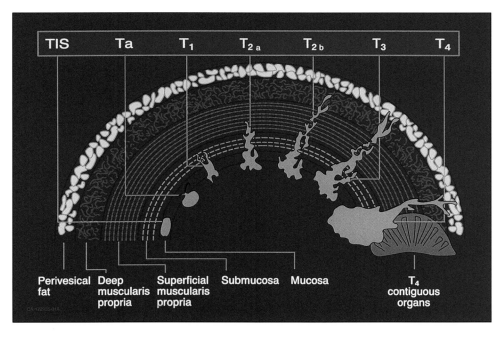

Figure 9.10 TNM staging of urothelial carcinoma of the urinary bladder.

1952). One of the most important tasks for staging in bladder biopsies and transurethral resections is determination of whether the muscularis propria has been invaded (Vicente-Rodriguez et al, 1994). It is important for the pathologist to avoid interpreting the muscularis mucosae bundles as muscularis propria (Angulo et al, 1995; Hasui et al, 1994) and interpreting fat cells in the lamina propria as extravesical tissue (Bochner et al, 1995).

Recent studies have emphasized the importance of the muscularis mucosa in substaging pT1 cancer. Younes et al (1991) subdivided the pT1 group into the following: T1a, invasion of connective tissue superficial to the muscularis mucosae; T1b, invasion to the level of the muscularis mucosae; and T1c, invasion through the level of the muscularis mucosae but superficial to the muscularis propria. These authors demonstrated that 75% of patients with T1a or T1b cancer survived at least 5 years, whereas only 11% of patients with T1c cancer survived. These results were confirmed by Hermann et al (1998). Conversely, other reports do not support the utility of the muscularis mucosa in substaging early invasive bladder cancer (Platz et al, 1996).

Cancer involves regional lymph nodes in 25% of cases in stages pT2 to pT4 and in rare pT1 cases. Implantation metastases after transurethral resection or biopsy and distant metastases in rare locations are more common in high-grade urothelial carcinoma (Andersen & Steven, 1995; Anderson et al, 1992; Arapontoni-Dadioti et al, 1995; Breul et al, 1992; Doval et al, 1994; Fabozzi et al, 1995; Fujita et al, 1994; Kakizaki et al, 1992; Pevarski et al, 1995; Stolla et al, 1994).

9.3.5 Prognosis of Urothelial Cancer

The prognosis for patients with invasive urothelial carcinoma is poor, with 5-year survival of <50% despite therapy (Lopez & Angulo, 1995).

Table 9.5 Factors predictive of recurrence and progression in urothelial carcinoma without muscle invasion

Number of tumors
Cancer size >5 cm diameter
Depth of invasion (lamina propria, muscularis mucosa)
Histologic grade
Coexistent dysplasia or carcinoma in situ
Recurrence at 3-month follow-up cystoscopy
Epidermal growth factor receptor expression
Loss of surface blood group antigens
Aneuploidy
p53 expression (probable, but still controversial)

Table 9.6 Factors predictive of survival in urothelial carcinoma with muscle invasion

Cancer size
Histologic grade
Depth of invasion
Pattern of invasion
Vascular/lymphatic invasion
Lymph node involvement
p53 expression (probable, but still controversial)

Numerous pathologic factors have been shown in select cohorts of patients with bladder cancer to correlate with recurrence, progression, and survival (Lapham et al, 1997) (Tables 9.5 and 9.6). The immune response to the tumor as measured by immunohistochemical staining for lymphocytes and antigen-presenting dendritic cells is useful in predicting recurrence (Lopez-Beltran et al, 1989). The number of papillary tumors also predicts recurrence but does not appear to be a significant determinant of invasive cancer. Patients with single foci of papillary cancer develop recurrence after transurethral resection in 45% of cases; however, patients who develop a second tumor have an 84% risk of developing a third tumor. Tumors larger than 5 cm in diameter also increase the risk of muscle invasion (Heney et al, 1983; Read-

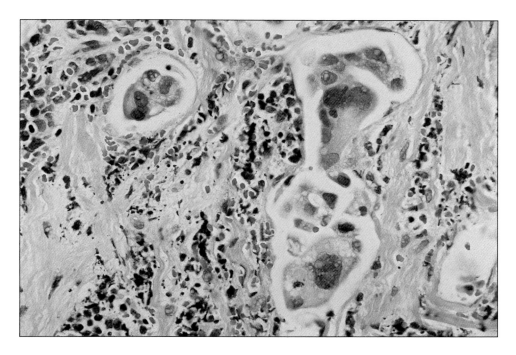

Figure 9.11 Vascular/lymphatic invasion by high-grade urothelial carcinoma.

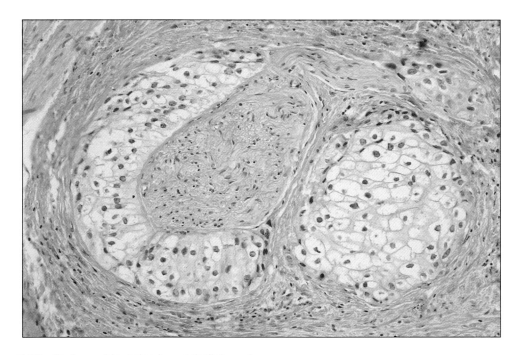

Figure 9.12 Perineural invasion by urothelial carcinoma.

(a)

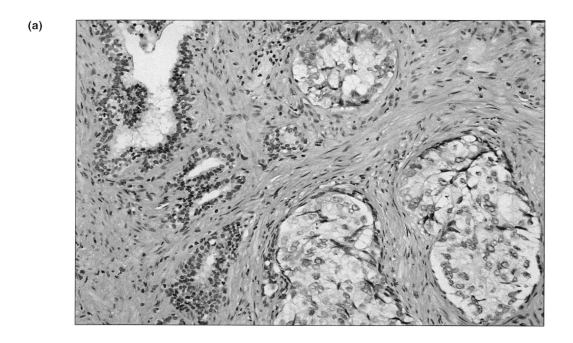

(b)

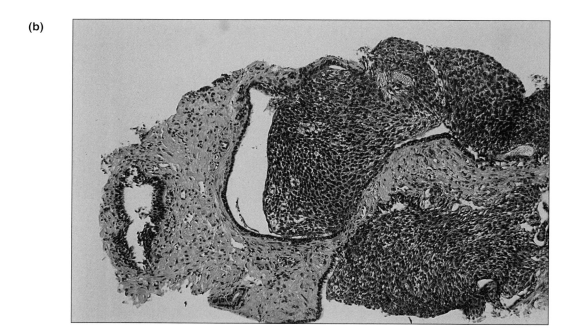

Figure 9.13 Prostatic duct involvement by contiguous spread of urothelial carcinoma of the bladder. **(a):** Low-grade urothelial carcinoma; **(b):** high-grade urothelial carcinoma.

144

ing et al, 1995). Tumor recurrence more than 4 years after resection of the primary tumor is an ominous sign (Holmäng et al, 1995; Morris et al, 1995). It is an important goal to exclude dysplasia or carcinoma in situ in the adjacent mucosa or elsewhere in the bladder, because the presence of one of these is a significant factor predictive of recurrence and invasion (Coloby et al, 1994; Kiemeney et al, 1994; Thrasher et al, 1994). Molecular biologic factors are discussed in Chapter 15.

9.3.5.1 Vascular/Lymphatic Invasion

The presence of vascular/lymphatic invasion is predictive of poor outcome, and this finding should be included in the pathology report, according to the Cancer Committee of the College of American Pathologists (Fig 9.11) (Hammond & Henson, 1996; Lopez & Angulo, 1995). Identification of vascular/lymphatic invasion may be difficult and can be confused with artifactual clefting around nests of invasive carcinoma, including perineural invasion (Fig 9.12) (Lopez & Angulo, 1995). The incidence of vascular/lymphatic invasion is variable, reportedly as high as 7% of cases. Immunohistochemical studies directed against endothelial cells that employ Ulex Europeus lectin, factor VIII, CD 31, or CD 34 may be of value in identifying vascular/lymphatic invasion, although less than 40% of cases with vascular/lymphatic invasion by routine examination can be confirmed immunohistochemically (Deen & Ball, 1994). Vascular invasion is an important predictor of patient outcome regardless of tumor grade (Jaeger et al, 1995; Lopez & Angulo, 1995).

9.3.5.2 Prostatic Involvement by Urothelial Cancer

Prostatic involvement by urothelial carcinoma is common (Fig 9.13) (Cheville et al, 1998; Esrig et al, 1996; Sakamoto et al, 1993; Solsona et al, 1995).

In patients with muscle-invasive bladder cancer, the prostate is involved in up to 50% of cases, and the frequency is even higher in those who have multifocal carcinoma in situ of the bladder. Prostatic involvement is classified into three groups (Hardeman & Soloway, 1988): (1) carcinoma confined to the prostatic urethral lining, (2) carcinoma extending into ducts and acini but confined by the basement membrane, and (3) cancer that invades the prostatic stroma. Metastases are most likely with prostatic stromal invasion (Solsona et al, 1995). The presence of prostatic urethral carcinoma in situ indicates a high risk for urethral recurrence after radical surgery (Sakamoto et al, 1993; Solsona et al, 1995; Tobisu et al, 1991). Prostatic stromal invasion is a strong predictor of poor patient survival (Cheville et al, 1998; Solsona et al, 1995), with 55% overall survival rate at 5 years (Esrig et al, 1996).

REFERENCES

Abou Farha KM, Janknegt RA, Kester AD, et al. Value of immunohistochemical laminin staining in transitional cell carcinoma of human bladder. *Urol Int.* 1993;50:133–140.

Amin MB, Ro JY, Lee KM, et al. Lymphoepithelioma-like carcinoma of the urinary bladder. *Am J Surg Pathol.* 1994;18:466–473.

Andersen JR, Steven K. Implantation metastases after laparoscopic biopsy of bladder cancer. *J Urol.* 1995;153:1047–1048.

Anderson RS, el-Mahdi AM, Kuban DA, et al. Brain metastases from transitional cell carcinoma of urinary bladder. *Urology.* 1992;39:17–20.

Angulo JC, Lopez JI, Grignon DJ, et al. Muscularis mucosa differentiates two populations with different prognosis in stage T1 bladder cancer. *Urology.* 1995;45:47–53.

Arapontoni-Dadioti P, Panayiotides J, Kalkandi P, et al. Metastases of malignant melanoma to transitional cell carcinoma of the urinary bladder. *Eur J Surg Oncol.* 1995;21:92–93.

Bergkvist A, Ljungquist A, Moberger G. Classification of bladder tumors based on cellular pattern. *Acta Chir Scand.* 1965;130:371–378.

Bostwick DG. Natural history of early bladder cancer. *J Cell Biochem.* 1992;16I(suppl):31–38.

Breul J, Block T, Breidenbach H, et al. Implantation metastases after a suprapubic catheter in a case of bladder cancer. *Eur Urol.* 1992;22:86–88.

Briggs NC, Young TB, Gilchrist KW, et al. Age as a predictor of an aggressive clinical course for superficial bladder cancer in men. *Cancer.* 1992;69:1445–1451.

Carbin BE, Ekman P, Gustafson H, et al. Grading of human urothelial carcinoma based on nuclear atypia and mitotic frequency, I: histological description. *J Urol.* 1991;145:968–971.

Chen SS, Chen KK, Lin ATL, et al. The significance of tumor grade in predicting disease progression in stage Ta transitional cell carcinoma of the urinary bladder. *Br J Urol.* 1996;78:209–212.

Cheville JC, Dundore PA, Bostwick DG, et al. Transitional cell carcinoma of the prostate: Clinicopathologic study of 50 cases. *Cancer.* 1998;82:703–707.

Choi HK, Vasko J, Bengtsson E, et al. Grading of transitional cell bladder carcinoma by texture analysis of histological sections. *Analyt Cell Pathol.* 1994;6:317–343.

Cohen MB, Waldman FM, Carroll PR, et al. Comparison of five histopathologic methods to assess cellular proliferation in transitional cell carcinoma of the urinary bladder. *Hum Pathol.* 1993;24:772–778.

Coloby PJ, Kakizoe T, Tobisu K, et al. Urethral involvement in female bladder cancer patients: Mapping of 47 consecutive cystourethrectomy specimens. *J Urol.* 1994;152:1438–1442.

Deen S, Ball RY. Basement membrane and extracellular interstitial matrix components in bladder neoplasia—evidence of angiogenesis. *Histopathology.* 1994;25:475–481.

Doval DC, Naresh KN, Sabitha KS, et al. Carcinoma of the urinary bladder metastic to the oral cavity. *Ind J Cancer.* 1994;31:8–11.

El Ouakdi M, Njeh M, Smaoui S, et al. T1 bladder tumors. Can they be considered superficial? *J Urol (Paris).* 1991;97:33–35.

Epstein JI, Amin MB, Reuter V, et al. WHO/ISUP consensus classification of urothelial (transitional cell) neoplasms of the urinary bladder. *Am J. Surg Pathol* 1998;22:1435-1448.

Esrig D, Elmajian D, Groshen S, et al. Accumulation of nuclear p53 and tumor progression in bladder cancer. *N Engl J Med.* 1994;331:1259–1264.

Esrig D, Freeman JA, Elmajian DA. Transitional cell carcinoma involving the prostate with a proposed staging classification for stromal invasion. *J Urol.* 1996;156:1071–1076.

Fabozzi SJ, Newton JR Jr, Moriarty RP, et al. Malignant pericardial effusion as initial solitary site of metastases from transitional cell carcinoma of the bladder. *Urology.* 1995;45:320–322.

Farrow GM, Utz DC. Observations on microinvasive transitional cell carcinoma of the urinary bladder. *Clin Oncol.* 1982;1:609–615.

Farrow GM, Utz DC, Rife CC. Morphological and clinical observations of patients with early bladder cancer treated with total cystectomy. *Cancer Res.* 1976;36:2495–2501.

Farrow GM, Utz DC, Rife CC, et al. Clinical observations on 69 cases of in situ carcinoma of the urinary bladder. *Cancer Res.* 1977;37:2794–2798.

Friedell GH, Hawkins I, Heney N, et al. Minimal papillary urinary bladder cancer. *Clin Oncol.* 1982;1:599–608.

Friedell GH, Soloway MS, Hilgar AG, et al. Summary of the workshop on carcinoma in situ of the bladder. *J Urol.* 1986;136:1047–1048.

Fujita K, Sakamoto Y, Fujime M, et al. Two cases of inflammatory skin metastases from transitional cell carcinoma of the urinary bladder. *Urol Int.* 1994;53:114–116.

Gospodarowitz MK. Staging of bladder cancer. *Sem Surg Oncol.* 1994;10:51–59.

Hammond EH, Henson DE. Practice protocol for the examination of specimens removed from patients with carcinoma of the urinary bladder, ureter, renal pelvis, and urethra. *Arch Pathol Lab Med.* 1996;120:1103–1110.

Hardeman SW, Soloway MS. Transitional cell carcinoma of the prostate: Diagnosis, staging, and management. *World J Urol.* 1998;6:170–174.

Hartveit F, Maehle BO, Thunold S. Koilocytosis in neoplasia of the urinary bladder. *Br J Urol.* 1992;69:46–48.

Hasui Y, Osada Y, Kitada S, et al. Significance of invasion to the muscularis mucosae on the progression of superficial bladder cancer. *Urology.* 1994;43:528–531.

Helpap B, Loesevitz L, Bulatko A. Nucleolar and argyrophilic nucleolar organizer region counts in urothelial carcinomas with special emphasis on grade II tumors. *Virchows Arch.* 1994;425:265–269.

Hemstreet GP III, Rollins S, Jones P, et al. Identification of a high risk subgroup of grade 1 transitional cell carcinoma using image analysis based deoxyribonucleic acid ploidy analysis of tumor tissue. *J Urol.* 1991;146:1525–1529.

Heney NM, Ahmed S, Flanagan MJ, et al. Superficial bladder cancer: progression and recurrence. *J Urol.* 1983;130:1083–1086.

146

Hermann GG, Horn T, Steven K. The influence of the level of lamina propria and the prevalence of P53 nuclear accumulation on survival in stage T1 transitional cell bladder cancer. *J Urol.* 1998;159:91–94.

Holmäng S, Hedelin H, Anderstrom C, et al. The relationship among multiple recurrences, progression and prognosis of patients with stages TA and T1 transitional cell cancer of the bladder followed for at least 20 years. *J Urol.* 1995;153:1823–1827.

Itoku KA, Stein BS. Superficial bladder cancer. *Hematol Oncol Clin North Am.* 1992;6:99–116.

Jaeger TM, Weidner N, Chew K, et al. Tumor angiogenesis correlates with lymph node metastases in invasive bladder cancer. *J Urol.* 1995;154:69–71.

Jakse G, Loidl W, Seeber G, et al. Stage T1, grade 3 transitional cell carcinoma of the bladder: an unfavorable tumor. *J Urol.* 1987;137:39–43.

Jarkrans T, Vasko J, Bentgsson E, et al. Grading of transitional cell bladder carcinoma by image analysis of histological sections. *Anal Cell Pathol.* 1995;8:135–158.

Jewett HJ. Carcinoma of the bladder: influence of depth of infiltration on the 5-year results following complete extirpation of the primary growth. *J Urol.* 1952;67:672.

Jordan AM, Weingarten J, Murphy WM. Transitional cell neoplasms of the urinary bladder: can biologic potential be predicted from histologic grading? *Cancer.* 1987;60:2766–2774.

Kakizaki H, Abe Y, Sugano O, et al. A hundred cases of multiple primary neoplasms in association with genitourinary cancer. *Jpn J Urol.* 1992;83:1841–1846.

Kakizoe T, Tobisu K, Mizunati T, et al. Analysis by step sectioning of early invasive bladder cancer with special reference to G3.pT1 disease. *Jpn J Cancer Res.* 1992;83:1354–1358.

Kaubisch S, Lum BL, Reese J, et al. Stage T1 bladder cancer: grade is the primary determinant for risk of muscle invasion. *J Urol.* 1991;146:28–31.

Kiemeney LA, Witjes JA, Heijbroek RP, et al. Predictability of recurrent and progressive disease in individual patients with primary superficial bladder cancer. *J Urol.* 1993;150:60–64.

Kiemeney LA, Witjes JA, Heijbroek RP, et al. Dysplasia in normal-looking urothelium increases the risk of tumor progression in primary superficial bladder cancer. *Eur J Cancer.* 1994;30A:1621–1625.

Koch M, Hill GB, McPhee MS. Factors affecting recurrence rates in superficial bladder cancer. *J Natl Cancer Inst.* 1986;76:1025–1029.

Koss LG. Tumors of the urinary bladder. In: *Atlas of Tumor Pathology* (2d ser, fascicle 11). Washington, DC: Armed Forces Institute of Pathology; 1975: 19–38.

Kruger S, Muller H. Correlation of morphometry, nucleolar organizer regions, proliferating cell nuclear antigen and Ki67 antigen expression with grading and staging in urinary bladder carcinomas. *Br J Urol.* 1995;75:480–484.

Lapham RL, Grignon D, Ro JY. Pathologic prognostic parameters in bladder urothelial biopsy, transurethral resection, and cystectomy specimens. *Sem Diagn Pathol.* 1997;14:109–122.

Lerman RI, Hutter RVP, Whitmore WF Jr. Papilloma of the urinary bladder. *Cancer.* 1970;25:333–342.

Lipponen PK, Eskelinen MJ. How to count mitosis in bladder cancer grading? *Anticancer Res.* 1991;11:825–829.

Lipponen PK, Eskelinen MJ, Jauhiainen K, et al. Tumor infiltrating lymphocytes as an independent prognostic factor in transitional cell bladder cancer. *Eur J Cancer.* 1992;29A:69–75.

Lipponen PK, Eskelinen MJ, Jauhiainen K, et al. Grading of superficial bladder cancer by quantitative mitotic frequency analysis. *J Urol.* 1993a;149:36–41.

Lipponen PK, Eskelinen MJ, Jauhiainen K, et al. Prognostic factors in nodular transitional cell bladder tumors. *Scan J Urol Nephrol.* 1993b;27:205–210.

Lopez JI, Angulo JC. The prognostic significance of vascular invasion in stage T1 bladder cancer. *Histopathology.* 1995;27:27–33.

Lopez-Beltran A, Garcia-Clavo J, Reymundo C, et al. Significance of intracytoplasmic lumina (Bull's eye) in urothelial carcinoma of the bladder. *Acta Urol Esp.* 19986;10:99–102.

Lopez-Beltran A, Morales C, Reymundo C, et al. T-zone histiocytes and recurrence of papillary urothelial bladder carcinoma. *Urol Int.* 1989;44: 205–209.

Lopez-Beltran A, Croghan GA, Croghan I, et al. Prognostic factors in survival of bladder cancer. *Cancer.* 1992;70:799–807.

Mazzucchelli L, Bacchi M, Studer UE, et al. Invasion depth is the most important prognostic factor for transitional cell carcinoma in a prospective trial of radical cystectomy and adjuvant chemotherapy. *Int J Cancer.* 1994;57:15–20.

Melamed MR. Papillary tumors of the bladder. *J Cell Bichem (Suppl).* 1992;161:44–47.

Montie JE. Follow up after cystectomy for carcinoma of the bladder. *Urol Clin N Am.* 1994;21:639–643.

Morris SB, Gordon EM, Shearer RJ, et al. Superficial bladder cancer: for how long should a tumor-free patient have check cystoscopies? *Br J Urol.* 1995;75:193–196.

Mostofi FK. A study of 2678 patients with initial carcinoma of the bladder, I: survival rates. *J Urol.* 1956;75:480.

Mostofi FK, Sorbin LH, Torloni H. Histological typing of urinary bladder tumours. In: *International Classification of Tumours* (19th ed). Geneva, Switzerland: WHO; 1973.

Mukamel E, Simon D, Edelman A, et al. Metachronous bladder tumors in patients with upper urinary tract transitional cell carcinoma. *J Surg Oncol.* 1994;57:187–190.

Njeh M, Kechaou M, Jeribi M, et al. Bladder tumors in patients under 40 years of age. *Ann Urol.* 1994;28:268–269.

Pauwels RPE, Schapers RFM, Smeets AWGB, et al. Grading in superficial bladder cancer, 1: morphological criteria. *Br J Urol.* 1988;61:129–134.

Pevarski DJ, Mergo PJ, Ros, PR. Peritoneal carcinomatosis due to transitional cell carcinoma of the bladder: CT findings in two patients. *Am J Roentgenology.* 1995;164:929–930.

Platz CE, Cohen MB, Jones MP, et al. Is microstaging of early invasive cancer of the urinary bladder possible or safe? *Mod Pathol.* 1996;9:1035–1039.

Portillo JA, Val-Bernal JF, Garijo MF, et al. The value of nuclear area as prognostic factor in T1 papillary transitional cell carcinoma of the bladder. *Br J Urol.* 1992a;70:622–627.

Portillo JA, Val-Bernal JF, Garijo MF, et al. Prognostic correlation of morphometric values with survival in invasive transitional cell carcinoma of the bladder. *Br J Urol.* 1992b;70:628–633.

Reading J, Hall RR, Parmar MKB. The application of a prognostic factor anaysis for Ta.T1 bladder cancer in routine urological practice. *Br J Urol.* 1995;75:604–607.

Sakamoto N, Tsuneyoshi M, Naito S, et al. An adequate sampling of the prostate to identify prostatic involvement by urothelial carcinoma in bladder cancer patients. *J Urol.* 1993;149:318–321.

Sanchez de la Muela P, Rosell D, Aguera L, et al. Multivariate analysis of progression in superficial bladder cancer. *Br J Urol.* 1993;71:284–289.

Shapers RF, Pauwels RP, Wijnen JT, et al. A simplified grading method of transitional cell carcinoma of the urinary bladder: Reproducibility, clinical significance and comparison with other prognostic parameters. *Br J Urol.* 1994;73:625–631.

Shokeir AA. Bladder cancer following ileal ureter. Case report. *Scand J Urol Nephrol.* 1995;29:113–115.

Solsona E, Iborra A, Ricos JV, et al. The prostate involvement as prognostic factor in patients with superficial bladder tumors. *J Urol.* 1995;154:1710–1713.

Soto EA, Friedell GH, Tiltman AJ. Bladder cancer as seen in giant histologic sections. *Cancer.* 1977;39: 447–455.

Stolla V, Rossi D, Bladou F, et al. Subcutaneous metastases after coelioscopic lymphadenectomy for vesical urothelial carcinoma. *Eur Urol.* 1994;26:342–343.

Tachibana M, Miyakawa A, Deguchi N, et al. A new scoring system based on the histological behavior and proliferative activity of tumor cells for grading the malignant potential of bladder cancers. *Int J Urol.* 1994;1:37–42.

Takashi M, Sakata T, Murase T, et al. Grade 3 bladder cancer with lamina propria invasion -pT1-: characteristics of tumor and clinical course. *Nagoya J Med Sci.* 1991;53:1–8.

Thrasher JB, Frazier HA, Robertson JE, et al. Clinical variables which serve as predictors of cancer-specific survival among patients treated with radical cystectomy for transitional cell carcinoma of the bladder and prostate. *Cancer.* 1994;73:1708–1715.

Tobisu K, Tanaka Y, Mizutani T, et al. Transitional cell carcinoma of the urethra in men following cystectomy for bladder cancer: Multivariate analysis for risk factors. *J Urol.* 1991;146:1551–1553.

Torti FM, Lum BL. Superficial bladder cancer: risk of recurrence and potential role for interferon therapy. *Cancer.* 1987;59:613–616.

Torti FM, Lum BL, Aston B, et al. Superficial bladder cancer: the primacy of grade in the development of invasive disease. *J Clin Oncol.* 1987;5:125–130.

van Velthoven R, Petein M, Oosterlinck WJ, et al. Image cytometry determination of ploidy level, proliferative activity, and nuclear size in a series of 314 transitional cell bladder carcinomas. *Hum Pathol.* 1995;26:3–11.

Vicente-Rodriguez J, Laguna-Pes P, Salvador Byarri J, et al. Endoscopic biopsy in the staging of infiltrating tumor of the bladder. *Arch Esp Urol.* 1994;43:782–786.

Witjes JA, Kiemeney LA, Schaafsma HE, et al. The influence of review pathology on study outcome of a randomized multicenter superficial bladder cancer trial. Members of the Dutch South East Cooperative Urological. *Br J Urol.* 1994;73:172–176.

Yang GCH, Campbell WG Jr. Morphogenesis of inclusion bodies of urothelial carcinoma: A case study. *Mod Pathol.* 1996;9:566–570.

Younes M, Sussman J, True LD. The usefulness of the level of the muscularis mucosae in the staging of invasive transitional cell carcinoma of the urinary bladder. *Cancer.* 1991;66:543–548.

10
VARIANTS OF UROTHELIAL CARCINOMA

Urothelial carcinoma may present with a remarkably wide diversity of histologic patterns, some of which mimic other malignancies (Table 10.1). These variants frequently coexist, and diligent search is often of value in identifying the typical pattern of cancer. Transition forms are sometimes present but may be absent because of sampling variation, particularly in small specimens. The clinical outcome of some of these variants differs from typical urothelial carcinoma, so recognition is important. Other carcinomas of the bladder, including adenocarcinoma and neuroendocrine carcinoma, are discussed in Chapter 11.

Table 10.1 Variants of urothelial carcinoma

Nested
Micropapillary
Microcystic
Lymphoepithelioma-like
Lymphoma-like or plasmacytoma-like
Inverted papilloma-like
Urothelial carcinoma with syncytiotrophoblastic giant cells
Giant cell
Clear cell (glycogen-rich)
Sarcomatoid
Mixed differentiation
Carcinoma with tumor-associated stromal reaction

10.1 NESTED VARIANT

This rare pattern of urothelial carcinoma was first described as a tumor with a "deceptively benign" appearance that closely resembles Brunn's nests infiltrating the lamina propria (Fig 10.1) (Murphy & Deana, 1992; Talbert & Young, 1987). Some nests have small tubular lumens. Nuclei generally show little or no atypia, but invariably the tumor contains foci of unequivocal cancer with cells exhibiting enlarged nucleoli and coarse nuclear chromatin. This feature is most apparent in the deeper aspects of the cancer. Useful features in recognizing this lesion as malignant are the tendency for increasing cellular anaplasia in the deeper aspects of the lesion, its infiltrative nature, and the frequent presence of muscle invasion (Drew et al, 1996; Paik & Park, 1996; Talbert & Young, 1989). We recently encountered a case arising in association with nephrogenic metaplasia; the initial superficial biopsy was benign, but subsequent excision by the doubtful surgeon revealed the nested variant of urothelial carcinoma immediately beneath, with invasion of the muscularis propria.

The differential diagnosis of the nested variant of urothelial carcinoma includes prominent Brunn's nests, cystitis cystica and glandularis,

(a)

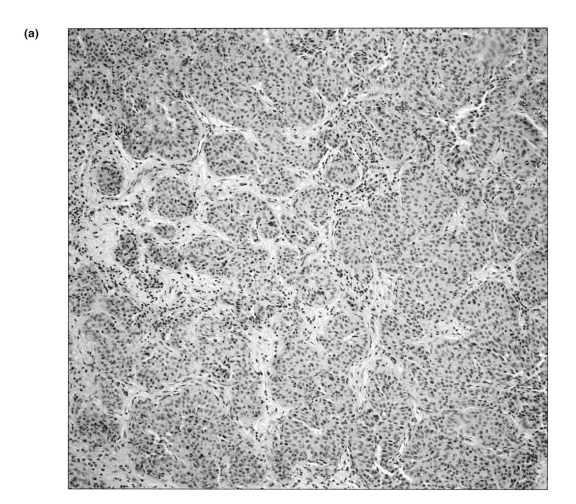

(b)

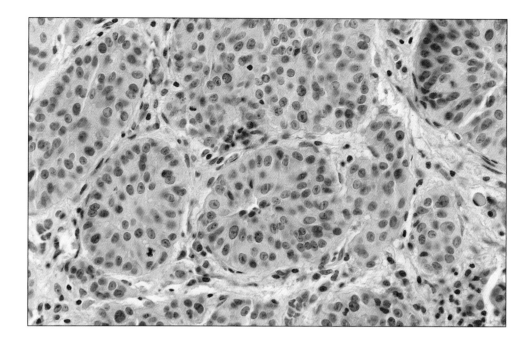

(c)

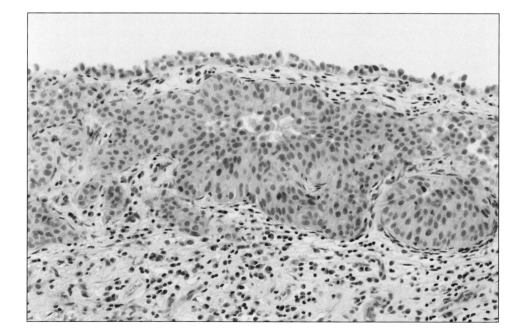

(d)

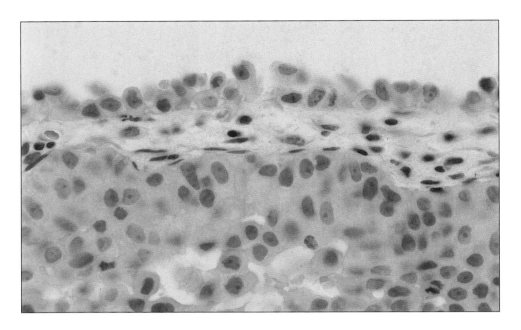

Figure 10.1 Nested variant of urothelial carcinoma. **(a):** The tumor is in contact with the overlying urothelium; **(b):** the deceptively benign appearance of cells in the superficial nests belies the malignant nature of this process; **(c, d):** Another case in which the biopsy reveals separation of the intact urothelium and cancer.

inverted papilloma, nephrogenic metaplasia, and paraganglionic tissue and paraganglioma. The presence of deep invasion is most useful in distinguishing carcinoma from benign proliferations, and nuclear atypia is also of value. Closely packed and irregularly distributed small tumor cell nests favor carcinoma. Inverted papilloma lacks a nested architecture; nephrogenic metaplasia typically has a mixed pattern, including tubular, papillary, and other components, and only rarely has deep muscle invasion in the urethra. The nested variant of carcinoma may mimic paraganglioma, but the prominent vascular network of paraganglioma, which surrounds individual nests, is not usually present in carcinoma.

10.2 MICROPAPILLARY CARCINOMA

The first description of micropapillary carcinoma consisted of 18 patients whose ages ranged from 47 to 81 years (mean: 67) with a male-to-female ratio of 5:1 (Amin et al, 1994a; Young & Zukerberg, 1991). Seven patients died of carcinoma. The micropapillary component is found in association with noninvasive papillary urothelial carcinoma, consisting of slender delicate filiform processes or small papillary clusters of tumor cells; when present in invasive carcinoma, it is composed of infiltrating tight clusters of micropapillary aggregates that are often within lacunae (Fig 10.2). Vascular and lymphatic invasion is common, and most cases show invasion of the muscularis propria or deeper, often with metastases. The presence of a surface micropapillary component in bladder biopsy specimens with cancer is an unfavorable prognostic feature, and deeper biopsies may be useful to determine the level of muscle invasion. The main differential consideration is serous micropapillary ovarian carcinoma in women or mesothelioma in both genders (Amin et al, 1994a).

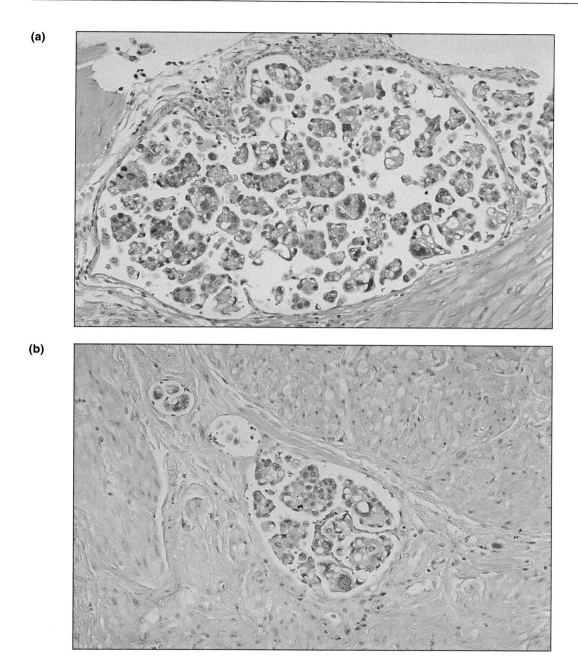

Figure 10.2 **(a):** Micropapillary variant of urothelial carcinoma; **(b):** the papillae are present within microvascular spaces in the deep muscularis propria.

153

10.3 MICROCYSTIC CARCINOMA

The microcystic variant of invasive low-grade or high-grade urothelial carcinoma is characterized by the formation of microcysts, macrocysts, or tubular structures (Fig 10.3) (Young & Zukerberg, 1991). The cysts and tubules may be empty or contain necrotic debris or mucin that stains with periodic acid-Schiff stain with diastase predigestion. This variant of cancer may be confused with benign proliferations such as florid polypoid cystitis cystica and glandularis and nephrogenic metaplasia. The presence of significant nuclear atypia at least focally and areas of typical invasive urothelial carcinoma allow accurate separation. Adenocarcinoma is the most difficult differential consideration, but the lining cells in microcystic urothelial carcinoma are urothelial.

10.4 LYMPHOEPITHELIOMA-LIKE CARCINOMA

Carcinoma that histologically resembles lymphoepithelioma of the nasopharynx has recently been described in the urinary bladder, with fewer than 30 cases reported (Fig 10.4) (Amin et al, 1994b; Homang et al, 1998; Young and Eble, 1993). Cases in the urinary bladder are more common in men than in women (10:3 ratio) and occur in late adulthood (range: 52–81 years; mean: 69 years) (Dinney et al, 1993). Most patients present with hematuria. The tumor is solitary and usually involves the dome, posterior wall, or trigone, often with a sessile growth pattern. Histologically, it may be pure or mixed with typical urothelial carcinoma, the latter being focal and inconspicuous in some instances. Glandular and squamous differentiation may be seen. The tumor is composed of nests, sheets, and cords of undifferentiated cells with large pleomorphic nuclei and prominent nucleoli. The cytoplasmic borders are poorly defined, imparting a syncytial appearance. The

background consists of a prominent lymphoid stroma that includes lymphocytes, plasma cells, histiocytes, and occasional neutrophils or eosinophils. It is rarely associated with dysplasia elsewhere in the bladder. Epstein-Barr virus infection has not been identified in lymphoepithelioma-like carcinoma of the bladder, although it is frequent in cases from the head and neck region (Gulley et al, 1995).

The major differential diagnostic considerations are poorly differentiated urothelial carcinoma with lymphoid stroma, poorly differentiated squamous cell carcinoma, and lymphoma. The presence of recognizable urothelial or squamous cell carcinoma does not exclude lymphoepithelioma-like carcinoma; rather, the diagnosis is based on finding areas typical of lymphoepithelioma reminiscent of that in the nasopharynx. Differentiation from lymphoma may be difficult, but the presence of a syncytial pattern of large malignant cells with a dense polymorphous lymphoid background is an important clue. Immunohistochemistry reveals cytokeratin immunoreactivity in the malignant cells, confirming their epithelial nature. It is possible to overlook the malignant cells in the background of inflamed bladder mucosa and misdiagnose the condition as florid chronic cystitis. The clinical significance of lymphoepithelioma-like carcinoma rests with the apparent chemosensitivity of this tumor.

10.5 LYMPHOMA-LIKE OR PLASMACYTOMA-LIKE CARCINOMA

Zukerberg et al (1991) described two cases of bladder carcinoma that diffusely permeated the bladder wall and were composed of cells with a monotonous appearance mimicking lymphoma. The tumor cells were medium-sized, with eosinophilic cytoplasm and eccentric nuclei producing a plasmacytoid appearance. Typical urothelial carcinoma was present in one case. The epithelial nature of the malignancy was con-

(a)

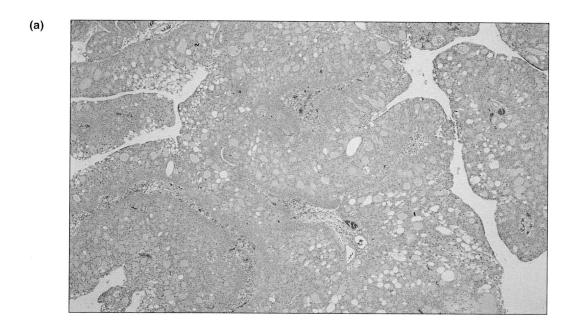

(b)

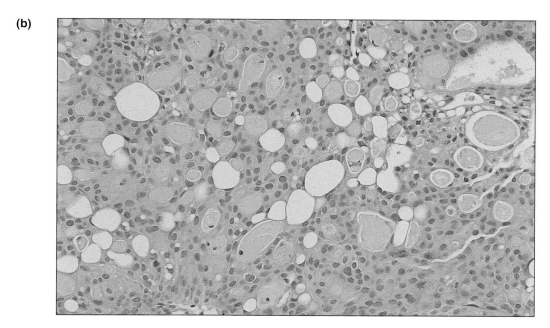

(c)

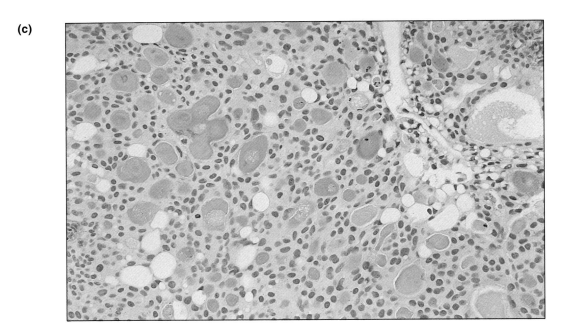

Figure 10.3 **(a, b):** Microcystic variant of urothelial carcinoma; **(c):** there are numerous psammoma bodies.

(a)

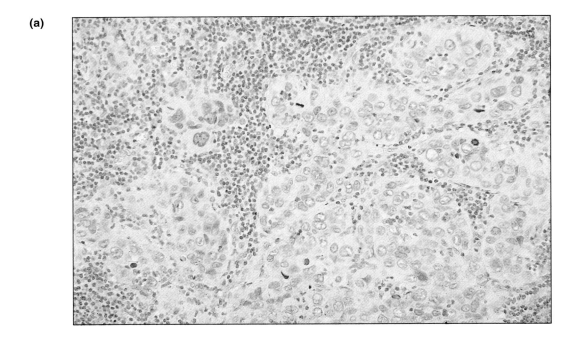

(b)

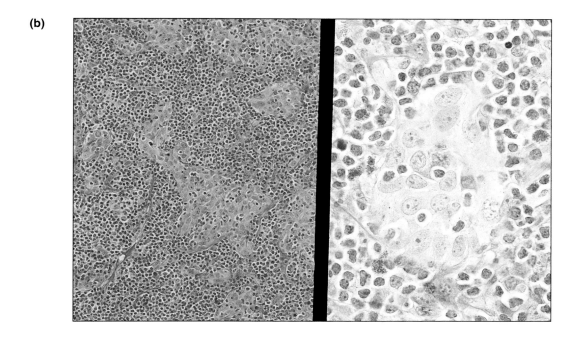

(c)

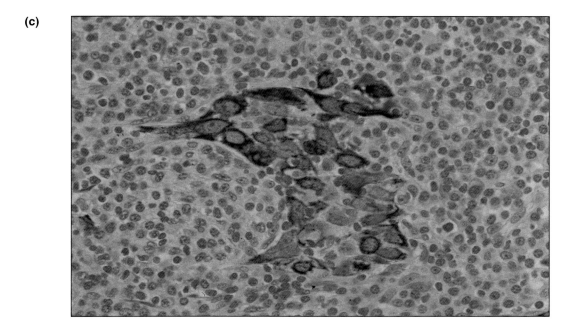

Figure 10.4 **(a, b):** Lymphoepithelioma-like variant of urothelial carcinoma. Discrete or irregular islands of malignant urothelial cells punctuate sheets of lymphocytes. **(c):** The epithelial component displays intense immunoreactivity for broad-spectrum keratin AE1/AE3.

firmed by immunoreactivity for cytokeratin and carcinoembryonic antigen and negative staining for lymphoid markers. A similar bladder tumor with prominent plasmacytoid pattern presented as a scalp metastasis mimicking multiple myeloma (Sahin et al, 1991).

Differential diagnostic considerations include lymphoma (plasmacytoid type) and multiple myeloma. Identification of an epithelial component confirms the diagnosis, but immunohistochemistry using CD45 (leucocyte common antigen) or keratins may be useful.

10.6 INVERTED PAPILLOMA-LIKE CARCINOMA

The potential for misinterpretation of urothelial carcinoma with endophytic growth as inverted papilloma is high (Amin et al, 1997; Cameron & Lupton, 1976; Talbert & Young, 1989). By definition, this variant of urothelial carcinoma has significant nuclear pleomorphism, mitotic figures, and architectural abnormalities consistent with low- or high-grade urothelial carcinoma (Fig 10.5). In most cases, the overlying epithelium has similar abnormalities and often contains typical urothelial carcinoma. We have seen rare cases of inverted papilloma-type carcinoma with minimal cytologic and architectural abnormalities that had high mitotic activity and have noted that distinction from the nested variant of urothelial carcinoma may be difficult or impossible in such instances, similar to the conclusions of Terai et al (1996). An exophytic papillary or invasive component is often associated with the inverted element. However, in cases of inverted papilloma fragmented during transurethral resection, a pseudoexophytic pattern may result. The stromal "cores" in this instance are wider and more variable than the fibrovascular cores of true papillary neoplasms. In some instances, both inverted papilloma and inverted papilloma-type carcinoma are intimately mixed (Goertchen et al, 1994). In rare cases of typical inverted papilloma associated with an exophytic papillary carcinoma, both diagnoses should be reported.

10.7 UROTHELIAL CARCINOMA WITH SYNCYTIOTROPHOBLASTIC GIANT CELLS

Giant cells are present in about 12% of cases of urothelial carcinoma, occasionally producing substantial amounts of immunoreactive β-human chorionic gonadotropin (HCG), indicative of syncytiotrophoblastic differentiation (Fig 10.6) (Campo et al, 1989; Fowler et al, 1992; Gramatico et al, 1993; Seidal et al, 1993; Shah et al, 1986; reviewed in Bastacky et al, 1997). The number of HCG-immunoreactive cells is inversely associated with cancer grade (Yamase et al, 1985). Secretion of HCG into the serum may be associated with a poor response to radiation therapy (Martin et al, 1989). The most important differential diagnostic consideration is choriocarcinoma; most but not all cases previously reported as primary choriocarcinoma of the bladder represent urothelial carcinoma with syncytiotrophoblasts (Cho et al, 1992) (see also Chapter 13).

10.8 GIANT CELL PATTERN OF CARCINOMA

Malignant giant cells in urothelial carcinoma, when present in great numbers, portend a poor prognosis, similar to giant cell carcinoma in the lung (Fig 10.6). The giant cells display cytokeratin and vimentin immunoreactivity. The differential diagnosis includes giant cells associated with HCG production, osteoclast-type giant cells in invasive high-grade urothelial carcinoma, and sarcomatoid carcinoma (Serio et al, 1995).

10.9 CLEAR CELL (GLYCOGEN-RICH) CARCINOMA

Up to two-thirds of cases of urothelial carcinoma have foci of clear cell change resulting

(a)

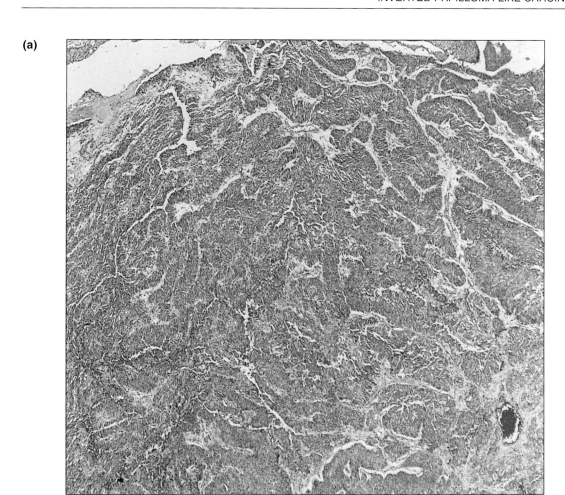

(b)

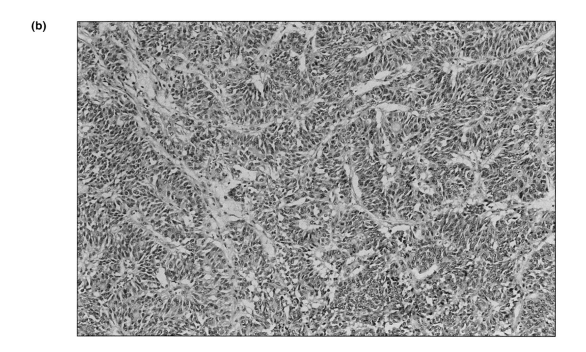

(c)

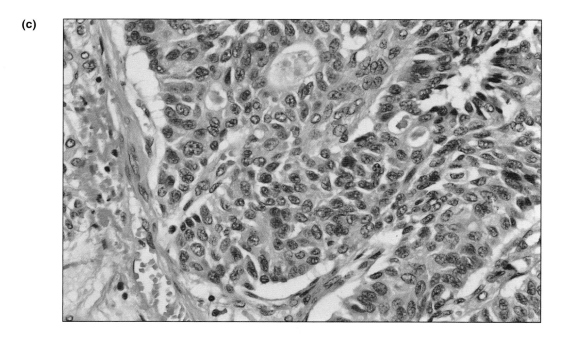

Figure 10.5 Inverted papilloma-like variant of urothelial carcinoma.

(a)

(b)

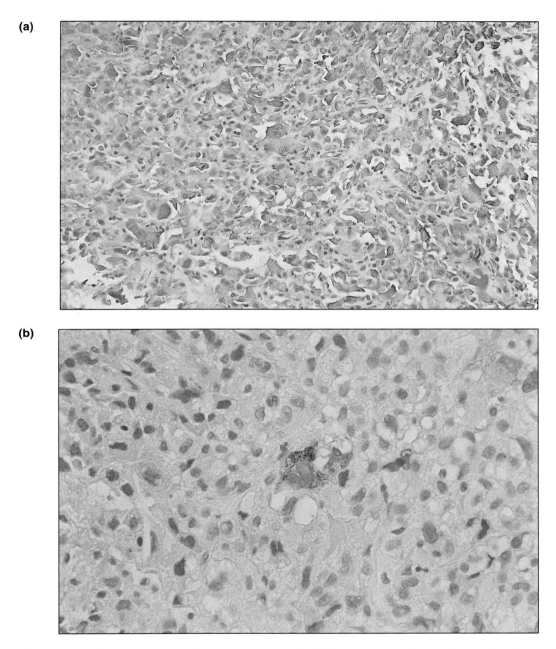

Figure 10.6 Numerous giant cells are present in this high-grade urothelial carcinoma. **(a):** Most cells are immunoreactive for keratin AE1/AE3; **(b):** scattered giant cells contained HCG.

from abundant glycogen. The glycogen-rich clear cell "variant" of urothelial carcinoma, recently described, appears to represent the extreme end of the morphologic spectrum, consisting predominantly or exclusively of cells with abundant clear cytoplasm (Fig 10.7) (Braslis et al, 1997; Kotliar et al, 1995; Young and Eble, 1991). Recognition of this pattern avoids confusion with clear cell adenocarcinoma. The amount of glycogen is directly related to cancer grade.

10.10 SARCOMATOID CARCINOMA (CARCINOSARCOMA; METAPLASTIC CARCINOMA; UROTHELIAL CARCINOMA WITH HETEROLOGOUS DIFFERENTIATION)

Rare cancers of the urinary bladder contain a mixture of malignant epithelial and spindle cell components (Figs 10.8 and 10.9) (Fossa, 1992; Lahoti et al, 1994; Lopez-Beltran et al, 1998;

Perrett et al, 1998). As with other organs, various terms have been used for these neoplasms, including *carcinosarcoma, sarcomatoid carcinoma, pseudosarcomatous transitional cell carcinoma, malignant mesodermal mixed tumor, spindle cell carcinoma, giant cell carcinoma,* and *malignant teratoma* (Jones & Young, 1994; Torenbeek et al, 1994). Some authors lump all of these tumors under the term "sarcomatoid carcinoma" or "carcinosarcoma" (Dundore et al, 1995). We prefer to limit the use of the term *sarcomatoid carcinoma* to those cases without heterologous elements in the spindle cell component and use *carcinosarcoma* for cases with heterologous elements in the spindle cell component (Lopez-Beltran et al, 1998; Sen et al, 1985). These two categories have similar clinical characteristics, including patient age, gender, presentation, and outcome.

Sarcomatoid carcinoma affects males more frequently than females (1.5:1), with a mean age of 66 years (range: 41–84 years). The most fre-

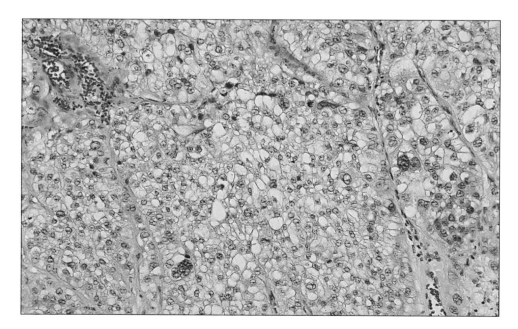

Figure 10.7 Clear cell variant of urothelial carcinoma. The cytoplasmic vacuoles contain abundant glycogen.

162

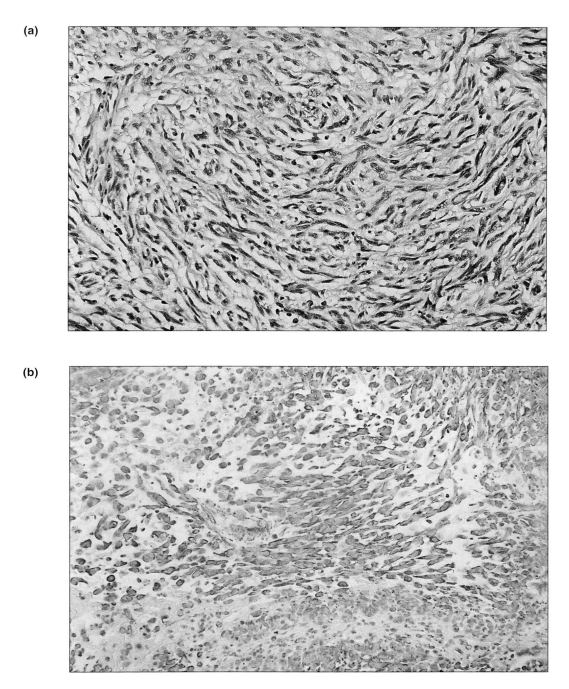

Figure 10.8   **(a):** Sarcomatoid variant of urothelial carcinoma; **(b):** these cells display keratin AE1/AE3 immunoreactivity.

163

(a)

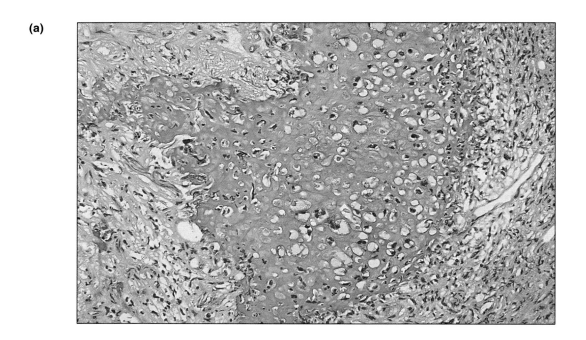

(b)

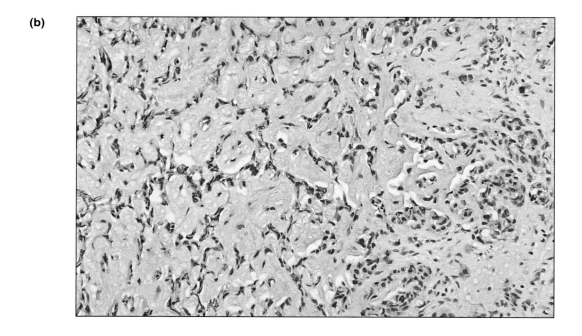

(c)

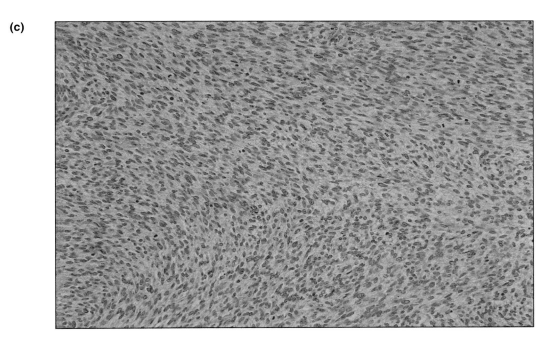

Figure 10.9 Sarcomatoid variant of urothelial carcinoma. Heterologous elements include osteosarcoma (**a**), myxoid sarcoma (**b**), and spindle cell malignancy suggestive of leiomyosarcoma (**c**).

quent presenting signs and symptoms are hematuria, dysuria, nocturia, acute urinary retention, and lower abdominal pain (Lopez-Beltran et al, 1998; Young et al, 1988). Macroscopically, sarcomatoid carcinoma is usually exophytic, nodular, polypoid, or pedunculated. Rarely, it appears as a sessile mass. In our study of more than two dozen cases, the tumors measured up to 11 cm in diameter (Lopez-Beltran et al, 1998).

Microscopically, sarcomatoid carcinoma contains a mixture of carcinoma and malignant spindle cells. The epithelial component is most often urothelial but may be squamous or rarely adenocarcinoma or small cell carcinoma. Carcinoma in situ is present in 30% of cases and occasionally is the only apparent epithelial component (Lopez-Beltran et al, 1997; Young et al,1988). In 15% of cases, immunohistochemistry is required to demonstrate the epithelial nature of the spindle cells. In most cases, the spindle cell component consists of solid sheets of cells in poorly formed fascicles, sometimes

with a myxoid stroma. Most commonly, the tumors are composed of a variable mixture of solid, myxoid, and sclerosing foci. The merging of the epithelial and spindle cell components is a useful diagnostic clue but is not a constant finding. In some cases, the epithelial element appears as discrete nests in a background of malignant spindle cells.

The spindle cells usually express cytokeratin at least focally, and we prefer keratin AE1/AE3 and CAM 5.2. However, the lack of keratin immunoreactivity should not be used to exclude the possibility of sarcomatoid carcinoma (Jones & Young, 1997). Epithelial membrane antigen is expressed less consistently. Intense coexpression of vimentin in the spindle cell component is commonly observed. Occasionally, the spindle cells express focal immunoreactivity for muscle-specific actin but are negative for desmin (Torenbeek et al, 1994). Ultrastructural studies may be useful in about 15% of cases that are negative for immunohistochemistry, particularly in those with only a spindle cell component (Torenbeek et al, 1994).

The major differential diagnostic consideration is urothelial carcinoma with pseudo-sarcomatous stroma (Bannach et al, 1993), a rare entity with reactive stroma that is cellular and displays cytologic atypia. The stroma may be myxoid with stellate or multinucleated cells or cellular and spindled with fascicle formation. Immunohistochemically, the stromal cells of pseudosarcomatous reaction show fibroblastic and myofibroblastic differentiation and invariably are cytokeratin negative (Bannach et al, 1993). In cases with exclusively spindle cells, the main differential diagnostic consideration is sarcoma, particularly leiomyosarcoma. The rarity of primary bladder sarcoma warrants that any malignant spindle cell tumor in the urinary bladder in an adult should be considered sarcomatoid carcinoma until proven otherwise. Extensive sectioning of the tumor and surrounding mucosa may reveal carcinoma in situ or focal invasive carcinoma.

Sarcomatoid carcinoma with prominent myxoid and sclerosing stroma may be mistaken for inflammatory pseudotumor, but this is an uncommon problem (Jones & Young, 1997). This cancer is typically rubbery or gelatinous and may have extensive myxoid areas. The spindle cells are invariably atypical, at least focally, with hyperchromatic pleomorphic nuclei, coarse chromatin, and enlarged nucleoli. Abnormal mitotic figures are frequent. Inflammatory pseudotumor is typically immunoreactive for vimentin and muscle-specific antigen and, occasionally, desmin. The spindle cells may display keratin immunorectivity in some cases, apparently as a result of shared epitopes by keratin and actin.

10.11 UROTHELIAL CARCINOMA WITH MIXED DIFFERENTIATION

About 20% of cases of urothelial carcinoma contain areas of glandular or squamous differentiation (Sakamoto et al, 1992; Vik et al, 1998).

These cases may have a less favorable response to therapy than pure urothelial carcinoma (Akdas & Turkeri, 1991; Ayala & Ro, 1989; Lopez-Beltran et al, 1988; Ro et al, 1992). Of 91 patients with metastatic carcinoma, cancer progressed despite intensive chemotherapy in 83% with mixed adenocarcinoma and 46% with mixed squamous cell carcinoma, whereas it progressed in <30% of patients with pure urothelial carcinoma (Ro et al, 1992). Low-grade urothelial carcinoma with focal squamous differentiation has a higher recurrence rate.

When small cell carcinoma is present in association with urothelial carcinoma, even focally, it portends a poor prognosis. The pathologist should carefully examine all sections of urothelial carcinoma to exclude this possibility, because small cell carcinoma is an important finding and usually dictates different therapy. Unlike other forms of mixed differentiation that are often considered histologic novelties, small cell carcinoma dominates and should be highlighted in the diagnosis because of its clinical importance.

10.12 TUMOR-ASSOCIATED STROMAL REACTIONS

Urothelial carcinoma may be associated with a variety of stromal reactions that mimic sarcoma.

10.12.1 Pseudosarcomatous Stromal Reaction

Urothelial carcinoma and other tumors may have a cellular pseudosarcomatous stroma, which rarely displays sufficient cellularity, cytologic atypia, and spindle cell proliferation to raise serious concern about sarcomatoid carcinoma (Figs 10.10 and 10.11) (Bannach et al, 1993; Mahadevia et al, 1989). The stroma is variable in appearance and may be myxoid or arranged in spindle cell fascicles, usually punctuated by stellate or multinucleated cells (Roth, 1980). The stromal cells reveal immunohistochemical evi-

(a)

(b)

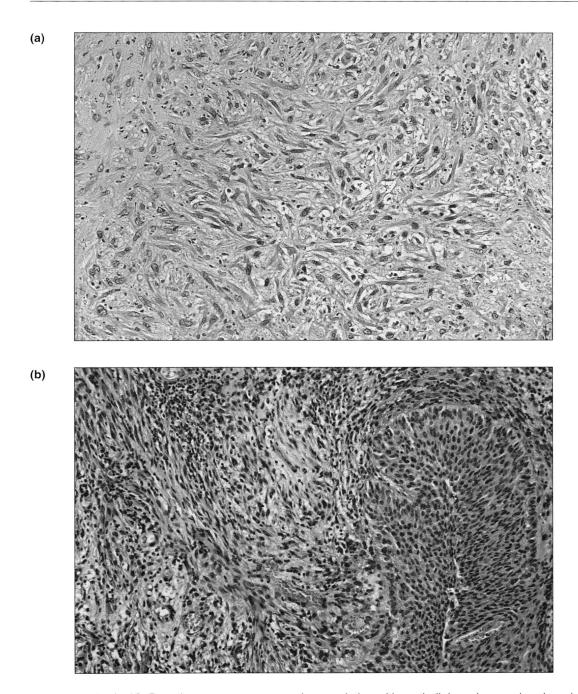

Figure 10.10   (a, b): Pseudosarcomatous stroma in association with urothelial carcinoma elsewhere in the bladder.

(a)

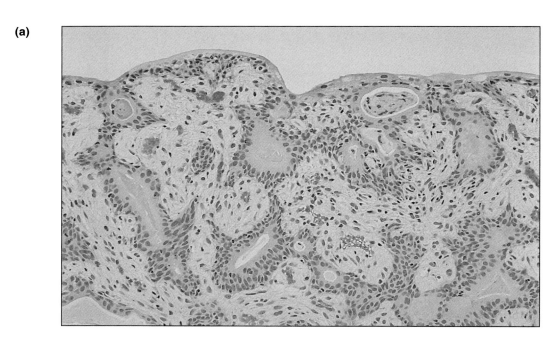

(b)

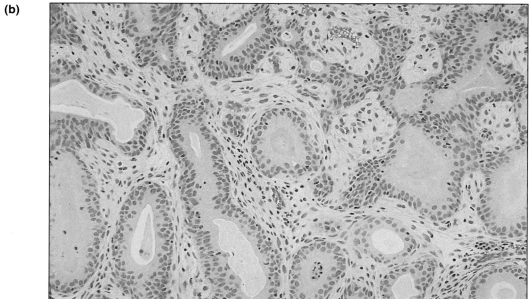

Figure 10.11 (a, b): Pseudosarcomatous stroma in a fibroepithelial polyp.

(a)

(b)

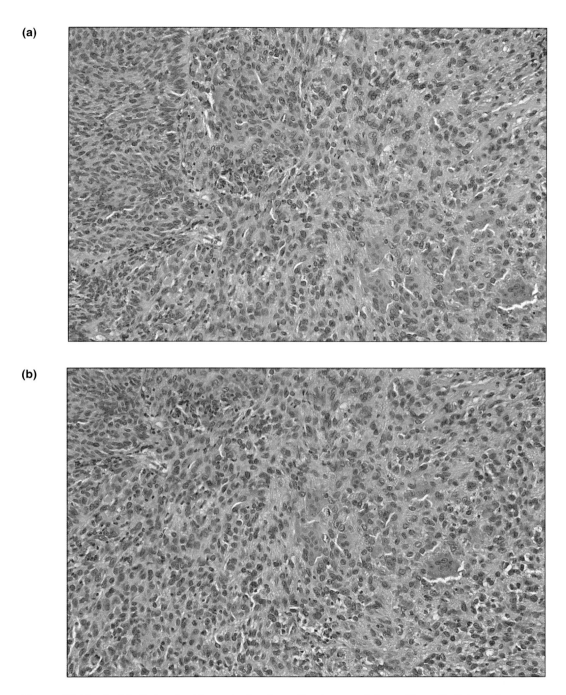

Figure 10.12   (a, b): Osteoclast-type giant cell reaction in association with urothelial carcinoma.

dence of fibroblastic and myofibroblastic differentiation and invariably are cytokeratin negative. Squamous cell carcinoma of the bladder may also have a pseudosarcomatous stroma (Kobayashi et al, 1994).

10.12.2 Tumor-Associated Osseous and Chondroid Metaplasia

Osseous metaplasia is present in some cases of urothelial carcinoma and its metastases (Eble & Young, 1991; Kinouchi et al, 1995; Lopez-Beltran et al, 1994), and this should be differentiated from osteosarcoma. This finding has also been described in metastatic urothelial carcinoma (Kinouchi et al, 1995). The metaplastic bone is histologically benign, with a normal lamellar pattern, and is usually adjacent to areas of hemorrhage (Lam, 1995). The cells in the adjacent stroma are cytologically benign (Eble & Young, 1991).

10.12.3 Osteoclast-Like Giant Cell Reaction

Zukerberg et al (1990) described the presence of osteoclast-like giant cells in two cases of invasive high-grade urothelial carcinoma, both of which had a sarcomatoid spindle cell component. The giant cells had abundant eosinophilic cytoplasm and numerous small, round, regular nuclei and displayed immunoreactivity for vimentin and tartrate-resistant acid phosphatase but not for epithelial markers (Fig 10.12). Similar tumors have been described as giant cell reparative granuloma and giant cell tumor. The giant cells probably reflect a stromal response to the tumor. The presence of osteoclast-like giant cells is not related to prognosis.

10.12.4 Tumor-Associated Inflammation and Eosinophilia

An inflammatory cell response in the stroma adjacent to the invasive tumors is relatively common. This response usually takes the form of a lymphocytic infiltrate with a variable ad-

mixture of plasma cells. Generally, this cellular reaction is mild to moderate, but occasionally it may be dense. Sometimes, a neutrophilic response is observed, with or without extensive eosinophilic infiltrate (Fenney et al, 1994; Flamm, 1992; Liponen et al, 1992; Sarma 1970), suggesting that, in the absence of a cellular response, the carcinoma is likely to be more aggressive in its behavior. The number of eosinophils may be a useful predictive factor for cancer-specific survival (Flamm, 1992).

Exclusion of lymphoepithelioma-like carcinoma of the urinary bladder is mandatory in cases with extensive inflammation in the stroma.

REFERENCES

Akdas A, Turkeri L. The impact of squamous metaplasia in transitional cell carcinoma of the bladder. *Int Urol Nephrol.* 1991;23:333–336.

Amin MB, Gomez JA, Young RH. Urothelial transitional cell carcinoma with endophytic growth patterns: a discussion of patterns of invasion and problems associated with assessment of invasion in 18 cases. *Am J Surg Pathol.* 1997;21:1057–1068.

Amin MB, Ro JY, El-Sharkawy T, et al. Micropapillary variant of transitional cell carcinoma of the urinary bladder. Histologic pattern resembling ovarian papillary serous carcinoma. *Am J Surg Pathol.* 1994a;18:1224–1232.

Amin MB, Ro JY, Lee KM, et al. Lymphoepithelioma-like carcinoma of the urinary bladder. *Am J Surg Pathol.* 1994b;18:466–473.

Ayala AG, Ro JY. Premalignant lesions of the urothelium and transitional cell tumors. In: Young RH, ed. *Pathology of the urinary bladder.* Philadelphia, PA: Churchill Livingstone; 1989.

Bannach B, Grignon DJ, Shum DT. Sarcomatoid transitional cell carcinoma vs pseudosarcomatous stromal reaction in bladder carcinoma: an immunohistochemical study. *J Urol Pathol.* 1993;1:105–113.

Bastacky S, Dhir R, Nangia AK, et al. Choriocarcinomatous differentiation in a high-grade urothelial carcinoma of the urinary bladder: case report and literature review. *J Urol Pathol.* 1997;6:223–234.

Braslis KG, Jones A, Murphy D. Clear-cell transitional cell carcinoma. *Aust N Z J Surg.* 1997;67:906–908.

Cameron KM, Lupton CH. Inverted papilloma of the lower urinary tract. *Br J Urol.* 1976;48:567–577.

Campo E, Algaba F, Palacin A. Placental proteins in high grade urothelial neoplasms: An immunohistochemical study of human chorionic gonadotropin, human placental lactogen, and pregnancy specific Beta-1-specific glycoprotein. *Cancer.* 1989;63:2497–2504.

Cho JH, Yu E, Kim KH, et al. Primary choriocarcinoma of the urinary bladder: a case report. *J Korean Med Sci.* 1992;7:369–372.

Dinney CP, Ro JY, Babaian RJ, et al. Lymphoepithelioma of the bladder: a clinicopathological study of 3 cases. *J Urol.* 1993;149:840–841.

Drew PA, Furman J, Civantos F, et al. The nested variant of transitional cell carcinoma: an aggressive neoplasm with innocuous histology. *Mod Pathol.* 1996;9:989–994.

Dundore PA, Cheville JC, Nascimento AG, et al. Carcinosarcoma of the prostate. Report of 21 cases. *Cancer.* 1995;76:1035–1042.

Eble JN, Young RH. Stromal osseous metaplasia in carcinoma of the bladder. *J Urol.* 1991;145:823–825.

Feeney D, Quesada ET, Sirbasku DM, et al. Transitional cell carcinoma in a tuberculous kidney: a case report and review of the literature. *J Urol.* 1994;151:989–991.

Flamm J. Tumor-associated tissue inflammatory reaction and eosinophilia in primary superficial bladder cancer. *Urology.* 1992;40:180–185.

Fossa S. Rare and unusual tumors of the genitourinary tract. *Curr Op Oncol.* 1992;4:463–468.

Fowler AL, Hall E, Rees G. Choriocarcinoma arising in transitional cell carcinoma of the bladder. *Br J Urol.* 1992;70:333–334.

Goertchen R, Seidenschnur A, Stosiek P. Clinical pathology of inverted papillomas of the urinary bladder. A complex morphologic and catamnestic study. *Pathologe.* 1994;15:279–285.

Gramatico D, Grignon DJ, Eberwein P, et al. Transitional cell carcinoma of the renal pelvis with choriocarcinomatous differentiation: immunohistochemical and immunoelectron microscopic assesment of human chorionic gonadotropin production by transitional cell carcinoma of the urinary bladder. *Cancer.* 1993;71:1835–1841.

Gulley ML, Amin MB, Nicholls JM, et al. Epstein-Barr virus is detected in undifferentiated nasopharyngeal carcinoma but not in lymphoepithelioma-like carcinoma of the urinary bladder. *Hum Pathol.* 1995;26:1207–1215.

Hölmang S, Borghede G, Johansson SL. Bladder carcinoma with lymphoeipthlioma-like differentiation: a report of cases. *J Urol.* 1998;159:779–182.

Jones EC, Young RH. Nonneoplastic and neoplastic spindle cell proliferations and mixed tumors of the urinary bladder. *J Urol Pathol.* 1994;2:105–134.

Jones EC, Young RH. Myxoid and sclerosing sarcomatoid transitional cell carcinoma of the urinary bladder: a clinicopathologic and immunohistochemical study of 25 cases. *Mod Pathol.* 1997;10:908–916.

Kinouchi T, Hanafusa T, Kuroda M, et al. Ossified cystic metastasis of bladder tumor to abdominal wound after partial cystectomy. *J Urol.* 1995;153:1049–1050.

Kobayashi M, Hashimoto S, Hara Y, et al. Squamous carcinoma with pseudosarcomatous stroma of the renal pelvis and ureter: a case report. *Acta Urol Jpn.* 1994;40:55–59.

Kotliar SN, Wood CG, Schaeffer AJ, Oyasu R. Transitional cell carcinoma exhibiting clear cell features. A differential diagnosis for clear cell adenocarcinoma of the urinary tract. *Arch Pathol Lab Med.* 1995;119:79–81.

Lahoti C, Schinella R, Rangwala AF, et al. Carcinosarcoma of urinary bladder: report of 5 cases with immunohistologic study. *Urology.* 1994;43:389–393.

Lam KY. Chondroid and osseous metaplasia in carcinoma of the bladder. *J Urol Pathol.* 1995;3:255–262.

Lipponen PK, Eskelinen MJ, Jauhiainon K, et al. Tumour infiltrating lymphocytes as an independent prognostic factor in transitional cell bladder cancer. *Eur J Cancer.* 1992;29A:69–75.

Lopez-Beltran A, Martin J, Garcia J, et al. Squamous and glandular differentiation in urothelial bladder carcinomas. Histopathology, histochemistry and immunohistochemical expression of carcinoembryonic antigen. *Histol Histopathol.* 1988;3:63–68.

Lopez-Beltran A, Nogales F, Donne CH, et al. Adenocarcinoma of the urachus showing extensive calcification and stromal osseous metaplasia. *Urol Int.* 1994;53:110–113.

Lopes-Beltran A, Pacelli A, Rothenberg HJ, et al. Carcinosarcoma and sarcomatoid carcinoma of the bladder: clinicopathological study of 41 cases. *J Urol.* 1998;159:1497–1503.

Mahadevia PS, Alexander JE, Rojas-Corona R, et al. Pseudosarcomatous stromal reaction in primary and metastatic urothelial carcinoma. A source of diagnostic difficulty. *Am J Surg Pathol.* 1989;13:782–790.

Martin JE, Jenkins BJ, Zuk RJ. Human chorionic gonadotropin expression and histological findings as predictor of response to radiotherapy in carcinoma of the bladder. *Virchows Arch A.* 1989; 414:273–277.

Murphy WM, Deana DG. The nested variant of transitional cell carcinoma: a neoplasm resembling proliferation of Brunn's nests. *Mod Pathol.* 1992;5:240–243.

Paik S-S, Park M-H. The nested variant of transitional cell carcinoma of the urinary bladder. *Br J Urol.* 1996;78:793–794.

Perrett L, Chaubert P, Hessler D, et al. Primary heterologous carcinosarcoma (metaplastic carcinoma) of the urinary bladder: a clinicopathologic immunohistochemical and ultrastructural analysis of eight cases and a review of the literature. *Cancer.* 1998;82:1535–1549.

Ro JY, Staerkel GA, Ayala AG. Cytologic and histologic features of superficial bladder cancer. *Urol Clin N Am.* 1992;19:435–453.

Roth JA. Reactive pseudosarcomatous response in urinary bladder. *Urology.* 1980;16:635.

Sahin AA, Myhre M, Ro JY. Plasmocytoid transitional cell carcinoma: report of a case with initial presentation mimicking multiple myeloma. *Acta Cytol.* 1991;35:277–280.

Sakamoto N, Tsuneyoshi M, Enjoji M. Urinary bladder carcinoma with a neoplastic squamous component: a mapping study of 31 cases. Histopathology 1992; 21: 135-41.

Sarma KP. The role of lymphoid reaction in bladder cancer. *J Urol.* 1970;104:843–849.

Seidal T, Breborowicz J, Malmstrom PU. Immunoreactivity to human chorionic gonadotropin in urothelial carcinoma: correlation with tumor grade, stage, and progression. *J Urol Pathol.* 1993; 1:397–410.

Sen SE, Malek RS, Farrow GM, et al. Sarcoma and carcinosarcoma of the urinary bladder in adults. *J Urol.* 1985;133:29–30.

Serio G, Zampatti C, Ceppi M. Spindle and giant cell carcinoma of the urinary bladder: a clinicopathological light microscopic and immunohistochemical study. *Br J Urol.* 1995;75:167–172.

Shah VM, Newman J, Crocker J, et al. Ectopic beta-human chorionic gonadotropin production by bladder urothelial neoplasia. *Arch Pathol Lab Med.* 1986;110:107–111.

Talbert ML, Young RH. Carcinomas of the urinary bladder with deceptively benign-appearing foci. A report of three cases. *Am J Surg Pathol.* 1989; 13:374–381.

Terai A, Tamaki M, Hayashida H, et al. Bluky transitional cell carcinoma of bladder with inverted proliferation. *Int J Urol.* 1996;3:316–319.

Torenbeek R, Blomjous CE, de Bruin PC, et al. Sarcomatoid carcinoma of the urinary bladder. Clinicopathologic analysis of 18 cases with immunohistochemical and electron microscopic findings. *Am J Surg Pathol.* 1994;18:241–249.

Yamase HT, Wurzel RS, Nieh PT, Gondos B. Immunohistochemical demonstration of human chorionic gonadotropin in tumors of the urinary bladder. *Ann Clin Lab Sci.* 1985;15:414–417.

Young RH, Eble JN. Unusual forms of carcinoma of the urinary bladder. *Hum Pathol.* 1991;22:948–965.

Young RH, Eble JN. Lymphoepithelioma-like carcinoma of the urinary bladder. *J Urol Pathol.* 1993;1:63–68.

Young RH, Wick MR, Mills SE. Sarcomatoid carcinoma of the urinary bladder. A clinicopathologic analysis of 12 cases and review of the literature. *Am Clin Pathol.* 1988;90:653–661.

Young RH, Zukerberg LR. Microcystic transitional cell carcinomas of the urinary bladder: a report of four cases. *Am J Clin Pathol.* 1991;96:635–639.

Zukerberg LR, Harris NL, Young RH. Carcinomas of the urinary bladder simulating malignant lymphoma. *Am J Surg Pathol.* 1991;15:569–576.

Zukerberg LR, Armin AR, Pisharodi L, et al. Transitional cell carcinoma of the urinary bladder with osteoclast-type giant cells: a report of two cases and review of the literature. *Histopathology.* 1990; 17:407–411.

11
OTHER CARCINOMAS

11.1 ADENOCARCINOMA

Primary adenocarcinoma of the bladder accounts for <1% of bladder cancers (Grignon et al, 1991a) and should be distinguished from adenocarcinoma arising in the urachus (Grignon et al, 1991a; Lopez-Beltran et al, 1994a). It occurs at any age but is most common after the fifth decade of life, with a male predominance (male-to-female ratio of 2.5:1). Patients present with hematuria, irritative voiding symptoms, and, rarely, mucousuria. The cancer is often advanced, with metastases in up to 40% of patients at the time of diagnosis (Grignon et al, 1991a). Intestinal metaplasia coexists in up to 67% of patients, and most cancers arising in association with exstrophy are adenocarcinomas (Bullock et al, 1987); nonetheless, the association of metaplasia and adenocarcinoma in the bladder has recently been challenged (Corica et al, 1997) (Chapter 6). Occasional cases of adenocarcinoma arise within a diverticulum (Lam et al, 1992). Other associations with adenocarcinoma include pelvic lipomatosis and *Schistosomiasis haematobium* infection.

Adenocarcinoma may appear as an exophytic, papillary, solid, sessile, ulcerating, or infiltrative mass. The signet-ring cell variant frequently shows diffuse thickening of the bladder wall, producing a linitis plastica-like appearance (Grignon et al, 1991a). Cold cup biopsies of the urothelial mucosa may be unrevealing.

There are seven main histologic patterns of adenocarcinoma of the bladder (Grignon et al, 1991a) (Table 11.1). This discussion excludes any case containing a dominant urothelial carcinoma component, and we prefer to classify such cases as mixed urothelial carcinoma with glandular differentiation; this distinction is probably semantic and academic.

Nonurachal adenocarcinoma, in contrast with urachal adenocarcinoma, is staged using the standard AJCC-TNM or Marshall modification of the Jewett staging system. As with other urinary bladder neoplasms, stage is considered the most significant predictive factor.

11.1.1 Adenocarcinoma Not Otherwise Specified

Adenocarcinoma not otherwise specified refers to a cancer that does not fit into one of the other categories. Remarkably, this and the colonic

Table 11.1 Histologic patterns of adenocarcinoma of the urinary bladder

Adenocarcinoma not otherwise specified
Colonic (enteric)
Mucinous (colloid)
Signet-ring cell
Clear cell
Hepatoid
Mixed

pattern are the most common forms of adenocarcinoma.

11.1.2 Colonic (Enteric or Intestinal-type) Pattern of Adenocarcinoma

The colonic pattern is composed of pseudostratified columnar cells forming glands, often with central necrosis, typical of colonic adenocarcinoma (Fig 11.1). Paneth cells and argentaffin cells may be present (Fish et al, 1994). The distinction from florid cystitis glandularis depends on architectural and cytologic differences, but these may be subtle.

11.1.3 Mucinous (Colloid) Adenocarcinoma

The mucinous (colloid) pattern consists of single tumor cells or nests floating in extracellular mucin (Fig 11.2). This pattern is unusual in isolation and usually coexists with the colonic pattern of adenocarcinoma. Florid cystitis glandularis with mucin extravasation has been previously mistaken for mucinous carcinoma according to a recent review by Young and Bostwick (1996). The complete absence of atypical cells within or at the periphery of the extravasated mucin strongly favors a benign diagnosis, although caution is urged in small or limited specimens (Jacobs et al, 1997). Endocervicosis is another benign mimic that rarely has mucin pools, sometimes eliciting an inflammatory response that is very uncommon in adenocarcinoma.

11.1.4 Signet-Ring Cell Adenocarcinoma

The signet-ring cell pattern of bladder adenocarcinoma consists of a diffuse infiltrate of distinctive cells involving the bladder wall (Fig 11.3). It is uncommon, with <100 reported cases (Muthuphei, 1994; Torenbeek et al, 1996; Yorukoglu et al, 1994) and accounts for 0.6% of primary bladder tumors in western Sweden (Holmäng et al, 1997). We concur with the requirement of Grignon and colleagues (1991b) that there be at least a focal component of diffuse linitis plastica-like growth and no element of urothelial carcinoma to qualify as a signet-ring cell pattern. Biopsies reveal diffuse permeation by solitary signet-ring cells or nests with single cytoplasmic vacuoles or foamy multivacuolated cytoplasm. In some cases, the cytoplasm is pale and eosinophilic, with the nucleus compressed at one end, a pattern referred to as "monocytoid."

Signet-ring cell adenocarcinoma has an extremely poor prognosis, with <13% 5-year survival compared with 33% in cancer with a mixed pattern (urothelial and signet-ring cells). Radiation therapy and systemic chemotherapy are ineffective in most cases (Holmäng et al, 1996).

11.1.5 Clear Cell Adenocarcinoma

The clear cell pattern is composed of papillary and tubular structures with cytologic features identical to mesonephric adenocarcinoma (Fig 11.4). It is very rare in the bladder (Young & Scully, 1985) and only slightly more common in the urethra (Meis et al, 1987). Macroscopically, clear cell adenocarcinoma is typically solid or papillary and located in the trigone or posterior wall. Microscopically, it invariably has a tubular component, often with cystic dilatation. The lining cells are flat, cuboidal, or columnar, and characteristic "hobnail" cells are at least focally present. There is typically significant

(a)

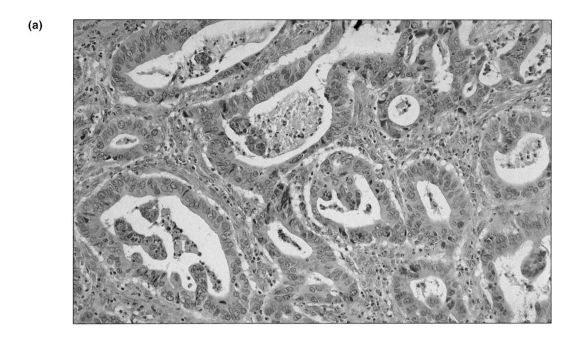

(b)

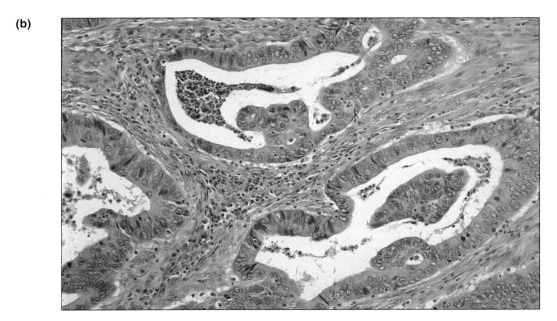

Figure 11.1   (a, b): Colonic pattern of adenocarcinoma arising in the bladder.

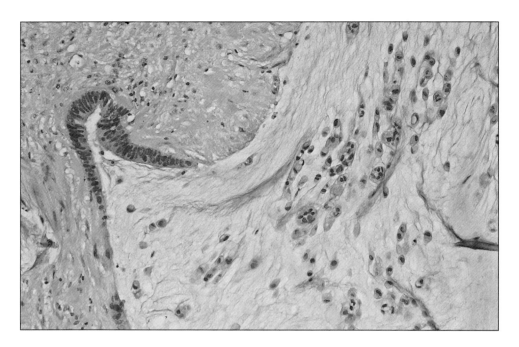

Figure 11.2   Mucin pool with malignant cells in the mucinous pattern of adenocarcinoma of the bladder.

nuclear pleomorphism with frequent mitotic figures. The cytoplasm is clear because of abundant glycogen and focal cytoplasmic and luminal mucin (Schultz et al, 1984).

The major differential diagnostic considerations are nephrogenic metaplasia (see Table 6.1) and metastatic clear cell carcinoma. Nephrogenic metaplasia is typically small, consisting of a papillary and tubular proliferation with minimal cytologic atypia; it may infiltrate the muscular wall, and the presence of this feature should not be used as a diagnostic criterion for malignancy. A clinical history of trauma or instrumentation may be helpful in identifying nephrogenic metaplasia. Metastatic clear cell carinoma should be excluded in female patients and requires clinical correlation. Renal cell carcinoma rarely metastasizes to the bladder and should be excluded; recognition of the typical sinusoidal vascular pattern, lack of tubular differentiation, absence of mucin, and clinical features should resolve this problem (Young & Scully, 1985).

11.1.6   Hepatoid Adenocarcinoma

Adenocarcinoma with a hepatoid pattern has been described in the stomach, ovary, pancreas, papilla of Vater, renal pelvis, and, recently, in the bladder (Sinard et al, 1994; Yamada et al, 1994). Strict morphologic criteria at all sites include formation of cords of polygonal cells separated by sinusoids or evidence of bile production and bile canaliculi formation. All reported cases are at least focally positive for alpha fetoprotein (AFP) and diffusely positive for α_1-antitrypsin and albumin; carcinoembryonic antigen is positive in about half of cases, sometimes in a canalicular pattern.

Hepatoid adenocarcinoma of the bladder was identified in an 89-year-old woman and consisted of urothelial carcinoma in situ, adenocarcinoma, and cancer with hepatocellular differentiation. These diverse findings were confirmed histologically, ultrastructurally, and immunohistochemically with AFP, resulting in a final diagno-

(a)

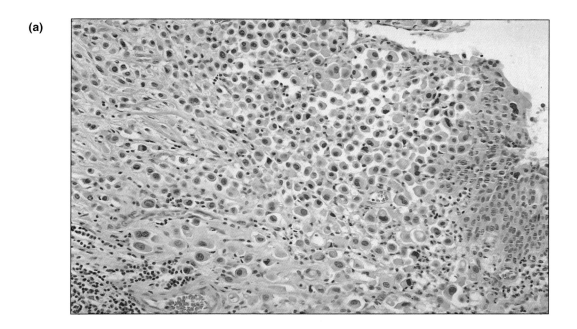

(b)

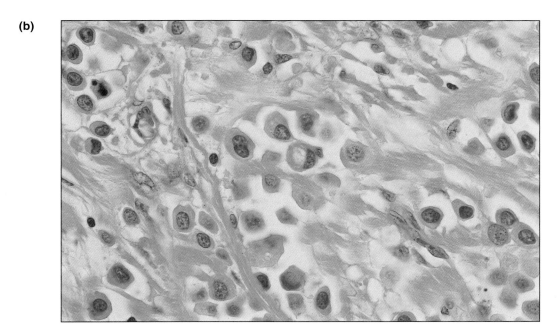

Figure 11.3 (a, b): Signet-ring cell pattern of adenocarcinoma of the urinary bladder with infiltration of the muscularis propria.

(a)

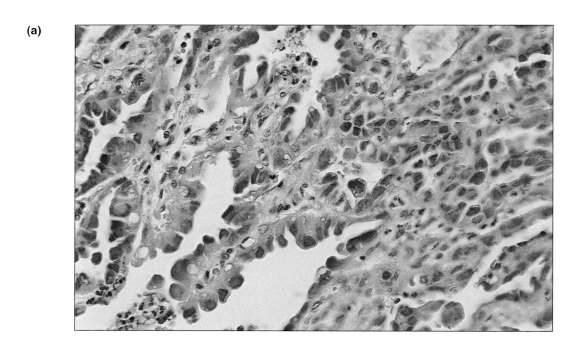

(b)

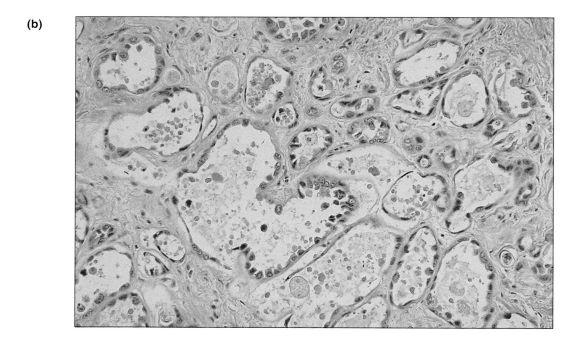

(c)

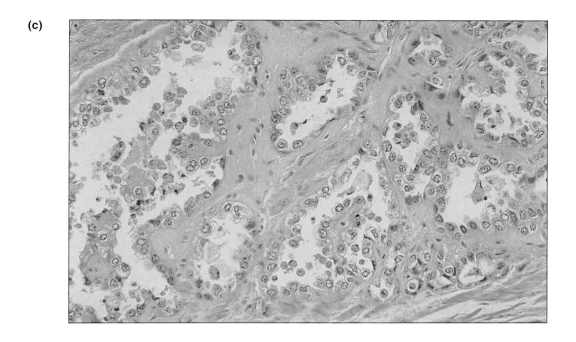

(d)

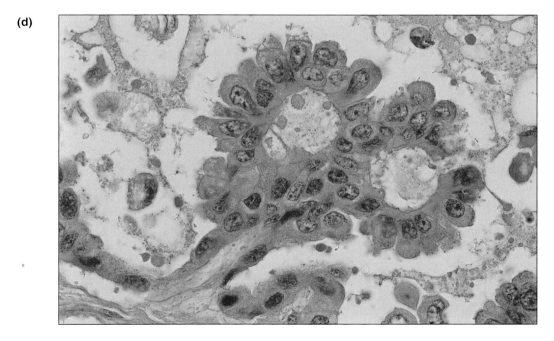

Figure 11.4   (a, b, c, d): Clear cell pattern of adenocarcinoma of the bladder.

sis of undifferentiated carcinoma with hepatoid features (Yamada et al, 1994). Another case was identified in a 68-year-old woman; the carcinoma was positive for AFP, carcinoembryonic antigen, and epithelial membrane antigen, and the cancer cells displayed focal intracytoplasmic hyaline globules and bile production. Tumor cells were large, polygonal, and poorly differentiated, arranged in solid sheets and focally formed glands. The cells showed prominent cytoplasmic clearing, although some had granular eosinophilic cytoplasm. Most contained a single large eosinophilic nucleolus. Cancer recurred at 3 years (Sinard et al, 1994).

Three cancers enter the differential diagnosis of hepatoid pattern of adenocarcinoma: adenocarcinoma with AFP production, germ cell tumor with hepatoid foci, and metastatic hepatocellular carcinoma. Adenocarcinoma with AFP production alone does not qualify as a hepatoid pattern if it fails to fulfill the strict criteria noted above. Such cases, including an AFP-producing nonhepatoid urachal adenocarcinoma, usually stain weakly for AFP; alpha-1-antitrypsin staining is diffuse or absent, and carcinoembryonic antigen immunoreactivity is not canalicular but membranous (Lertprasertsuke & Tsutsumi, 1991). Hepatoid foci were first described in yolk sac tumor of the testis and sex cord-stromal tumor of the ovary, but, to our knowledge, this has not been described in association with a bladder tumor. Metastases to the bladder are almost always associated with widespread disseminated cancer and can usually be excluded by clinical investigation.

11.1.7 Mixed Pattern of Adenocarcinoma

The mixed pattern refers to an adenocarcinoma composed of two or more patterns.

11.1.8 Differential Diagnosis of Adenocarcinoma

The differential diagnosis of bladder adenocarcinoma is extensive. Benign mimics must be excluded, including florid cystitis cystica and cystitis glandularis with mucin extravasation (Young & Bostwick, 1996). These lesions may produce pseudopapillary or polypoid lesions, but the benign cytology of the lining cells and lack of invasion are important distinguishing features. In unusual cases, extracellular mucin is present, and careful evaluation for malignant cells is necessary. Also, it is important to know the location in the bladder of the worrisome tissue, recognizing that cystitis glandularis of the intestinal type usually arises in the bladder neck or trigone. Villous adenoma rarely occurs in the urinary bladder and shows cytologic and architectural abnormalities of adenomatous epithelium without stromal invasion. Nephrogenic metaplasia must be distinguished from adenocarcinoma, particularly the clear cell pattern, which may be difficult in small or distorted superficial biopsies. Endocervicosis is a difficult problem in small biopsy samples but lacks the cytologic atypia of adenocarcinoma.

11.2 NEUROENDOCRINE CARCINOMA (CARCINOID AND SMALL CELL CARCINOMA)

11.2.1 Carcinoid (Low-Grade Neuroendocrine Carcinoma)

Rarely, carcinoid tumor without an associated urothelial carcinoma may involve the bladder (Chin et al, 1992; Walker et al, 1992). An organoid growth pattern is invariably present, and tumor cells have abundant cytoplasm that is immunoreactive for neuron-specific enolase, chromogranin, and synaptophysin. Cytokeratin is demonstrable in most cases, often with a "dot-like" pattern of expression (Lertprasertsuke & Tsutsumi, 1991). Ultrastructural studies reveal typical neurosecretory granules. One case was associated with a typical inverted papilloma (Stanfield et al, 1994). Metastatic carcinoid should be ruled out before diagnosing a case as primary in the bladder.

11.2.2   Small Cell Carcinoma (High-Grade Neuroendocrine Carcinoma)

Small cell carcinoma represents about 0.5% of bladder malignancies (Abbas et al, 1995; Ali et al, 1997; Holmäng et al, 1995). It develops much more frequently in men than women (ratio: 4:1), and the patient age ranges from 20 to 85 years (mean: 66 years). Hematuria, dysuria, and symptoms of bladder irritability are common (Abbas et al, 1995; Holmäng et al, 1995). Patients often present with locally advanced or metastatic cancer. Paraneoplastic syndromes rarely occur, including ectopic adrenocorticotropic hormone production, hypercalcemia, and hypophosphatemia.

There are no specific gross features that separate small cell carcinoma from other carcinomas of the bladder. Tumors range in size from 2 cm to 10 cm in diameter and may be polypoid or solid. They can develop at any location, including the dome and within diverticula (Lopez et al, 1994).

Small cell carcinoma of the bladder is histologically identical to its counterpart in the lung and other sites (Figs 11.5–11.7). It may consist of either the oat cell or intermediate cell pattern, and these patterns may coexist. The oat cell type consists of a relatively uniform population of cells with scant cytoplasm, hyperchromatic nuclei with dispersed chromatin, and absent or inconspicuous nucleoli. The intermediate cell type has more abundant cytoplasm, larger nuclei with less hyperchromasia, and a similar chromatin pattern and nucleolar features. In some cases, the intermediate pattern of small cell carcinoma consists of elongate or spindle cells. Both types have extensive necrosis, prominent nuclear molding, frequent mitotic figures, and may have DNA encrustation of blood vessel walls. A single case with large cell neuroendocrine carcinoma pattern has been

described, and the presence of scattered cells with "monstrous nuclei" has been reported (Grignon et al, 1991c). Some cases are mixed with other histologic patterns, but the small cell pattern is clinically dominant, invariably indicating rapid growth and poor prognosis. Urothelial carcinoma (papillary or nonpapillary) is most common, but glandular, squamous, and spindle cell differentiation have also been observed (Abbas et al, 1995). The adjacent urothelium frequently has dysplasia or urothelial carcinoma in situ.

The immunohistochemical findings in small cell carcinoma of the urinary bladder are presented in Table 11.2 (Abbas et al, 1995) and are largely typical of counterparts at other sites.

Primary peripheral neuroectodermal tumor of the urinary bladder is exceedingly rare (Hurwitz et al, 1980). One case occurred in a patient after renal transplantation (Banerjee et al, 1997).

11.3   SQUAMOUS CELL CARCINOMA

The prevalence of squamous cell carcinoma of the bladder is widely variable around the world and is highest in areas that are endemic for schistosomiasis, accounting for up to 73% of bladder cancers in those countries (Horner et al, 1991). In nonendemic areas, such as the United States and Europe, squamous cell carcinoma comprises 1%–7% of bladder cancers. Patients range in age from 30 to 90 years (mean: 65.5 years), although it occurs at a younger age when associated with schistosomiasis. Squamous cell carcinoma is more common in men than women (ratio: 2:1).

Patients typically present with hematuria and lower urinary tract irritative symptoms, and the majority have advanced cancer at the time of diagnosis (Shaaban et al, 1997). Often, there is a long history of bladder irritation caused by infections, calculi, indwelling catheters, intermittent self-catheterization, or urinary retention. One case arose 17 months after

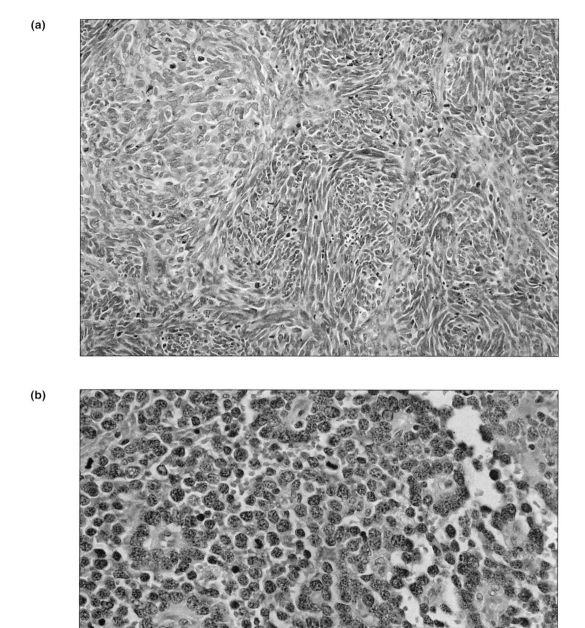

Figure 11.5   (a, b): Small cell carcinoma with spindle cells and rosette-like formations.

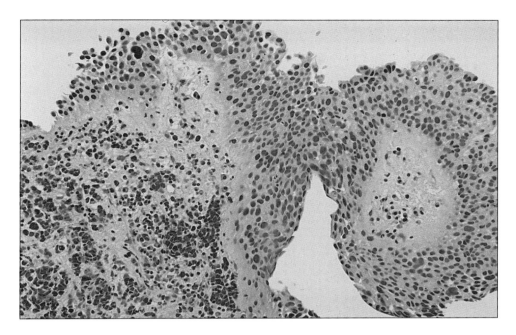

Figure 11.6 Small cell carcinoma (bottom left) and urothelial carcinoma in situ.

treatment of urothelial carcinoma in situ with bacillus Calmette-Guérin. Some patients have an underlying neurogenic bladder or a bladder diverticulum (Bickel et al, 1991; Kaye et al, 1992). Keratinizing squamous metaplasia may be an important risk factor for the development of squamous cell carcinoma, with cancer occurring from 3 months to 30 years after the diagnosis of metaplasia (mean: 12 years) (Benson et al, 1984). Squamous metaplasia is present in the adjacent epithelium in 17% to 60% of cases not associated with schistosomiasis (Benson et al, 1984). Rarely, squamous cell carcinoma induces hypercalcemia (Yoshida et al, 1994).

Macroscopically, squamous cell carcinoma is usually bulky, polypoid, solid, and necrotic, often filling the bladder lumen, although it may be flat, irregular, ulcerated, and infiltrating. Necrotic material and keratin debris are usually present on the surface. There is an apparent propensity for the lateral wall and trigone. The tumor may be well differentiated, consisting of circumscribed islands of squamous cells with extensive keratinization, prominent intercellular bridges, and minimal nuclear pleomorphism, while poorly differentiated cancer displays marked nuclear pleomorphism and focal evidence of squamous differentiation (Fig 11.8). Verrucous carcinoma is a rare and unique variant (see below).

Grading is similar to that at other sites and is based on the extent of keratinization and degree of nuclear pleomorphism (Sharfi et al, 1992). Grade correlates with stage and patient outcome, although results have not been consistent.

The diagnosis of squamous cell carcinoma of the bladder is usually not difficult. The major differential diagnostic consideraton of squamous cell carcinoma is urothelial carcinoma with extensive squamous differentiation. In areas not endemic for schistosomiasis, such tumors should be carefully studied for a urothelial component, including urothelial carcinoma in situ (Sharfi et al, 1992); if found, the tumor is best classified as a urothelial carcinoma with

(a)

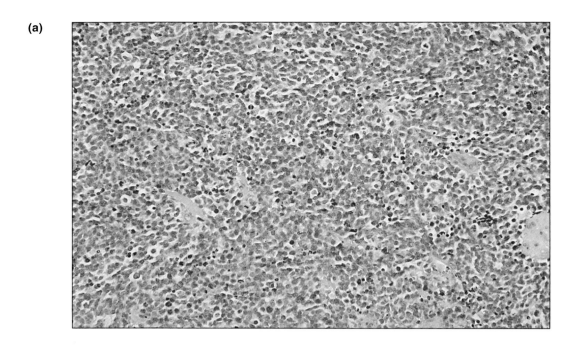

(b)

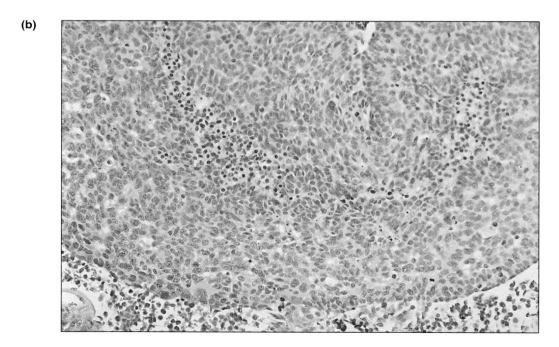

Figure 11.7 Small cell carcinoma of the urinary bladder. **(a):** Solid pattern; **(b):** solid pattern with rosette-like formations.

Table 11.2 Immunohistochemistry of small cell carcinoma of the urinary bladder (Abbas et al, 1995)

Antibody	Cases Staining (%)
Neuron-specific enolase (NSE)	90
Neurofilament	84
Human milk fat globulin	67
Epithelial membrane antigen (EMA)	63
Keratin AE1/AE3; CAM 5.2	61
Carcinoembryonic antigen (CEA)	50
Synaptophysin	46
CD 15 (Leu -M1)	43
Chromogranin	41
Serotonin	38
CD 57 (Leu-7)	35
S-100 protein	34
Vasoactive intestinal peptide (VIP)	17
Vimentin	17
Adrenocorticotropin hormone (ACTH)	9

squamous differentiation. The presence of keratinizing squamous metaplasia, especially if associated with dysplasia, favors the diagnosis of squamous cell carcinoma. Secondary invasion of the bladder by squamous cell carcinoma of the cervix or other contiguous primary sites should be excluded (Sharfi et al, 1992). Condyloma acuminatum is also a consideration but is usually easily distinguished by prominent koilocytotic changes. Squamous papilloma of the bladder is extremely rare.

The most important prognostic indicator for squamous cell carcinoma is stage. The biological behavior of squamous cell carcinoma is different from that of urothelial carcinoma. In most patients, death results from local recurrence rather than metastatic cancer, and metastases show a striking predilection for bone (Horner et al, 1991). Five-year survival after surgery varies from 35% to 48% (Richie et al, 1976; Utz et al, 1973).

11.3.1 Verrucous Carcinoma

Verrucous carcinoma is a rare, low-grade, clinically indolent form of squamous cell carcinoma

that is usually reported in association with *Schistosomiasis* infection. It is composed of well differentiated squamous mucosa with complex papillary and exophytic growth and invasive bulbous broad rete ridges (Fig 11.9). It may co-exist with squamous metaplasia and typical poorly differentiated squamous cell carcinoma (Oida et al, 1997). Sebaceous differentiation has recently been described in an unusual case, appearing as collections of CEA-immunoreactive clear cells with peculiar glandular spaces at the base (Michal et al, 1997).

Local recurrence is frequent, but this cancer does not metastasize early (if ever) to regional lymph nodes. Verrucous carcinoma often undergoes transformation to aggressive anaplastic carcinoma after radiation therapy, so this treatment should be avoided. Condyloma acuminatum is the most common and important differential diagnostic consideration.

11.4 CARCINOMA OF THE URACHUS

Malignancy of the urachus is rare and carries a poor prognosis (Lane, 1976). The incidence of urachal carcinoma varies from 0.07% to 0.7% of bladder cancers in North America and Europe but is as high as 1.2% in Japan (Ghazizadeh et al, 1983). Most urachal malignancies involve the urinary bladder, creating the difficult problem of classification and separation from primary tumors of the bladder, particularly those at the dome. Criteria for separating adenocarcinoma of the urinary bladder and urachus are summarized in Tables 11.3 and 11.4 (Mostofi et al, 1955; Wheeler & Hill, 1954). Ultimately, advanced cancer in the dome of the bladder may not be distinguishable as of vesical or urachal origin. Unless the evidence of urachal origin is strong for urothelial and squamous cell carcinomas in this area, they are generally assumed to be of bladder mucosal origin. Similar criteria are applied for a sarcoma arising in the dome of the bladder

(a)

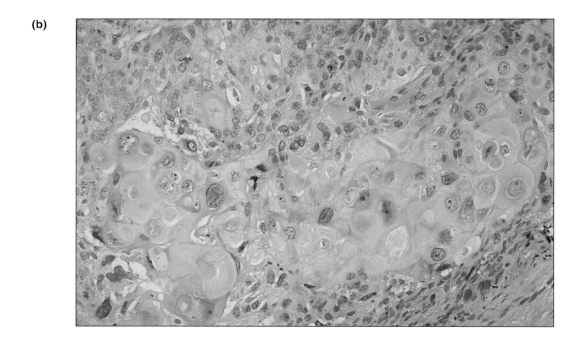

(b)

(c)

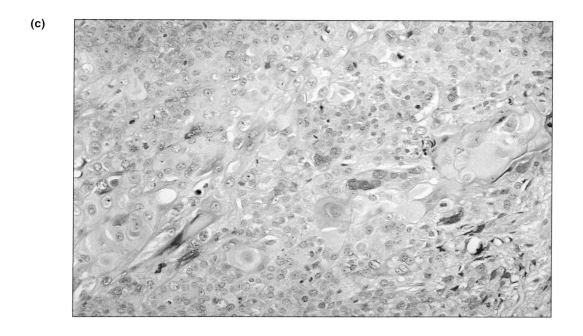

(d)

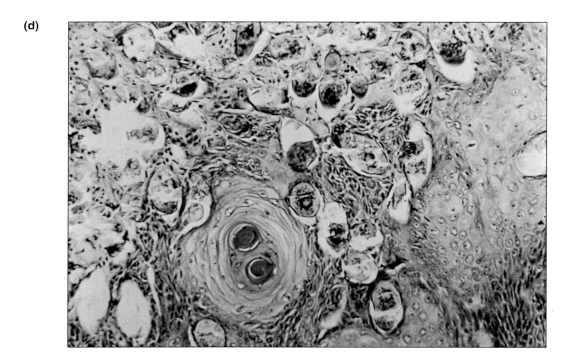

Figure 11.8   (a, b, c): Squamous cell carcinoma of the urinary bladder (not associated with schistosomiasis); **(d):** Low-grade squamous cell carcinoma with schistosomal eggs.

(a)

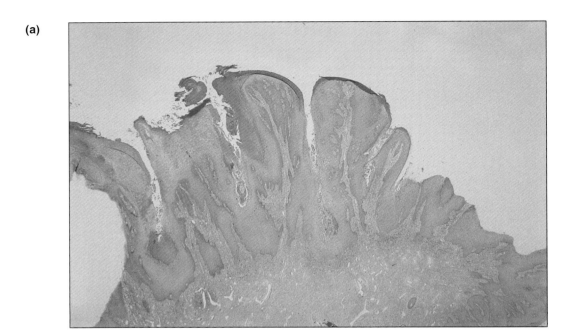

(b)

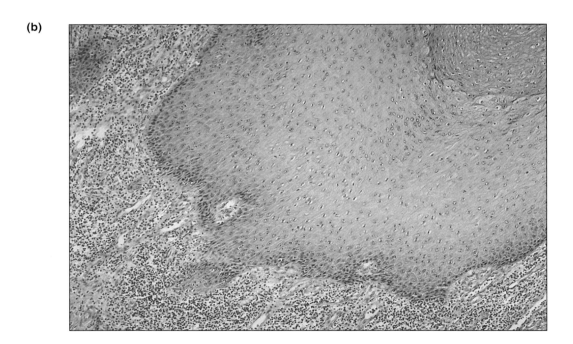

Figure 11.9 Verrucous carcinoma of the bladder. **(a):** The tumor appears as broad exophytic fronds of squamous mucosa. **(b):** The epithelium is remarkably well differentiated, with evidence of koilocytotic change. There is chronic inflammation at the interface with the stroma.

Table 11.3 Diagnostic criteria for urachal origin of adenocarcinoma

Cancer located in the dome or anterior wall of the bladder
Absence of cystitis cystica or cystitis glandularis in dome
Predominant involvement of the muscularis propria by cancer rather than the lamina propria (submucosa). The vesical mucosal surface may be intact or ulcerated
Urachal remnant connected with cancer
Presence of a suprapubic mass
Cancer infiltrating through the bladder wall, with contiguous spread through the space of Retzius in the anterior abdominal wall
Sharp demarcation between the cancer and the overlying urothelium of the bladder dome

Table 11.4 Criteria to distinguish urachal and nonurachal adenocarcinoma of the bladder

Location in bladder dome or anterior wall
Cancer is chiefly intramural, with deep ramifications in the bladder wall
Absence of intestinal metaplasia in urothelium
Other primary sites excluded

Table 11.5 Staging of urachal adenocarcinoma

Stage I	Carcinoma confined to the urachal mucosa
Stage II	Invasion confined to the urachus
Stage III	Local extension
Stage IIIA	Extension into urinary bladder
Stage IIIB	Extension into abdominal wall
Stage IIIC	Extension into the peritoneum
Stage IIID	Extension into other viscera
Stage IV	Metastasis
Stage IVA	Metastasis to regional lymph nodes
Stage IVB	Metastasis to distant sites

(Hayman, 1984). The staging of urachal carcinoma is similar regardless of histologic subtype (Table 11.5) (Sheldon et al, 1984).

11.4.1 Urachal Adenocarcinoma

Adenocarcinoma is the most common cancer of the urachus, accounting for 85%–90% of cases (Ghazizadeh et al, 1983; Loening et al, 1978; Mattelaer et al, 1997; Petersen, 1992; Sheldon et al, 1984). More than 70% of cases arise in patients between 20 and 84 years, with a male-to-female ratio of 3:1 (Ghazizadeh et al, 1983; Sheldon et al, 1984). Presenting symptoms include hematuria, irritative voiding symptoms, abdominal pain, a suprapubic mass, and occasional mucinuria. At cystoscopy, the tumor protrudes from the dome or anterior surface of the bladder as a polypoid or papillary mass, some-

times creating a gelatinous or bloody discharge from the urachal orifice (Sheldon et al, 1984; Vergos et al, 1992). Transurethral biopsy is often helpful in establishing the diagnosis.

Radiographically, adenocarcinoma creates a filling defect in the dome of the bladder. Stippled calcifications are strongly suggestive of a neoplasm of urachal origin (Lopez-Beltran et al, 1994b). Urachal adenocarcinoma has a poorer survival rate than adenocarcinoma of the bladder.

Macroscopically, urachal adenocarcinoma is often extensive, infiltrating the bladder wall musculature and extending superiorly toward the abdominal wall in the space of Retzius. The cancer may be gelatinous depending on the amount of mucin production, and the mucosal surface is often ulcerated. The cancer may be partially or extensively calcified (Lopez-Beltran et al, 1994b).

Microscopically, urachal adenocarcinoma has a varied appearance (Figs 11.10 and 11.11). Most tumors are mucinous (Burnett et al, 1991). Nonmucinous types often resemble adenocarcinoma of the colon, but other types include colloid carcinoma, signet-ring cell carcinoma, and high-grade poorly differentiated adenocarcinoma. Osseous metaplasia of the stroma may be present (Lopez-Beltran et al, 1994b; Okamoto et al, 1993).

Signet-ring cell adenocarcinoma of the urachus is considered by many authors as a sepa-

(a)

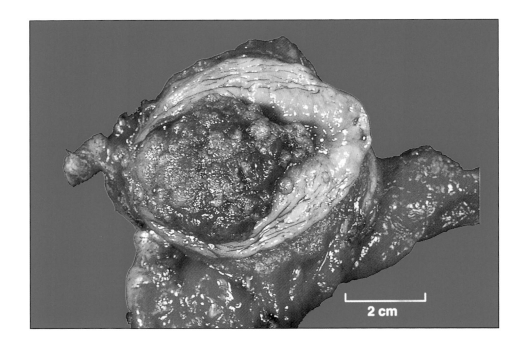

(b)

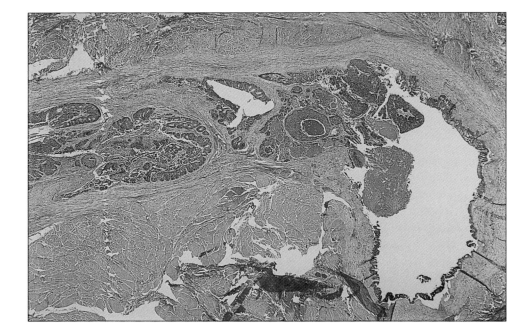

(c)

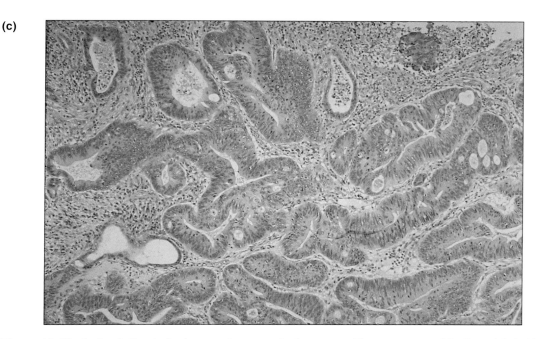

Figure 11.10 **(a, b, c):** Urachal adenocarcinoma, colonic pattern. (Case courtesy of Dr. Bernd Scheithauer, Mayo Clinic, Rochester, MN.)

rate histopathologic subtype of adenocarcinoma because of its distinctive morphology (Alonso-Gorrea et al, 1985). Most cases are mixed with typical adenocarcinoma, and the signet-ring cells may be present within glands or in mucus lakes of typical colloid carcinoma. The diffusely infiltrative pattern resembles linitis plastica (Johnson et al, 1985). Pure signet-ring cell pattern accounts for <10% of cases of urachal adenocarcinoma (Petersen, 1992). Inclusion criteria for signet-ring cell carcinoma of the urachus are similar to those for the bladder, including at least a focal component of diffuse linitis plastica-like growth and the absence of urothelial carcinoma (Grignon et al, 1991c). The male-to-female ratio (3:1) is similar to that of a typical urachal adenocarcinoma, and the patient mean age varies from 48 to 54 years (Grignon et al, 1991a, 1991b). Local recurrence is frequent and usually precedes metastasis. Sites of recurrence include the pelvis and urinary bladder, wound, and abdomi-

nal wall. The most common sites for metastases in descending order are lymph nodes, lung, peritoneum, omentum, mesentery, liver, bone, and small intestine.

Urachal adenocarcinoma may display neuroendocrine differentiation. One case consisted of a composite of colonic-type adenocarcinoma and large-cell neuroendocrine carcinoma (Abenoza et al, 1987). The normal urachus also contains argyrophilic cells (Satake et al, 1984). Immunohistochemical studies reveal expression of chromogranin, serotonin, somatostatin, neuron-specific enolase, and carcinoembryonic antigen in cases with neuroendocrine differentiation (Johnson et al, 1985; Melamed et al, 1987). Urachal adenocarcinoma and bladder adenocarcinoma display immunoreactivity for a colonic epithelial protein recognized by monoclonal antibody 7E12H12, unlike urothelial carcinoma (Pantuck et al, 1997).

Differential diagnostic considerations include metastasis or contiguous spread from

(a)

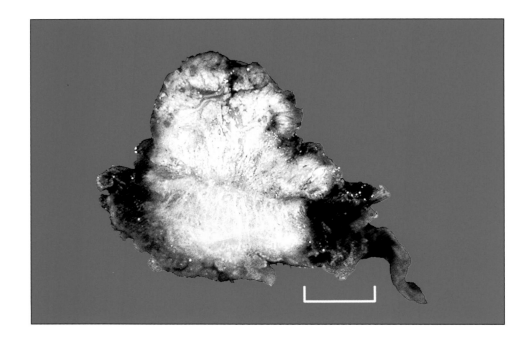

(b)

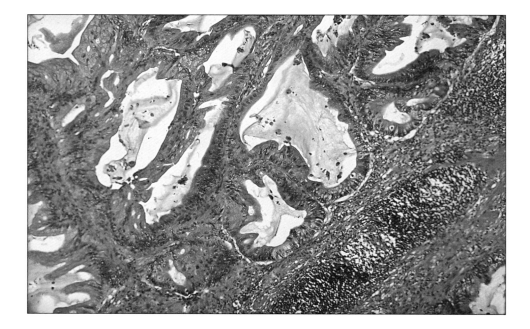

(c)

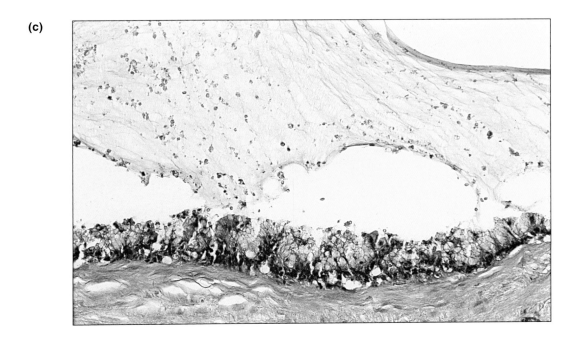

(d)

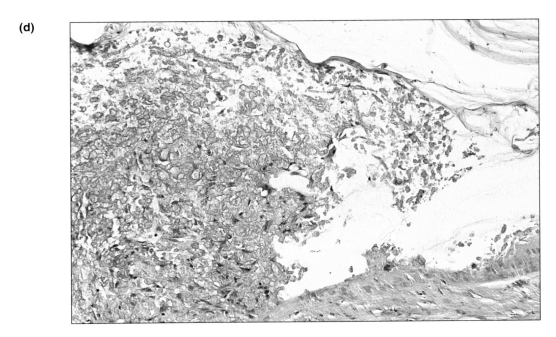

Figure 11.11 Urachal adenocarcinoma, colonic type. Note abundant mucin.(a)Gross appearance of exophytic mass;ruler indicates 2cm;(b)typical adenocarcinoma in muscular wall of bladder; (c)in some areas,there was marked cystic dilatation with luminal mucin;(d)in this focus, the lining of the cyst is lost.

colorectal adenocarcinoma; this is usually easily distinguished clinically (Kitami et al, 1987; Wheeler & Hill, 1954; Whitehead & Tessler, 1971). Unlike colonic adenocarcinoma, urachal and urinary bladder cancers do not produce sulfated acid mucopolysaccharides (Tiltman & Maytom, 1977). Unusual metastases from urachal adenocarcinoma include involvement of the orbit and the ovary (Giordano, 1995; Young, 1995). Malignant lymphoma may also rarely simulate signet-ring cell carcinoma of the urachus (Siegel & Napoli, 1991).

11.4.2   Urachal Squamous Cell Carcinoma

Squamous cell carcinoma accounts for about 4% of urachal cancers. Mean patient age is 50 years (range: 27–77 years), with a higher incidence in men. The cancer may be supravesical or intramural and is typical squamous cell carcinoma, similar to that in the urinary bladder (Jimi et al, 1986; Lin et al, 1983).

11.4.3   Urachal Urothelial Carcinoma

Urothelial carcinoma of the urachus comprises about 3% of urachal cancers (Fisher, 1958). It occurs mainly in patients over 40 years of age who present with typical symptoms of hematuria and pain. The histologic findings are similar to those of urothelial carcinoma occurring in the bladder. Urachal carcinoma may also contain mixed differentiation, including one case with adenocarcinoma, squamous cell carcinoma, and urothelial carcinoma (Kitami et al, 1987). A metachronous urothelial carcinoma of the bladder and urachus has also been reported (Satake et al, 1995).

REFERENCES

Abbas F, Civantos F, Benedetto P, Soloway MS. Small cell carcinoma of the bladder and prostate. Urology. 1995;46:617–630.

Abenoza P, Manivel C, Fraley EE. Primary adenocarcinoma of the urinary bladder. Clinicopathologic study of 16 cases. Urology. 1987;29:9–14.

Ali SZ, Reuter VE, Zakowski MF. Small cell neuroendocrine carcinoma of the urinary bladder. A clinicopathologic study with emphasis on cytologic features. Cancer. 1997;79:356–361.

Alonso-Gorrea M, Mompo-Sanchis JA, Jorda-Cuevas M, et al. Signet ring cell adenocarcinoma of the urachus. Eur Urol. 1985;11:282–284.

Banerjee SS, Eyden BP, McVey RJ, et al. Primary peripheral primitive neuroectodermal tumour of urinary bladder. Histopathology. 1997;30:486–490.

Benson RC Jr, Swanson SK, Farrow GM. Relationship of leukoplakia to urothelial malignancy. J Urol. 1984;131:507–511.

Bickel A, Culkin DJ, Wheeler JS Jr. Bladder cancer in spinal cord injury patients. J Urol. 1991;146:1240–1242.

Bullock PS, Thoni DE, Murphy WM. The significance of colonic mucosa (intestinal metaplasia) involving the urinary tract. Cancer. 1987;59:2086–2090.

Burnett AL, Epstein JI, Marshall FF. Adenocarcinoma of urinary bladder: classification and management. Urology. 1991;37:315–321.

Chin NW, Marinescu AM, Fani K. Composite adenocarcinoma and carcinoid tumor of urinary bladder. Urology. 1992;40:249–252.

Corica FA, Husmann DA, Churchill BM, et al. Intestinal metaplasia is not a strong risk factor for bladder cancer: study of 53 cases with long term follow-up. Urology. 1997;50:427–431.

Fish DE, Rose DS, Adamson A, et al. Neoplastic Paneth cells in a mucinous adenocarcinoma of the bladder. Br J Urol. 1994;73:105–106.

Fisher ER. Transitional-cell carcinoma of the urachal apex. Cancer. 1958;11:245–254.

Ghazizadeh M, Yamamoto S, Kurokawa K. Clinical features of urachal carcinoma in Japan: review of 157 patients. Urol Res. 1983;11:235–238.

Giordano GG. Orbital metastasis from a urachal tumor [letter]. Arch Ophthalmol. 1995;113:413–415.

Grignon DJ, Ro JY, Ayala AG, et al. Primary adenocarcinoma of the urinary bladder. A clinicopathologic analysis of 72 cases. Cancer. 1991a;69:2165–2172.

Grignon DJ, Ro JY, Ayala AG, et al. Primary signet-ring cell carcinoma of the urinary bladder. Am J Clin Pathol. 1991b;95:13–20.

Grignon DJ, Ro JY, Ayala AG, et al. Small cell carcinoma of the urinary bladder. A clinicopathologic analysis of 22 cases. Cancer. 1991c;69:527–536.

Hayman J. Carcinoma of the urachus. Pathology. 1984;16:167–171.

Holmäng S, Borghede G, Johansson SL. Primary small cell carcinoma of the bladder: a report of 25 cases. *J Urol.* 1995;153:1820–1822.

Holmäng S, Borghede G, Johansson SL. Primary signet ring cell carcinoma of the bladder: a report on 10 cases. *Scand J Urol Nephrol.* 1996;31:145–148.

Horner SA, Fisher HA, Barada JH, et al. Verrucous carcinoma of the bladder. *J Urol.* 1991;145:1261–1263.

Hurwitz R, Fitzpatrick T, Ackerman I, et al. A neuroectodermal tumor in the bladder. *J Urol.* 1980;124:417–419.

Jacobs LB, Brooks JD, Epstein JI. Differentiation of colonic metaplasia from adenocarcinoma of urinary bladder. *Hum Pathol.* 1997;28:1152–1157.

Jimi A, Munaoka H, Sato S-I, et al. Squamous cell carcinoma of the urachus: a case report and review of the literature. *Acta Pathol Jpn.* 1986;36:945–949.

Johnson DE, Hodge GB, Abdul-Karim FW, et al. Urachal carcinoma. *Urology.* 1985;26:218–221.

Kaye MC, Levin HS, Montague DK, et al. Squamous cell carcinoma of the bladder in a patient on intermittent self-catheterization. *Clev Clin J Med.* 1992;59:645–646.

Kitami K, Masuda M, Chiba K, et al. Carcinoma of the urachus with variable pathological findings: report of a case and review of the literature. *Hinyokika Kiyo.* 1987;33:1459.

Holmäng S, Borghede G, Johansson SL. Primary small cell carcinoma of the bladder: a report of 25 cases. *J Urol.* 1995;153:1820–1822.

Holmäng S, Borghede G, Johansson SL. Primary signet ring cell carcinoma of the bladder: a report on 10 cases. *Scand J Urol Nephrol.* 1997;31:145–148.

Lam KY, Ma L, Nicholls J. Adenocarcinoma arising in a diverticulum of the urinary bladder. *Pathology.* 1992;24:40–42.

Lane V. Prognosis in carcinoma of the urachus. *Eur J Urol.* 1976;2:282–283.

Lertprasertsuke N, Tsutsumi Y. Neuroendocrine carcinoma of the urinary bladder: case report and review of the literature. *Jpn J Clin Oncol.* 1991;21:203–210.

Lin R-Y, Rappoport AE, Deppisch LM, et al. Squamous cell carcinoma of the urachus. *J Urol.* 1983;118:1066–1067.

Loening SA, Jacobo E, Hawtrey CE, et al. Adenocarcinoma of the urachus. *J Urol.* 1978;119:68–73.

Lopez JI, Angulo JC, Flores N, et al. Small cell carcinoma of the urinary bladder. A clinicopathological study of six cases. *Br J Urol.* 1994;73:43–49.

Lopez-Beltran A, Croghan GA, Croghan I, et al. Prognostic factors in bladder cancer. A pathologic, immunohistochemical, and DNA flow-cytometric study. *Am J Clin Pathol.* 1994a;102:109–114.

Lopez-Beltran A, Nogales F, Donne CH, et al. Adenocarcinoma of the urachus showing extensive calcification and stromal osseous metaplasia. *Urol Int.* 1994b;53:110–113.

Mattelaer P, Wolff JM, Jung P, et al. Adenocarcinoma of the urachus: 3 case reports and a review of the literature. *Acta Urol Belg.* 1997;65:63–67.

Michal M, Sulc M, Mukensnabl P. Verrucous carcinoma of the urinary bladder associated with sebaceous differentiation. *J Urol Pathol.* 1997;6:153–158.

Meis JM, Ayala AG, Johnson DE. Adenocarcinoma of the urethra in women. A clinicopathologic study. *Cancer.* 1987;60:1038–1052.

Melamed MR, Farrow GM, Haggitt RC. Urologic neoplasms. In: *Proceedings of the 50th annual anatomic pathology slide seminar of the American Society of Clinical Pathologists.* Chicago: ASCP Press; 1987.

Mostofi FK, Thomson RV, Dean AL. Mucous adenocarcinoma of the urinary bladder. *Cancer.* 1955;8:741–751.

Muthuphei MN. Primary signet-ring cell carcinoma of the bladder. A case report. *S Afr J Surg.* 1994;32:107–108.

Oida Y, Yasuda M, Kajiwara H, et al. Double squamous cell carcinomas, verrucous type and poorly differentiated type, of the urinary bladder unassociated with bilharzial infection. *Pathol Int.* 1997;47:651–654.

Okamoto K, Fukuyama T, Okamoto E, et al. Adenocarcinoma of the urachus associated with stromal osseous metaplasia. *Urol Int.* 1993;51:240–243.

Pantuck AJ, Bancila E, Das KM, et al. Adenocarcinoma of the urachus and bladder expresses a unique colonic epithelial epitope: an immunohistochemical study. *J Urol.* 1997;158:1722–1727.

Richie JP, Waisman J, Skinner DG, Dretler SP. Squamous carcinoma of the bladder: treatment by radical cystectoma. *J Urol.* 1976;115:670–672.

Satake I, Nakagomi K, Tari K, et al. Metachronous transitional cell carcinoma of the urachus and bladder. *Br J Urol.* 1995;75:244–246.

Satake T, Takeda A, Matsuyama M. Argyrophil cells in the urachal epithelium and urachal adenocarcinoma. *Acta Pathol Jpn.* 1984;34:1193–1197.

Schultz RE, Bloch MJ, Tomaszewski JE, et al. Mesonephric adenocarcinoma of the bladder. *J Urol.* 1984;132:263–265.

Shaaban AA, Orkubi SA, Said MT, et al. Squamous cell carcinoma of the urinary bladder. *Ann Saudi Med.* 1997;17:115–119.

Sharfi AR, el Sir S, Beleil O. Squamous cell carcinoma of the urinary bladder. *Br J Urol.* 1992;69:369–371.

Sheldon CA, Clayman RV, Gonzalez R, et al. Malignant urachal lesions. *J Urol.* 1984;131:1–8.

Siegel RJ, Napoli VM. Malignant lymphoma of the urinary bladder. A case with signet-ring cells simulating urachal adenocarcinoma. *Arch Pathol Lab Med.* 1991;115:635–637.

Sinard J, Macleay L Jr, Melamed J. Hepatoid adenocarcinoma in the urinary bladder. Unusual localization of a newly recognized tumor type. *Cancer.* 1994;73:1919–1925.

Stanfield BL, Grimes MM, Kay S. Primary carcinoid tumor of the bladder arising beneath an inverted papilloma. *Arch Pathol Lab Med.* 1994;118:666–667.

Tiltman AJ, Maytom PAM. Adenocarcinoma of the urinary bladder, histochemical distinction between urachal and metastatic carcinomas. *SA Mediese Tydskrif.* 1977;51:74–75.

Torenbeek R, Koot RA, Blomjous CE, et al. Primary signet-ring cell carcinoma of the urinary bladder. *Histopathology.* 1996;28:33–40.

Utz DC, Schmitz SE, Fugelso PD, Farrow GM. A clinicopathologic evaluation of partial cystectomy for carcinoma of the urinary bladder. *Cancer.* 1973;32:1075–1077.

Vergos M, Messina MH, Lhomme Desages B, et al. Cancer of the urachus. A rare form of tumors of the bladder. *J Urol.* 1992;98:56–59.

Walker BF, Someren A, Kennedy JC, et al. Primary carcinoid tumor of the urinary bladder. *Arch Pathol Lab Med.* 1992;116:1217–1220.

Wheeler JD, Hill WT. Adenocarcinoma involving the urinary bladder. *Cancer.* 1954;7:119–127.

Whitehead ED, Tessler AN. Carcinoma of the urachus. *Br J Urol.* 1971;43:468–476.

Yamada K, Fujioka Y, Ebihara Y, et al. Alpha-fetoprotein producing undifferentiated carcinoma of the bladder. *J Urol.* 1994;152:958–960.

Yorukoglu K, Gencbay A, Cakalagaoglu F, et al. Primary signet-ring cell carcinoma of the bladder. *Br J Urol.* 1994;73:210–211.

Yoshida T, Suzumiya J, Katakami H, et al. Hypercalcemia caused by PTH-rP associated with lung metastasis from urinary bladder carcinoma: an autopsied case. *Intern Med.* 1994;33:673–676.

Young RH. Urachal adenocarcinoma metastatic to the ovary simulating primary mucinous adenocarcinoma of the ovary: report of a case. *Virchows Arch.* 1995;426:529–532.

Young RH, Bostwick DG. Florid cystitis glandularis of intestinal type with mucin extravasation: a mimic of adenocarcinoma. *Am J Surg Pathol.* 1996;20:1462–1468.

Young RH, Scully RE. Clear cell adenocarcinoma of the bladder and urethra. A report of three cases and review of the literature. *Am J Surg Pathol.* 1985;9:816–826.

12

SOFT TISSUE TUMORS
AND TUMOR-LIKE CONDITIONS

12.1 TUMOR-LIKE CONDITIONS OF THE BLADDER

12.1.1 Postoperative Spindle Cell Nodule

Postoperative spindle cell nodule (PSCN) is an uncommon lesion in the lower genitourinary tract. By definition, it develops within 3 months of a surgical procedure, and most urinary bladder cases follow a transurethral resection (Biyani et al, 1996; Guillon & Costa, 1989; Huang et al, 1990; Jones et al, 1993; Proppe et al, 1984).

Macroscopically, PSCN appears as a friable vegetant mass. Microscopically, it consists of intersecting fascicles of spindle cells that often display conspicuous numbers of mitotic figures, but none are atypical (Fig 12.1). There is usually a delicate network of small blood vessels, patchy or dense, with acute and chronic inflammation, small foci of hemorrhage, mild to moderate edema, and focal myxoid change in the stroma. Reactive atypia may be present, but the cells do not exhibit marked cytologic abnormalities. The history of a recent operation is the major clue that this lesion represents an exuberant reactive proliferation. Outcome is invariably benign, and this lesion rarely, if ever, recurs (Proppe et al, 1984).

PSCN shows a marked resemblance to leiomyosarcoma (Biyani et al, 1996), but other sarcomas such as Kaposi's sarcoma should also be considered. PSCN is easily distinguished from intermediate- or high-grade leiomyosarcoma because of the absence of cytologic abnormalities but is most difficult to separate from low-grade leiomyosarcoma. Both may involve the muscularis propria, and both may display myxoid changes, although extensive and prominent myxoid changes favor leiomyosarcoma (Young, 1988; Young & Scully, 1987; Young et al, 1987). The clinical history is of great diagnostic utility, as is the distinctive delicate network of small blood vessels in PSCN. Immunohistochemistry is also of value (Table 12.1) (Wick et al, 1988). PSCN displays cytokeratin immunoreactivity in 80% of cases, whereas this is less common in leiomyosarcoma of the bladder. Ultrastructural studies of PSCN reveal a proliferation of myofibroblasts. In difficult cases, the distinction between these two processes depends on the clinical history.

197

Table 12.1 Immunohistochemistry of spindle cell lesions of the urinary bladder

Diagnosis	Keratin	EMA	Vimentin	Desmin	MSA
Postoperative spindle cell nodule	+	−	+	+	+
Inflammatory pseudotumor*	−	−	+	−	−[†]
Spindle cell carcinoma	+	+	+/−	−	−
Leiomyosarcoma	−	−	+	+/−	+
Rhabdomyosarcoma	−	−	+	+	+

EMA = epithelial membrane antigen; MSA = muscle-specific actin.
* Inflammatory myofibroblastic tumor.
[†] MSA positivity focal.

(a)

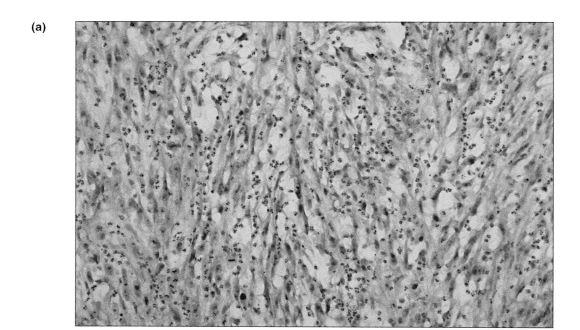

(b)

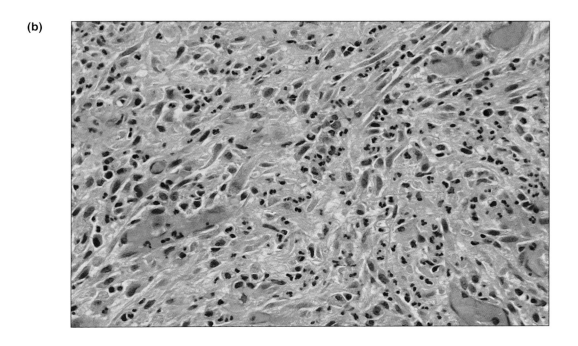

(c)

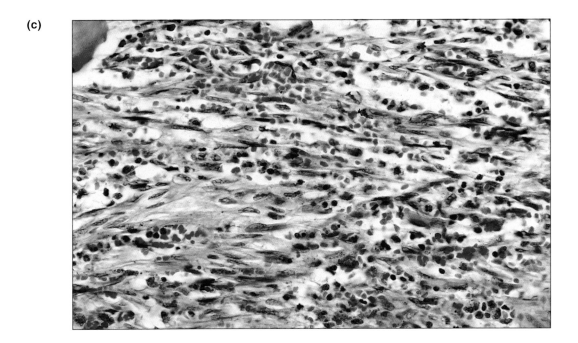

Figure 12.1 (a, b, c): Postoperative spindle cell nodule. Each of these tumors arose in patients within 3 months of a transurethral resection of the bladder.

12.1.2 Inflammatory Pseudotumor (Pseudosarcomatous Myofibroblastic Tumor; Inflammatory Myofibroblastic Tumor; Pseudosarcomatous Fibromyxoid Tumor)

Proliferative spindle cell lesions of the bladder that microscopically suggest sarcoma, but are benign, rarely occur in patients without a history of a previous surgical procedure (Angulo et al, 1994; Dietrick et al, 1992; Hughes et al, 1991; Jones et al, 1993; Lopez-Beltran et al, 1995; Nochomovitz & Orenstein, 1985). A variety of names have been used for this lesion; *inflammatory pseudotumor* is currently widely accepted (Angulo et al, 1995; Jufe et al, 1984; Khan, 1992; Lundgren et al, 1994; Ro et al, 1986, 1993). Inflammatory pseudotumor may occur at all ages, with a mean of about 30 years, and there is a female predominance (Hojo et al, 1995). Inflammatory pseudotumor may be mistaken for rhabdomyosarcoma in children and leiomyosarcoma or sarcomatoid carcinoma in adults (Lakshmanan et al, 1997; Lopez-Beltran et al, 1996; Mincione et al, 1995; Sandhu & Iacovou, 1997). Some cases occur after urinary tract infection, but most have no demonstrable etiology. Pathologists should be aware of this lesion and not misinterpret it as a spindle cell malignancy because of the important prognostic and therapeutic differences. However, we believe that many cases arising in the bladder, if followed long enough, will recur, similar to low-grade inflammatory fibrosarcoma. Most reported cases have been completely excised, so the outcome after partial resection is not known. Consequently, the long-term prognosis of inflammatory pseudotumor of the bladder should be considered uncertain.

Inflammatory pseudotumor is composed of proliferating myofibroblasts, fibroblastic cells, and endothelial cells set in an acid-mucopolysaccaride–rich stroma that suggests active granulation tissue, similar to nodular fasciitis (Figs 12.2–12.4) (Khan,1992). The tumor cells often have eosinophilic cytoplasm resembling myocytes. The nuclei of the fibroblastic and endothelial cells are ovoid, regular, and usually vesicular and normochromatic with dispersed chromatin. These cells may exhibit cellular and nuclear enlargement with prominent eosinophilic nucleoli, features attributable to reactive atypia. In such cases, it is usually possible to trace an orderly spectrum of cell types from typically benign cells to the atypical forms. Tumor cells do not show anaplasia and nuclear hyperchromasia, effectively excluding intermediate- and high-grade sarcoma. Multinucleated stromal cells may be present, which exhibit the nuclear and cytoplasmic characteristics noted above (Nochomovitz & Orenstein, 1985). The endothelial cells share some features with myofibroblasts and can be recognized by the formation of primitive neovascular channels. Mitotic figures are present in moderate numbers and are typical. A sparse infiltrate of chronic inflammatory cells may be present, including lymphocytes and plasma cells (Jones & Young, 1994). The background substance is usually abundant and may form pools and lakes of mucin (Nochomovitz & Orenstein, 1985). Infiltration into the muscularis propria is frequent and should not be considered as strong evidence of malignancy (Saavedra et al, 1990). Sarcomatoid carcinoma may have foci resembling an inflammatory pseudotumor, and caution is warranted when making a diagnosis using small or limited samples. Variants include cases with a storiform pattern or those with hyalinization that produces a sclerosing pattern. Ultrastructural studies demonstrate a predominance of myofibroblastic cells. Immunohistochemically, the spindle cells stain for vimentin and rarely for myogenic markers such as muscle-specific actin (Table 12.1). Imaging studies and flow cytometry reveal DNA diploid content (August et al, 1993; Lopez-Beltran et al, 1995).

(a)

(b)

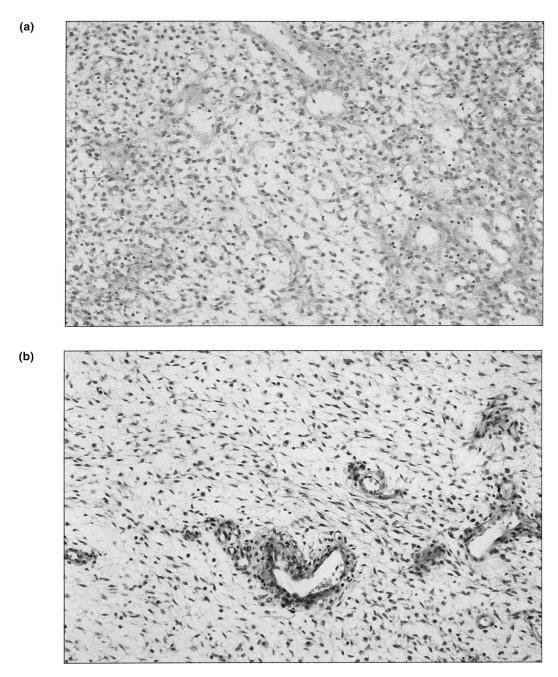

Figure 12.2 Inflammatory pseudotumor. **(a):** There is abundant acute and chronic inflammation admixed with the spindle cells, but **(b)** in some areas, the inflammation is sparse or absent.

(a)

(b)

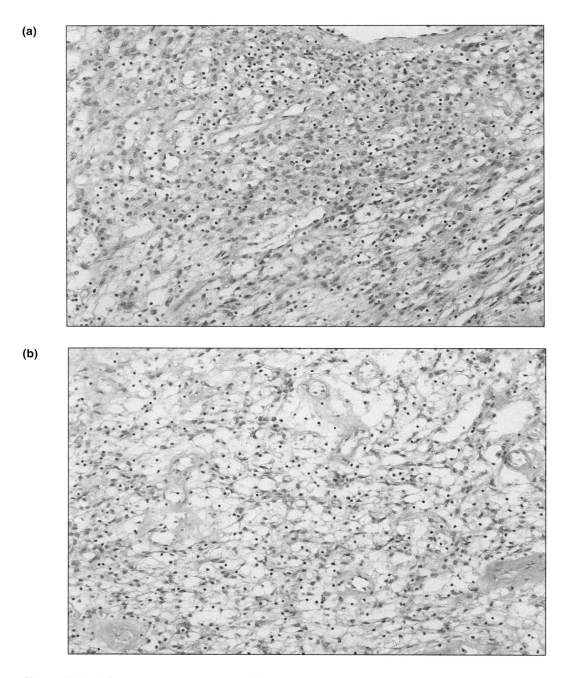

Figure 12.3 Inflammatory pseudotumor. **(a):** The tumor cells are triangular to ovoid, admixed with chronic inflammation. **(b)**: Elsewhere, tumor cells have vacuolated cytoplasm.

(a)

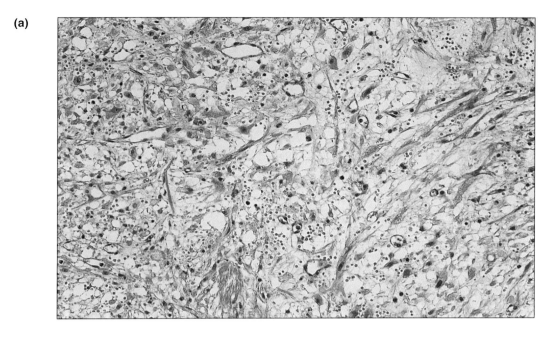

(b)

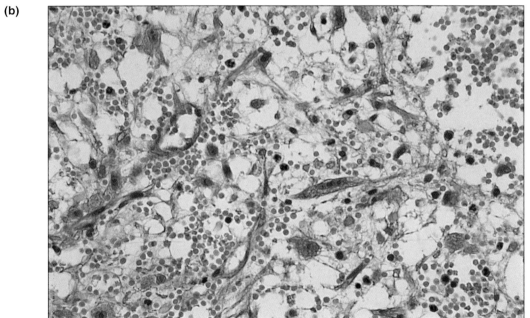

(c)

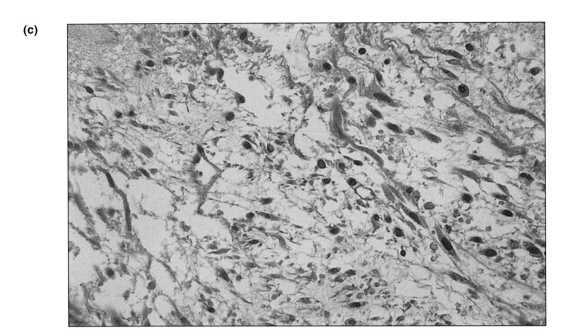

(d)

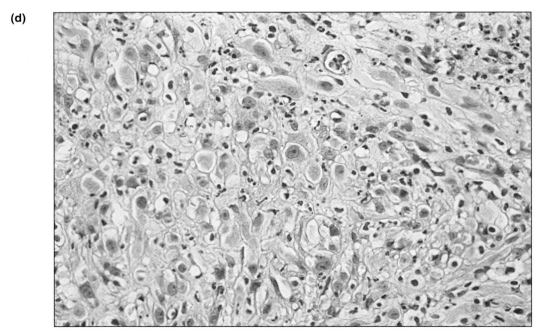

(e)

(f)

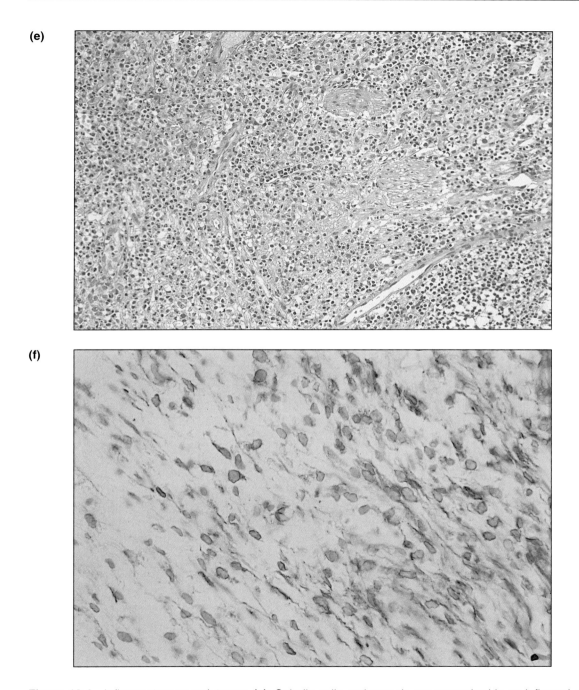

Figure 12.4 Inflammatory pseudotumor. **(a):** Spindle cells and vessels are enmeshed in an inflamed and edematous stroma. **(b):** At high magnification, atypical myofibroblasts are apparent, together with extravasated red blood cells. **(c):** Myxoid stroma. **(d):** In this focus, the myofibroblasts have epithelioid features that may be mistaken for an urothelial carcinoma. **(e):** Numerous mature lymphocytes create a pseudolymphomatous appearance; note the presence of eosinophils. **(f):** Intense vimentin immunoreactivity is observed in the spindle cells.

12.2 BENIGN SOFT TISSUE TUMORS

Benign soft tissue tumors are uncommon in the bladder; most are leiomyoma (35%), hemangioma, or neurofibroma. Benign soft tissue tumors account for <1% of primary bladder neoplasms (Melicow, 1955). Other benign soft tissue tumors are rare and include granular cell tumor, lymphangioma, benign fibrous histiocytoma, lipoma, fibroma, and ganglioneuroma (Suhler et al, 1994).

12.2.1 Leiomyoma

Leiomyoma of the urinary bladder is more common in women than men (2:1 ratio), and most tumors occur in adults. Patients may be asymptomatic, but most present with obstructive symptoms as a result of the size and proximity of the tumor to the bladder outlet (Loh et al, 1996). Bladder leiomyoma may coexist with paraurethral leiomyoma (Suhler et al, 1994).

Macroscopically, leiomyoma is submucosal in more than 60% of cases, producing a polypoid or pedunculated mass (Fig 12.5) (Bornstein et al, 1986). Less commonly, it arises within the bladder wall or in the subserosa. The overlying urothelium is usually intact. Most tumors are small, measuring 1–4 cm in diameter. Rarely, there may be multiple leiomyomata. The cut surface is typically circumscribed, with a whorled grey-white appearance.

Microscopically, the characteristic features of leiomyoma at other sites are present in the bladder, including fascicles of spindle cells with fusiform blunt-ended nuclei and eosinophilic cytoplasm (Knoll et al, 1986; Swartz et al, 1985). There is minimal cytologic atypia and few or no mitotic figures. One report recommended that a smooth muscle tumor of the bladder with few or no mitotic figures but an infiltrative pattern should be considered as low-grade leiomyosarcoma (Mills et al, 1989). These authors argued that the infiltrative pattern mitigates against a benign diagnosis. Focal myxoid change can also be found in leiomyoma, but prominant myxoid stroma is more common in leiomyosarcoma.

12.2.2 Hemangioma

Hemangioma of the urinary bladder accounts for 40% of benign soft tissue tumors (Caro & Brown, 1976; Mor et al, 1997; Radke et al, 1993). It occurs at any age but is more common prior to 30 years of age, with a slight male predominance. Most patients present with hematuria, irritative symptoms, pain, or urinary obstructive symptoms. Up to 30% of patients have a cutaneous hemangioma. Bladder hemangioma occurs in more than 5% of patients with Klippel-Trenaunay syndrome and may also arise in patients with Sturge-Weber syndrome.

Macroscopically, hemangioma appears as a purple, multilobulated, and sessile mass (Gottesman & Seale, 1983; Vicente-Rodriguez et al, 1986). It may be single (70% of cases) or multiple and can be superficial or extend through the full thickness of the bladder wall. The majority are small, measuring <2 cm in the greatest dimension.

Microscopically, hemangioma consists of vascular spaces containing blood and thrombi (Hendry & Vinnicombi, 1971). Depending on the pattern, hemangioma is variously classified as cavernous, capillary, venous, or racemose, with cavernous being most common in the bladder. Some are associated with lymphangioma (Chandna et al, 1987). One case of vesicular and cutaneous hemangiomatosis (blue rubber–bleb–nevus syndrome) was effectively treated by laser therapy in a 2-year-old girl (Hockley et al, 1989).

The major differential diagnostic consideration of bladder hemangioma is angiosarcoma, although that typically displays greater cytologic abnormalities and numerous mitotic figures. Involvement of the bladder by Kaposi's sarcoma in immunocompromised patients has also been described (Biermann et al, 1992).

(a)

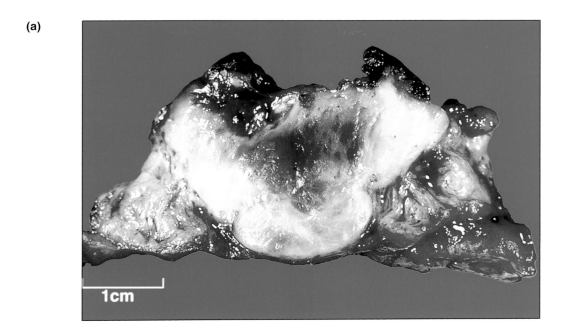

(b)

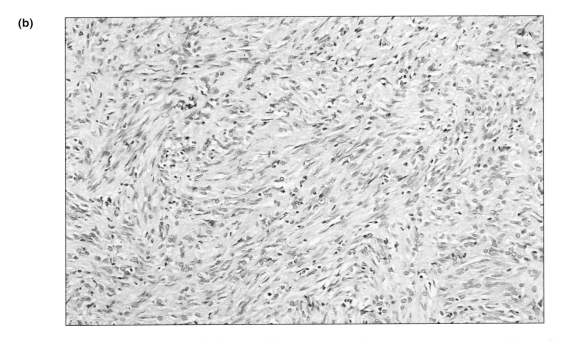

Figure 12.5 Leiomyoma of the bladder. **(a):** This large, centrally hemorrhagic tumor consists entirely of benign smooth muscle cells **(b)** without cytologic atypia, necrosis, or mitotic figures. The patient was alive and free of disease after 11 years.

12.2.3 Neurofibroma

Most cases of bladder neurofibroma occur in patients with Recklinghausen's disease, although rare sporadic cases also arise. In Recklinghausen's disease, the urinary bladder is the most frequent site of involvement in the genitourinary tract (Sane et al, 1991), and malignant degeneration has been reported (Hulsa, 1990). Neurofibroma can present at any age, including infancy, and is slightly more common in males. The majority of patients complain of hematuria, dysuria, or irritative symptoms. In some cases, there is concomitant involvement of other genitourinary sites, including the ureter, spermatic cord, penis, and scrotum. Malignant degeneration of bladder neurofibroma is rare, with only two reported cases, although the frequency in other sites varies from 13% to 29% (Hintsa et al, 1996).

Macroscopically, neurofibroma may be single or multiple, consisting of discrete variably sized nodules within the wall or submucosa that may be polypoid or pedunculated. It is usually small but may rarely measure up to several centimeters in diameter. It may also appear as a diffuse thickening in the bladder wall without discrete margins; this pattern corresponds to the plexiform variant characteristically associated with Recklinghausen's disease (Clark et al, 1977). In these patients, the tumor may extensively invade the bladder wall, ureters, and adjacent soft tissues.

Microscopically, neurofibroma of the bladder is identical to neurofibroma occurring elsewhere (Brooks & Scully, 1985). It is composed of fascicles of elongate spindle cells with thin, wavy nuclei set in a collagenized and fibrillar background. Small nerve fibers are usually present within the mass, and there may be myxoid changes. Wagner-Meissner bodies may also be present (Mooney et al, 1994).

The results of immunohistochemical studies in bladder neurofibroma are similar to results in other neurofibromas (Hasui et al, 1991); some cases are S-100 protein immunoreactive (Winfield & Catalona, 1985).

The differential diagnostic considerations for neurofibroma include other benign spindle cell lesions such as leiomyoma and inflammatory pseudotumor. A malignant peripheral nerve sheath tumor of the urinary bladder should also be considered (Dahm et al, 1995).

12.2.4 Neurilemmoma (Schwannoma)

Three cases of neurilemmoma have been described in the bladder, including in an incontinent 88-year-old woman with a 20-cm-diameter ancient neurilemmoma, in a 51-year-old woman with an enlarging pelvic mass and obstructive renal failure, and in a 19-year-old woman with recurrent urinary tract infections and a 1-cm-diameter mass medial to the ureteric orifice (Brown & Futter, 1997). Resection is curative. The histologic findings are similar to those of neurilemmoma at other sites, and there is intense cytoplasmic immunoreactivity in tumor cells for S-100 protein.

12.2.5 Paraganglioma (Pheochromocytoma)

Paraganglioma probably arises from normal paraganglionic tissue within the bladder wall (Fig 12.6) (Grignon et al, 1991). It appears at any age and is equally common in men and women. Rare cases are associated with neurofibromatosis (Burton et al, 1986), intestinal carcinoid (Lam & Chan, 1993), and, curiously, long-term dialysis (Misawa et al, 1993). Patients characteristically present with symptoms of catecholamine excess, including tachycardia, hypertension, and headaches. Hematuria is common, and paroxysmal hypertension with painless hematuria at the time of micturition is pathognomonic (Das et al, 1983). The diagnosis is usually confirmed by measurement of catecholamines and metabolites in urine and serum.

(a)

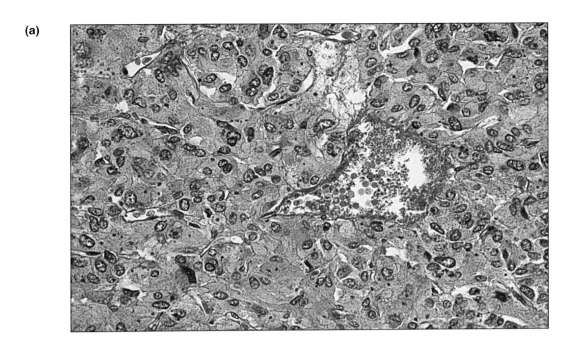

(b)

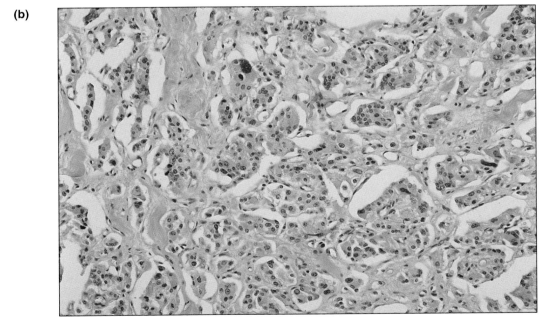

(c)

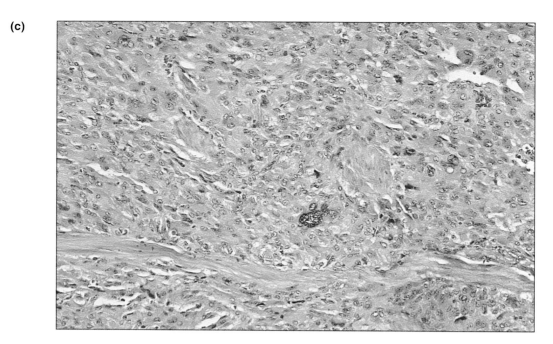

Figure 12.6 Pheochromocytoma (paraganglioma) of the bladder. **(a, b):** Discrete nests of tumor cells are typical, although other patterns, including **(c)** a spindle cell pattern may be encountered.

Grossly, paraganglioma is intramural, with a predilection for the trigone, anterior wall, and dome. The overlying mucosa may be intact or ulcerated. The tumor is usually circumscribed, lobulated, and pink to yellow-brown, ranging from 0.2 cm to 15 cm in diameter. Histologically, paraganglioma of the bladder is identical to its counterpart occurring elsewhere and is composed of cells arranged in discrete nests ("zellballen") separated by a prominent sinusoidal vascular network. The tumor cells have abundant pale eosinophilic or clear cytoplasm with central nuclei and finely dispersed chromatin, but there may be considerable variation in size with some nuclear atypia. Mitotic figures are usually infrequent, and necrosis is not prominent. In some cases, flattened sustentacular cells can be recognized around the cell nests. One case contained foci of ganglioneuroma (Grignon et al, 1991). Pathologic predictors of behavior for these tumors are not well defined (Boyle et al, 1996). Features associated with ag-gressive behavior in paraganglioma arising at other sites, including mitotic figures, necrosis, and vascular invasion, have not been studied in urinary bladder tumors. The development of malignant behavior has been associated with an increase in the numbers of mitotic figures (Grignon et al, 1991).

The most useful immunohistochemical features are the lack of immunoreactivity for cytokeratin, epithelial membrane antigen, and carcinoembryonic antigen and a positive reaction with antibodies to neuroendocrine markers, including neuron-specific enolase, chromogranin, synaptophysin, serotonin, somatostatin, and others. Sustentacular cells stain positively for S-100 protein (Moyana & Kontozoglu, 1988).

The main differential diagnostic consideration is invasive urothelial carcinoma, and the prominent sinusoidal vascular pattern of paraganglioma allows separation. The possibility of metastasis from another site should be considered, although this occurs in <15% of cases. The tendency for late and sometimes multiple recurrences of paraganglioma has been noted (Boyle et al, 1996; Grignon et al, 1991).

12.2.6 Solitary Fibrous Tumor

Solitary fibrous tumor, previously referred to as "localized fibrous mesothelioma," rarely arises within the bladder wall (Bainbridge et al, 1997; Mentzel et al, 1997). It is usually hyocellular and may have angiomatous and hemangiopericytoma-like areas. Variable amounts of hyalinized collagen are present; the spindle cells in the stroma have little or no atypia and very few or no mitotic figures. Myxoid stromal changes and cystic degeneration may be observed. Tumor necrosis is absent. Immunohistochemical studies are useful in separating solitary fibrous tumor from other soft tissue tumors of the bladder; it is characteristically immunoreactive for CD34 and negative for keratin and S-100 protein. Rare cells may display actin and muscle-specific actin, but this finding is inconsistent.

12.2.7 Other Benign Soft Tissue Tumors

Granular cell tumor of the urinary bladder (myoblastoma, Abrikossov's tumor) is rare, invariably arising in adults (Mouradian et al, 1974). There is an equal gender distribution, and all patients present with hematuria (Fletcher et al, 1985). All but one reported case has been benign. Macroscopically, granular cell tumor is circumscribed or encapsulated, appearing as yellow-white nodules measuring up to 12 cm in diameter. Histologically, the tumor is composed of spindle or polygonal cells with abundant coarsely granular eosinophilic cytoplasm. The granules are positive with PAS stain and resistant to diastase. This tumor is considered neurogenic (Schwann cell) in origin and is S-100 protein immunoreactive, similar to granular cell tumor elsewhere.

Ganglioneuroma of the bladder was described in a 17-year-old boy with a history of pyelonephritis (Wyman et al, 1950). The tumor was composed of ganglion cells set in a matrix suggestive of a plexiform neurofibroma. The patient did not have any other stigmata of Recklinghausen's disease. Unusual cases of bladder neurilemmoma have also been described, including epithelial neurilemmoma (Kindblom et al, 1998).

Lymphangioma of the bladder is very rare. One case arose in a 13-year-old boy with a history of painless hematuria (Bolkier et al, 1983). Macroscopically, the tumor measured about 10 cm in diameter. Microscopically, it was composed of typical cystic spaces of lymphangioma lined by flattened endothelial cells and separated by delicate connective tissue stroma containing scattered smooth muscle bundles (Chandna et al, 1987).

A bladder lipoma, composed of typically mature fat cells, was described in a 72-year-old woman (Alonso et al, 1982). An adenofibroma of the urinary bladder has also been described (Martin, 1936). Benign fibrous histiocytoma has also been reported in the bladder (Karol et al, 1977). Macroscopically, the tumors displays typical features, including a dense cellularity or collagenized stroma with fibroblastic cells arranged at least focally in a storiform pattern.

We recently encountered an unique case of aggressive angiomyxoma of the bladder arising in a young patient with Peutz-Jeghers syndrome (Fig 12.7).

12.3 MALIGNANT SOFT TISSUE TUMORS

Urinary bladder sarcoma accounts for <3% of primary bladder neoplasms (Kunze et al, 1994). In children, rhabdomyosarcoma is the most frequent bladder sarcoma (Hawkins & Camacho-Velazquez, 1987), whereas leiomyosarcoma is the most frequent in adults. Other unusual sarco-

(a)

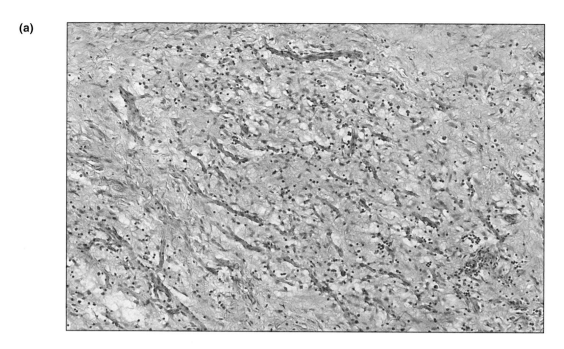

(b)

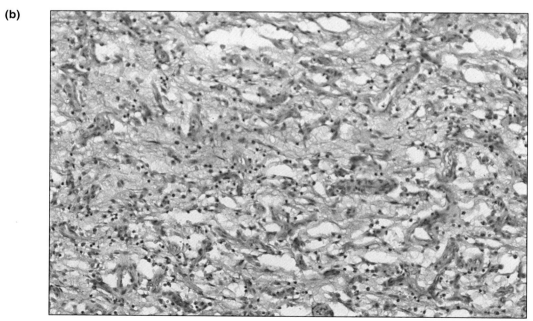

(c)

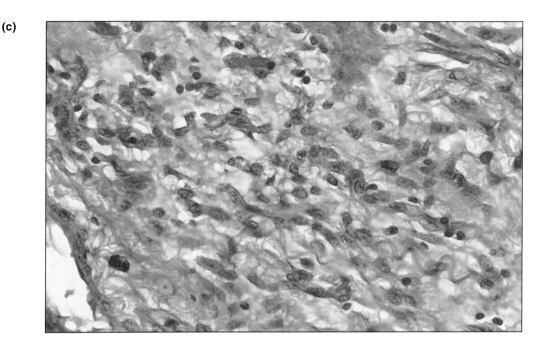

Figure 12.7 Aggressive angiomyxoma arising in the bladder in a patient with Peutz-Jeghers syndrome. **(a, b):** The tumor consists of spindle cells and stellate cells with thin- and thick-walled hyaline vessels in a myxoid stroma. **(c):** The tumor cells have little or no nuclear atypia and no mitotic activity. (Case courtesy of Dr. Aidan Carney, Mayo Clinic, Rochester, MN.)

mas arising in the urinary bladder include osteosarcoma, malignant fibrous histiocytoma, fibrosarcoma, angiosarcoma, malignant mesenchymoma, liposarcoma, and rhabdoid tumor. A chordoid sarcoma has also been described (Goertchen et al, 1984).

12.3.1 Rhabdomyosarcoma

Less than 10% of malignant tumors in children under age 15 years are rhabdomyosarcoma (Fleischmann et al, 1981). Rhabdomyosarcoma of the bladder is very rare in adults (Miettinen, 1988). In children, it occurs more frequently in boys than girls (3:2 ratio), and most tumors arise before the age of 5 years (Hawkins & Camacho-Velazquez, 1987). It usually causes hematuria and bladder neck obstruction.

Macroscopically, the characteristic finding is a polypoid mass filling the bladder lumen.

The mass may be single or multiple, producing in some instances a sarcoma botryoides (grape-like) appearance. The trigone is the most common location, although rare cases may originate at the bladder dome (Royal et al, 1996). Rhabdomyosarcoma is also discussed in Chapter 2.

Microscopically, most tumors are embryonal rhabdomyosarcoma with diffuse infiltration of small blue round cells with scant cytoplasm. In the sarcoma botryoides type, the cells are scattered in a loose myxoid stroma with condensation of rhabdomyoblasts beneath the urothelium, creating a cambium layer (Mostofi & Moss, 1952). Although rhabdoid or strap cells with cross-striations may be present, their presence is not necessary for diagnosis. In our experience, immunohistochemistry with desmin, vimentin, and muscle-specific actin is often of value. Ultrastructural studies may demonstrate

213

rhabdomyoblastic differentiation, but this technique is used in a minority of cases.

12.3.2 Leiomyosarcoma

Leiomyosarcoma is the most common sarcoma of the bladder in adults. Patients range in age from 7 to 81 years, with a mean age of 52 years; 10% of cases arise in patients under the age of 20 years. Several cases have developed after cyclophosphamide therapy for other conditions (Rowland & Eble, 1983; Seo et al, 1985). One patient had a family history of bone abnormalities; another patient had bilateral retinoblastoma as an infant, and one-third of patients had urothelial carcinoma (Chen, 1986). Patients usually present with hematuria and obstructive symptoms (Kunze et al, 1994; Sen et al, 1985).

Macroscopically, leiomyosarcoma is most often lobulated or polypoid and may be ulcerated and multifocal (Angulo et al, 1995). A mushroom shape at cystoscopy is typical. The tumors measure up to 13 cm in greatest dimension. Most have the typical appearance of leiomyosarcoma, composed of interweaving fascicles of spindle cells with long blunt-ended nuclei and eosinophilic cytoplasm (Fig 12.8). Nuclear pleomorphism is variable, as is the mitotic rate (Patterson & Barrett, 1983). Necrosis may be present (Van Thillo et al, 1991). Variants include myxoid leiomyosarcoma and epithelioid leiomyosarcoma (leiomyoblastoma).

Immunohistochemical studies usually reveal the absence of cytokeratin immunoreactivity and the presence of staining for vimentin and muscle-specific actin, but exceptions have been described; desmin is variably reactive. Ultrastructural studies reveal typical features of smooth muscle cells, including thin filaments with dense bodies and pinocytotic vesicles (Ozteke et al, 1992).

Leiomyosarcoma may coexist with urothelial carcinoma in situ, noninvasive papillary carcinoma, and invasive urothelial carcinoma, and these should be considered as examples of sarcomatoid carcinoma (carcinosarcoma) if they are intimately admixed. The differential diagnosis of spindle cell lesions in the bladder is extensive. If the tumor is malignant, the major considerations are other types of sarcoma and sarcomatoid carcinoma. Other sarcomas are distinguished by histologic features, immunohistochemical findings, and, if needed, ultrastructural findings. Sarcomatoid carcinoma may mimic high-grade leiomyosarcoma, but, in most cases, sampling reveals a recognizable epithelial component; in cases without identifiable carcinoma, immunohistochemistry is invaluable. Most cases of sarcomatoid carcinoma express cytokeratin at least focally in the spindle cell component and do not stain with muscle markers such as actin and desmin. This distinction is not merely academic; sarcomatoid carcinoma has a much poorer prognosis than leiomyosarcoma. Separation of leiomyoma from low-grade leiomyosarcoma may be difficult because of the lack of unequivocal criteria, similar to many other sites in the body. The presence of significant nuclear pleomorphism, a high mitotic rate, infiltrative growth, and necrosis suggest malignancy (Mills et al, 1989). In this report, the authors considered any tumor with five or more mitotic figures per 10 high-power fields as leiomyosarcoma and cautioned that tumors with even zero or one mitotic figure should be considered malignant if there is infiltrative growth. Caution is warranted in considering any mitotically active smooth muscle tumor of the bladder as benign. In difficult cases with overlapping features, it is best to report "smooth muscle tumor of uncertain malignant potential, favor leiomyoma (or favor low-grade leiomyosarcoma)."

12.3.3 Malignant Fibrous Histiocytoma

Malignant fibrous histiocytoma (MFH) typically presents with hematuria and lower abdominal

(a)

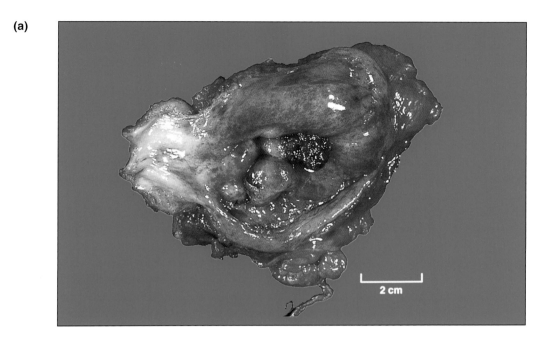

(b)

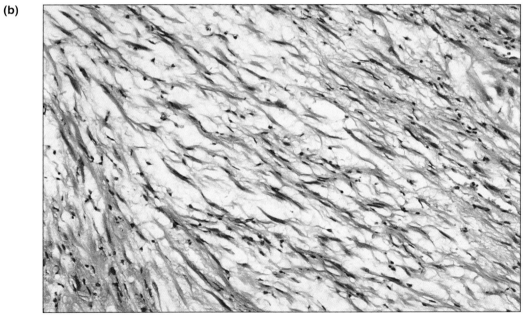

Figure 12.8 Myxoid leiomyosarcoma. **(a):** The bladder lumen is filled and distorted by a large necrotic mass. **(b):** The spindle cells are arranged in fascicles with a prominent myxoid stroma.

215

pain, and all reported cases were locally advanced (Harrison, 1986). Macroscopically, MFH is large, polypoid, and frequently necrotic (Fig 12.9). Variants include inflammatory, myxoid, and pleomorphic MFH (Hendriksen et al, 1982). The major differential diagnostic consideration is sarcomatoid carcinoma (Torenbeek et al, 1994) and giant cell carcinoma, both of which also are typically large and polypoid. Microscopically, sarcomatoid carcinoma frequently shows a storiform pattern, at least focally. One case of MFH coexisted with rhabdoid differentiation (Egawa et al, 1994).

12.3.4 Osteosarcoma

Primary osteosarcoma of the urinary bladder is extremely rare (Okada et al, 1997; Tzakas et al, 1994; Young & Rosenberg, 1985). Most cases occur in men (male:female ratio: 4.5:1) at an average age of 62 years. Presenting symptoms include hematuria, irritative symptoms, and an abdominal mass. Some patients have a previous history of radiation therapy (Young & Rosenberg, 1985).

Macroscopically, osteosarcoma is large, polypoid, and deeply infiltrative (Berenson et al, 1986). Microscopically, the tumor is a high-grade sarcoma with distinct osteoid production. Sarcomatoid carcinoma with osteosarcoma and urothelial carcinoma with osseous metaplasia must be considered in the differential diagnosis. In sarcomatoid carcinoma, the tumor contains an identifiable epithelial component. In urothelial carcinoma with osseous metaplasia, the bone is mature with a lamellar architecture and no cytologic atypia (Eble & Young, 1994). A rare case of osteoma of the bladder has been reported (Collings & Welebir, 1941).

12.3.5 Fibrosarcoma

The diagnosis of fibrosarcoma of the bladder is based on histologic features at other sites. In

two reported cases, the tumor was large, with one extensively involving the retroperitoneum and bladder (Keenan & Buchanan, 1979; Savir & Meiraz, 1980).

12.3.6 Malignant Mesenchymoma

Malignant mesenchymoma is a malignant tumor containing two or more unrelated differentiated tissue types in addition to the fibrosarcoma element. To date, there have been two accepted examples of this entity arising in the bladder. One included leiomyosarcoma and osteosarcoma, and the other included leiomyosarcoma, chondrosarcoma, and osteosarcoma (Terada et al, 1987). Both tumors were pedunculated and polypoid, measuring 3 cm and 18 cm in greatest diameter, respectively. One patient died of progressive disease 21 months after diagnosis, and the other one was alive at 18 months.

12.3.7 Angiosarcoma

Rare examples of primary angiosarcoma of the bladder have been reported, including the epithelioid variant (Figs 12.10 and 12.11) (Stroup & Chang, 1987). Occasional cases resemble Kaposi's sarcoma and may appear in patients with acquired immune deficiency syndrome. The major differential diagnostic consideration is hemangioma, which is much more common. Angiosarcoma of the bladder followed radiation therapy for cervical or prostate carcinoma has been reported (Morgan et al, 1989; Navon et al, 1997).

12.3.8 Hemangiopericytoma

Rare cases of hemangiopericytoma occur in the bladder (Burgess et al, 1993), three of which apparently arose in or near the urachus. All reported cases occurred in adults (four women and one man; age range: 29–50 years). One developed in a patient exposed to polyvinyl alco-

(a)

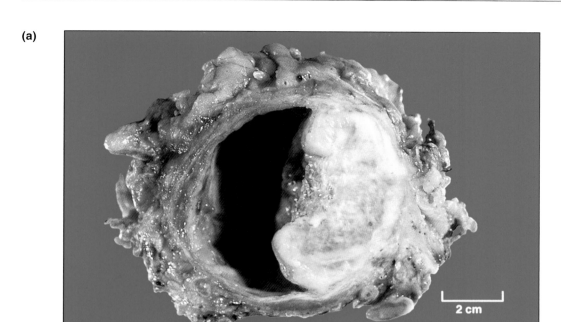

(b)

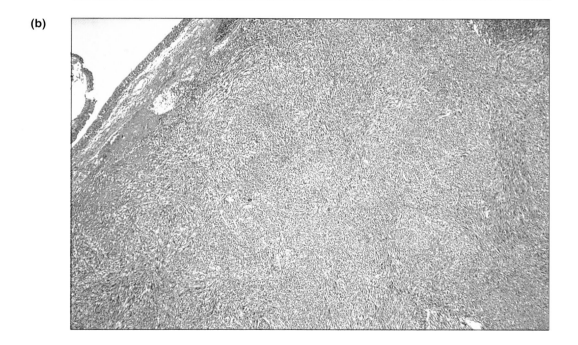

(c)

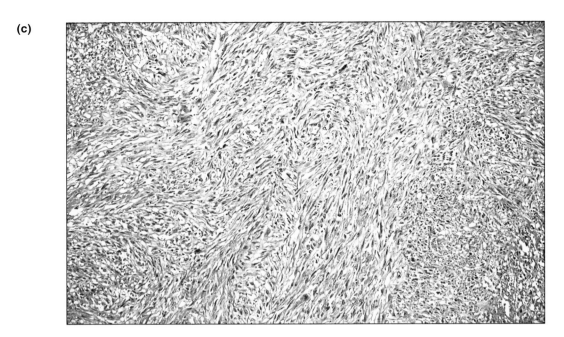

(d)

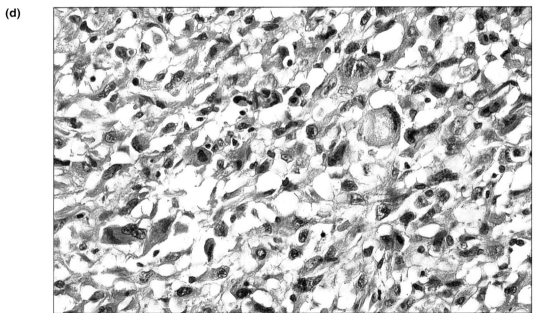

(e)

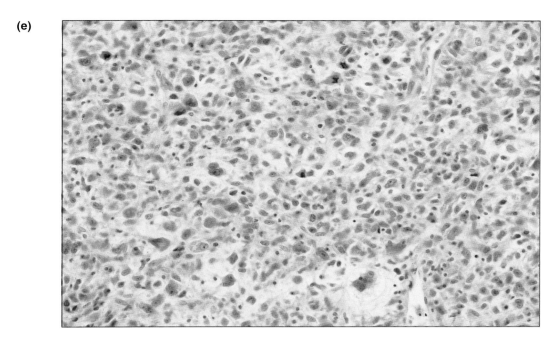

Figure 12.9 Malignant fibrous histiocytoma (high-grade sarcoma). **(a):** This whole mount of the bladder reveals a large fleshy mural mass on one side partially filling the lumen. **(b):** The sarcoma is transmural, with an overlying intact urothelium (top left). **(c):** The spindle cells are predominantly arranged in a storiform pattern. **(d):** There is prominent pleomorphism. **(e):** In another case, large multinucleate cells punctuate sheets of smaller tumor cells.

(a)

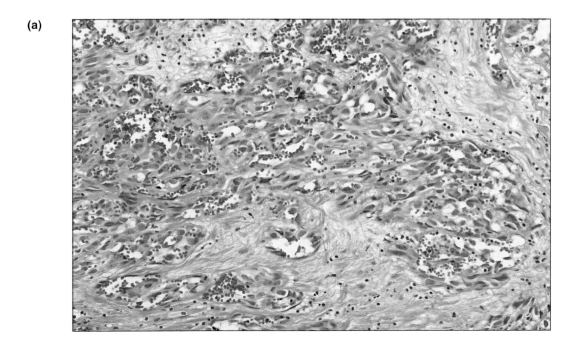

(b)

(c)

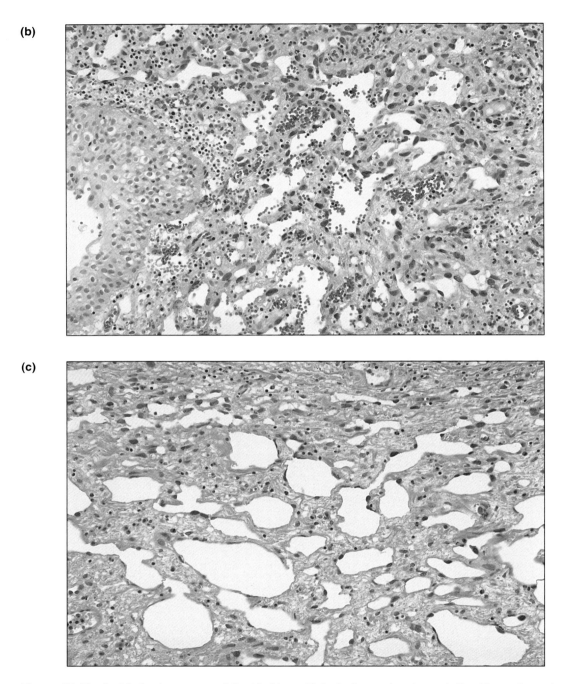

Figure 12.10   (a, b): Angiosarcoma of the bladder, with typical vascular channels lined by malignant endothelial cells. **(c):** The lumens are dilated and the malignant cells may be mistaken for reactive endothelial cells.

(a)

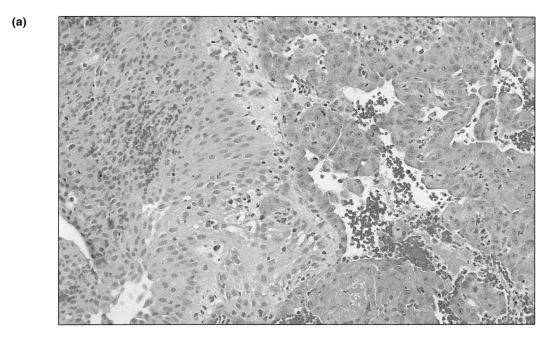

(b)

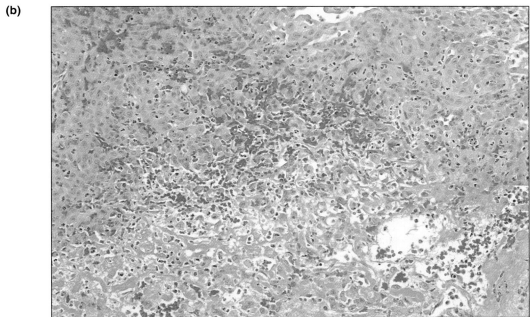

(c)

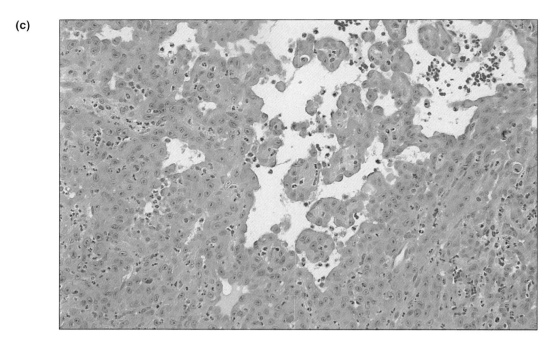

Figure 12.11 Epithelioid angiosarcoma of the urinary bladder. **(a):** The sarcoma (right) is present in intimate association with the urothelium (left), and concern was raised for possible sarcomatoid carcinoma. Elsewhere, **(b)** the angiosarcoma consists of closely packed vascular structures with extravasated red blood cells or **(c)** papillary tufts lined by malignant cells.

hol (Prout & Davis, 1977). Macroscopically, the tumor is solid, ovoid, and well circumscribed. Microscopically, typical features of hemangiopericytoma are present (Fig 12.12). Hemangiopericytoma-like areas can also be found in sarcomatoid carcinoma and leiomyosarcoma of the bladder, and these entities should be considered in the differential diagnosis.

12.3.9 Liposarcoma

A single case of myxoid liposarcoma developed in the bladder of a 36-year-old man. After a partial cystectomy, the patient was alive and free of tumor at 30 months (Rosi et al, 1983).

12.3.10 Rhabdoid Tumor

A small number of cases of primary rhabdoid tumor of the bladder have been reported (Egawa et al, 1994; Harris et al, 1987; McBride et al, 1994).

The first case arose in a 46-year-old woman. The growth contained a mixture of urothelial carcinoma, high-grade sarcoma, and rhabdoid tumor, apparently representing a case of sarcomatoid carcinoma (Egawa et al, 1994). The other cases developed in two girls aged 6 and 14 years, with typical histologic, immunohistochemical, and ultrastructural features of rhabdoid tumor (Harris et al, 1987; McBride et al, 1994). Key diagnostic features include characteristic rhabdoid morphology, constant expression of vimentin, and variable coexpression of cytokeratin. The patients are typically young, and ultrastructural features include whorled cytoplasmic intermediate filaments adjacent to the nucleus.

12.4 SOFT TISSUE TUMORS AND MIXED TUMORS OF THE URACHUS

Benign soft tissue tumors of the urachus are rare, including case reports of fibroma, lei-

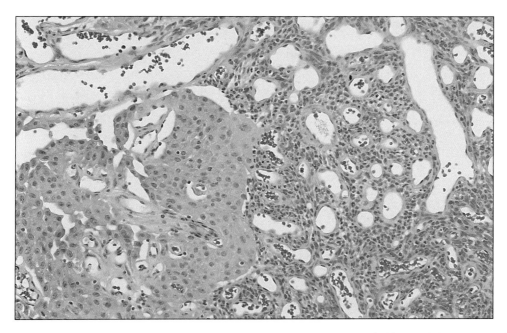

Figure 12.12 Hemangiopericytoma of the urinary bladder. The urothelium (left) stands in contrast with the tumor (right), which consists of a characteristic pattern of anastomosing vessels surrounded by tumor cells with indistinct cellular outlines.

omyoma, and hemangiopericytoma. Tumors composed of epithelial and mesenchymal elements have been reported as fibroadenoma (Loening & Richardson, 1974).

Sarcoma of the urachus comprises approximately 5% of urachal cancers (Butler & Rosenberg, 1959; Powley, 1961). It occurs in a younger population than carcinoma (range: 4 months to 51 years) with a mean age of 21 years. Sarcoma occurs equally in males and females, presenting with symptoms of pain, umbilical discharge, or irritative bladder symptoms; interestingly, hematuria has not been reported. Case reports include fibrosarcoma, hemangiopericytoma (Baglio & Crowson, 1964), rhabdomyosarcoma, and leiomyosarcoma (Noyes & Vinson, 1981).

REFERENCES

Alonso GM, Tramoyeres CA, Pastor SF, et al. Bladder lipoma: apropos of a case. *Arch Esp Urol.* 1982;35:381–383.

Angulo JC, Lopez JI, Flores N. Pseudosarcomatous myofibroblastic proliferation of the bladder: report of 2 cases and literature review. *J Urol.* 1994;151:1008–1012.

Angulo J, Sakr W, Oldford J, et al. Multifocal leiomyosarcoma of the urinary bladder. *J Urol Pathol.* 1995;3:377–384.

August CZ, Khazoum SG, Mutchnik DL. Inflammatory pseudotumor of the bladder: a case report with DNA content analysis. *J Urol Pathol.* 1993;1:211–216.

Baglio CM, Crowson CN. Hemangiopericytoma of urachus: report of a case. *J Urol.* 1964;91:660–661.

Bainbridge TC, Singh RR, Mentzel T, Katenkamp D. Solitary fibrous tumor of urinary bladder: report of two cases. *Hum Pathol.* 1997;28:1204–1206.

Berenson RJ, Flynn S, Freiha FS, et al. Primary osteogenic sarcoma of the bladder: case report and review of the literature. *Cancer.* 1986;57:350–355.

Biermann CW, Gasser TC, Rutishauser G. Kaposi's sarcoma of the urinary bladder after kidney transplantation. *Helv Chir Acta.* 1992;59:503–505.

Biyani CS, Sharma N, Nicol A, Heal MR. Postoperative spindle cell nodule of the bladder: a diagnostic problem. *Urol Int.* 1996;56:119–121.

Bolkier M, Ginesin Y, Lichtig C, et al. Lymphangioma of bladder. *J Urol.* 1983;129:1049–1050.

Bornstein I, Charboneau JW, Hartman GW. Leiomyoma of the bladder: sonographic and urographic findings. *J Ultrasound Med.* 1986;5:407–408.

Boyle M, Gaffney EF, Thurston A. Paraganglioma of the prostatic urethra. A report of 3 cases and a review of the literature. *Br J Urol.* 1996;77:445–448.

Brooks PT, Scally JK. Case report: bladder neurofibromas causing ureteric obstruction in von Recklinghausen's disease. *Clin Radiol.* 1985;36:537–538.

Brown IR, Futter NG. Primary neurilemmoma of the bladder. *Br J Urol.* 1997;79:132–133.

Burgess NA, Hudd C, Matthews PN. Two cases of haemangiopericytoma. *Br J Urol.* 1993;71:238–239.

Burton EM, Schellhammer PF, Weaver DL, et al. Paraganglioma of urinary bladder in patient with neurofibromatosis. *Urology.* 1986;27:550–552.

Butler DB, Rosenberg HS. Sarcoma of the urachus. *Arch Surg.* 1959;79:724–734.

Caro DJ, Brown JS. Hemangioma of bladder. *Urology.* 1976;8:479–481.

Chandna S, Bhatnagar V, Mitra DK, et al. Hemangiolymphangioma of the urinary bladder in a child. *J Ped Surg.* 1987;22:1051–1052.

Chen KTK. Coexisting leiomyosarcoma and transitional cell carcinoma of the urinary bladder. *J Surg Oncol.* 1986;33:36–38.

Clark SS, Marlett MM, Prudencia RF, et al. Neurofibromatosis of the bladder in children: case report and literature review. *J Urol.* 1977;118:654–656.

Collings CW, Welebir F. Osteoma of the bladder. *J Urol.* 1941;46:494–496.

Dahm P, Manseck A, Flössel C, et al. Malignant neurofibroma of the urinary bladder. *Eur Urol.* 1995;27:261–263.

Das S, Bulusu NV, Lowe P. Primary vesical pheochromocytoma. *Urology.* 1983;21:20–25.

Dietrick DD, Kabalin JN, Daniels GF Jr, et al. Inflammatory pseudotumor of the bladder. *J Urol.* 1992;148:141–144.

Eble JN, Young RH. Stromal osseous metaplasia in carcinoma of the bladder. *J Urol.* 1994;145:823–825.

Egawa S, Uchida T, Koshiba K, et al. Malignant fibrous histiocytoma of the bladder with focal rhabdoid tumor differentiation. *J Urol.* 1994;151:154–156.

Fleischmann J, Perinetti EP, Catalona WJ. Embryonal rhabdomyosarcoma of the genitourinary organs. *J Urol.* 1981;126:389–392.

Fletcher MS, Aker M, Hill JT, et al. Granular cell myoblastoma of the bladder. *Br J Urol.* 1985;57:109–110.

Goertchen R, Dominok G, Mobius G. Chordoid sarcoma of the urinary bladder. *Zentralbl Allg Pathol.* 1984;129:379–382.

Gottesman JE, Seale RH. Cavernous haemangioma of the bladder. *Br J Urol.* 1983;55:450–451.

Grignon DJ, Ro JY, Mackay B, et al. Paraganglioma of the urinary bladder: immunohistochemical, ultrastructural, and DNA flow cytometric studies. *Hum Pathol.* 1991;22:1162–1169.

Guillon J, Costa J. Pseudosarcomes post-operatoires du tractus genito-urinaire. Un piege diagnostique. Presentation de 4 observations dont 2 avec etude immunohistochemique et revue de la litterature. *Ann Pathol.* 1989;9:340–345.

Harris MH, Eyden BP, Joglekar VM. Rhabdoid tumor of the bladder: a histological, ultrastructural and immunohistochemical study. *Histopathology.* 1987;11:1083–1092.

Harrison GSM. Malignant fibrous histiocytoma of the bladder. *Br J Urol.* 1986;58:457–459.

Hasui Y, Osada Y, Kitada S, et al. Solitary retrovesical neurofibroma extending to the perineal region. *Urol Int.* 1991;46:90–92.

Hawkins HK, Camacho-Velazquez JV. Rhabdomyosarcoma in children: correlation of form and prognosis in one institution's experience. *Am J Surg Pathol.* 1987;11:531–536.

Hendriksen OB, Mogensen P, Engelholm AJ. Inflammatory fibrous histiocytoma of the urinary bladder. *Acta Pathol Microbiol Immunol Scand [A].* 1982;90:333–337.

Hendry WF, Vinnicombe J. Haemangioma of bladder in children and young adults. *Br J Urol.* 1971;43:209–216.

Hintsa A, Lindell O, Heikkila P. Neurofibromatosis of the bladder. *Scand J Urol Nephrol.* 1996;30:497–499.

Hockley NM, Bihrle R, Bennet RM 3rd, et al. Congenital genitourinary hemangiomas in a patient with Klippel-Trenaunay syndrome: management with the neodynium YAG laser. *J Urol.* 1989;141:940–941.

Hojo H, Newton WA Jr, Hamoudi AB, et al. Pseudosarcomatous myofibroblastic tumor of the urinary bladder in children: a study of 11 cases with review of the literature. An intergroup rhabdomyosarcoma study. *Am J Surg Pathol.* 1995;19:1224–1236.

Huang W-L, Ro JY, Grignon DJ, et al. Postoperative spindle cell nodule of the prostate and bladder. *J Urol.* 1990;143:824–826.

Hughes DF, Biggart JD, Hayes D. Pseudosarcomatous lesions of the urinary bladder. *Histopathology.* 1991;18:67–71.

Hulsa CA. Neurofibromatosis: bladder involvement with malignant degeneration. *J Urol.* 1990;144:742–743.

Jones EC, Clement PB, Young RH. Inflammatory pseudotumor of the urinary bladder: a clinicopathological, immunohistochemical, ultrastructural and flow cytometric study of 13 cases. *Am J Surg Pathol.* 1993;17:264–274.

Jufe R, Molinolo AA, Fefer SA, et al. Plasma cell granuloma of the bladder: a case report. *J Urol.* 1984;131:1175–1176.

Karol JB, Eason AA, Tanagho EA. Fibrous histiocytoma of the bladder. *Urology.* 1977;10:593–595.

Keenan RA, Buchanan JD. Fibrosarcoma of the bladder exhibiting endocrine characteristics of phaeochromocytoma. *J R Soc Med.* 1979;72:618–620.

Khan LB. Spindle cell and miscellaneous proliferative lesions of the urinary bladder. In: Nochomovitz LE, ed. *Bladder biopsy interpretation.* New York: Raven Press; 1992.

Kindblom LG, Meis-Kindblom JM, Havel G, et al. Benign epithelial schwannoma. *Am J Surg Pathol.* 1998;22:762–770.

Knoll LD, Segura JW, Scheithauer BW. Leiomyoma of the bladder. *J Urol.* 1986;136:906–908.

Kunze E, Theuring F, Kruger G. Primary mesenchymal tumors of the urinary bladder. A histological and immunohistochemical study of 30 cases. *Pathol Res Pract.* 1994;190:311–332.

Lakshmanan Y, Wills ML, Gearhart JP. Inflammatory (pseudosarcomatous) myofibroblastic tumor of the bladder. *Urology.* 1997;50:285–288.

Lam KY, Chan AC. Paraganglioma of the urinary bladder: an immunohistochemical study and report of an unusual association with intestinal carcinoid. *Aust N Z J Surg.* 1993;63:740–745.

Loening S, Richardson JR. Fibroadenoma of the urachus. *J Urol.* 1974;112:759–761.

Loh CS, Richards CJ, Jenkins BJ. Bladder neck leiomyoma causing obstructive renal failure. *Scand J Urol Nephrol.* 1996;30:495–496.

Lopez-Beltran A, Lopez-Ruiz J, Vicioso L. Inflammatory pseudotumors of the urinary bladder. *Urol Int.* 1995;55:173–176.

Lopez-Beltran A, Escudero AL, Cavazzana AO, et al. Sarcomatoid transitional cell carcinoma of the renal pelvis. A report of five cases with clinical, pathological, immunohistochemical and DNA ploidy analysis. *Pathol Res Pract.* 1996;192:1181–1296.

Lundgren L, Aldenborg F, Angervall L, et al. Pseudomalignant spindle cell proliferations of the urinary bladder. *Hum Pathol.* 1994;25:181–191.

Martin C. Pure fibroma of the bladder: report of a case. *Urol Cutan Rev.* 1936;40:542–546.

McBride JA, Ro JY, Hicks J, et al. Malignant rhabdoid tumor of the bladder in an adolescent. *J Urol Pathol.* 1994;2:255–264.

Melicow MM. Tumors of the urinary bladder: a clinico-pathological analysis of over 2500 specimens and biopsies. *J Urol.* 1955;74:498–521.

Mentzel T, Bainbridge TC, Katenkamp D. Solitary fibrous tumor: clinicopathological, immunohistochemical, and ultrastructural analysis of 12 cases arising in soft tissues, nasal cavity and nasopharynx, urinary bladder and prostate. *Virchows Arch.* 1997;430:445–453.

Miettinen M. Rhabdomyosarcoma in patients older than 40 years of age. *Cancer.* 1988; 62:2060–2065.

Mills SE, Bova GS, Wick MR, et al. Leiomyosarcoma of the urinary bladder. A clinicopathologic and immunohistochemical study of 15 cases. *Am J Surg Pathol.* 1989;13:480–489.

Mincione GP, Gasbarre M, Paglierani M, et al. Pseudosarcoma of the urinary bladder. *Pathologica.* 1995;87:554–558.

Misawa T, Shibasaki T, Toshima R, et al. A case of pheochromocytoma of the urinary bladder in a long-term hemodialysis patient. *Nephron.* 1993;64: 443–446.

Mooney J, Willis D, Benson GS, et al. Urinary bladder neurofibroma with Wagner-Meissner bodies. *J Urol Pathol.* 1994;2:283–290.

Mor Y, Hitchcock RJI, Zaidi SZ, et al. Bladder hemangioma as a cause of massive hematuria in a child. *Scand J Urol Nephrol.* 1997;31:305–307.

Morgan MA, Moutos DM, Pippitt CH Jr, et al. Vaginal and bladder angiosarcoma after therapeutic irradiation. *South Med J.* 1989;82:1434–1436.

Mostofi FK, Moss WH. Polypoid rhabdomyosarcoma: sarcoma botryoides of bladder in children. *J Urol.* 1952;67:681–685.

Mouradian JA, Coleman JW, McGovern JH, et al. Granular cell tumor (myoblastoma) of the bladder. *J Urol.* 1974;112:343–344.

Moyana TN, Kontozoglu T. Urinary bladder paragangliomas: an immunohistochemical study. *Arch Pathol Lab Med.* 1988;112:70–72.

Nochomovitz LE, Orenstein JM. Inflammatory pseudotumor of the urinary bladder: possible relationship to nodular fasciitis. Two case reports, cytologic observations, and ultrastructural observations. *Am J Surg Pathol.* 1985;9:366–373.

Noyes D, Vinson RK. Urachal leiomyosarcoma. *Urology.* 1981;17:279–281.

Okada E, Hasegawa Y, Takahashi K, et al. Primary osteosarcoma of the urinary bladder. *Int Urol Nephrol.* 1997;29:437–440.

Ozteke O, Demirel A, Aydin NE, et al. Bladder leiomyosarcoma: report of three cases. *Int Urol Nephrol.* 1992;24:393–396.

Patterson DE, Barrett DM. Leiomyosarcoma of urinary bladder. *Urology.* 1983;21:367–369.

Powley PH. Sarcoma of the urachus. *Br J Surg.* 1961;48:649–653.

Proppe KH, Scully RE, Rosai J. Postoperative spindle cell nodules of genitourinary tract resembling sarcomas. A report of eight cases. *Am J Surg Pathol.* 1984;8:101–108.

Prout MN, Davis HL Jr. Hemangiopericytoma of the bladder after polyvinyl alcohol exposure. *Cancer.* 1977;39:1328–1330.

Radke M, Waldschmidt J, Stolpe HJ, et al. Blue rubber-bleb-nevus syndrome with predominant urinary bladder hemangiomatosis. *Eur J Pediatr Surg.* 1993;3:313–316.

Ro JY, Ayala AG, Ordonez NG, et al. Pseudosarcomatous fibromyxoid tumor of the urinary bladder. *Am J Clin Pathol.* 1986;86:583–590.

Ro JY, El-Naggar AK, Amin MB, et al. Pseudosarcomatous fibromyxoid tumor of the urinary bladder and prostate: immunohistochemical, ultrastructural, and DNA flow cytometric analyses of nine cases. *Hum Pathol.* 1993;24:1203–1210.

Rosi P, Selli C, Carini M, et al. Myxoid liposarcoma of the bladder. *J Urol.* 1983;130:560–561.

Rowland RG, Eble JN. Bladder leiomyosarcoma and pelvic fibroblastic tumor following cyclophosphamide therapy. *J Urol.* 1983;130:344–346.

Royal SA, Hedlund GL, Galliani CA. Rhabdomyosarcoma of the dome of the urinary bladder. A difficult imaging diagnosis. *Am J Roentgen.* 1996;167:524–525.

Saavedra JA, Manivel JC, Essenfeld H, et al. Pseudosarcomatous myofibroblastic proliferations in children. *Cancer.* 1990;66:1234–1241.

Sandhu SS, Iacovou JW. Pseudotumor of the bladder. *J R Soc Med.* 1997;90:46–47.

Sane SY, Garpure SS, Borwankar SS. Neurogenic tumor of the urinary bladder (a case report). *J Postgrad Med.* 1991;37:115–116.

Savir A, Meiraz D. Malignant mesodermal (mesenchymal) tumors of the bladder. *Urology.* 1980;16:307–309.

Sen SE, Malek RS, Farrow GM, et al. Sarcoma and carcinosarcoma of the bladder in adults. *J Urol.* 1985;133:29–30.

Seo IS, Clark SA, McGovern FD, et al. Leiomyosarcoma of the urinary bladder: 13 years after cyclophosphamide therapy for Hodgkin's disease. *Cancer.* 1985;55:1597–1603.

Stroup RM, Chang YC. Angiosarcoma of the bladder: a case report. *J Urol.* 1987;137:984–985.

Suhler A, Masson JC, Pages C, et al. Bladder leiomyomas and fibromas. Apropos of 8 cases. *Ann Urol.* 1994;28:28–32.

Swartz DA, Johnson DE, Ayala AG, et al. Bladder leiomyosarcoma: a review of 10 cases with 5-year followup. *J Urol.* 1985;133:200–202.

Terada Y, Saito I, Morohoshi T, et al. Malignant mesenchymoma of the bladder. *Cancer.* 1987;60:858–860.

Torenbeek R, Blomjous CE, de Bruin PC, et al. Sarcomatoid carcinoma of the urinary bladder. Clinicopathologic analysis of 18 cases with immunohistochemical and electron microscopic findings. *Am J Surg Pathol.* 1994;18:241–249.

Tzakas K, Ioannidis S, Dimitriadis G, et al. Primary osteochondrosarcoma of the urinary bladder. *Br J Urol.* 1994;73:320–321.

Van Thillo EL, Casselman J, Defloor E. Leiomyosarcoma of urinary bladder. *Acta Urol Belg.* 1991;59:113–118.

Vicente-Rodriguez J, Garat JM, Perea C, et al. Hemangiomes vesicaux. *J Urol.* 1986;92:43–46.

Wick MR, Brown BA, Young RH, et al. Spindle cell proliferations of the urinary tract: an immunohistochemical study. *Am J Surg Pathol.* 1988;12:379–389.

Winfield HN, Catalona WJ. An isolated plexiform neurofibroma of the bladder. *J Urol.* 1985;134:542–543.

Wyman HE, Chappell BS, Jones WR Jr. Ganglioneuroma of the bladder. Report of a case. *J Urol.* 1950;63:526–532.

Young RH. Pseudoneoplastic lesions of the urinary bladder. *Pathol Ann.* 1988;23:67–87.

Young RH, Rosenberg AE. Osteosarcoma of the urinary bladder. Report of a case and review of the literature. *Cancer.* 1985;59:174–178.

Young RH, Scully RE. Pseudosarcomatous lesions of the urinary bladder, prostate gland, and urethra. A report of three cases and review of the literature. *Arch Pathol Lab Med.* 1987;111:354–358.

Young RH, Proppe KH, Dickersin GR, et al. Myxoid leiomyosarcoma of the urinary bladder. *Arch Pathol Lab Med.* 1987;111:359–362.

13

HEMATOLYMPHOID MALIGNANCIES AND OTHER RARE TUMORS

13.1 MALIGNANT LYMPHOMA AND LEUKEMIA

13.1.1 Malignant Lymphoma

The bladder is secondarily involved in up to 13% of cases of non-Hodgkin's lymphoma at autopsy (Clarke & Maxwell, 1991; Freeman et al, 1972; Kempton et al, 1997), and most patients have no bladder symptoms. Primary malignant lymphoma in the bladder is very rare, with less than 100 reported cases, accounting for only 0.2% of extranodal lymphomas (Kempton et al, 1997; Simpson et al, 1990). Up to 13% of patients with advanced lymphoma have involvement of the lower urinary tract at autopsy; however, only 1% of these are clinically apparent (Kempton et al, 1997). In an autopsy series of 1,467 extranodal lymphomas, only two were located in the bladder (Freeman et al, 1972). Most examples have been reported as single cases, and histologic classification has varied greatly, with only a small number having immunologic studies to phenotype the lymphoma (Kuhara et al, 1990; Ohsawa et al, 1993; Pawade et al, 1993; Siegelbaum et al, 1986). Most patients with primary lymphoma are women (fe-

male-to-male ratio: 6.5:1), with a median age of 64 years. Signs and symptoms include gross hematuria, dysuria, and irritative symptoms.

Cystoscopically, lymphoma appears as single or multiple masses that are sessile or polypoid. The mucosa overlying the mass is usually intact, and this is a useful diagnostic clue. The tissue specimen for examination usually comes from a biopsy or transurethral resection (Simpson et al, 1990). Histologically, the tumor consists of a diffuse infiltrate of lymphoid cells surrounding and permeating normal structures rather than replacing them (Fig 13.1). Lymphoepithelial lesions are often frequent. The most common types of lymphoma are mucosa-associated lymphoid tissue (MALT)-type lymphoma (Fig 13.2), diffuse large cell lymphoma, and small lymphocytic lymphoma (Kempton et al, 1997; Pawade et al, 1993). Less frequent types include follicular, plasmacytoid (Biancari et al, 1998), mantle zone, and monocytoid lymphoma (Abraham et al, 1993; Mourad et al, 1998; Ohsawa et al, 1993). Rare cases of lymphoma arise synchronously in association with adenocarcinoma and urothelial carcinoma.

Immunohistochemically, almost all bladder lymphomas are of B-cell origin and display

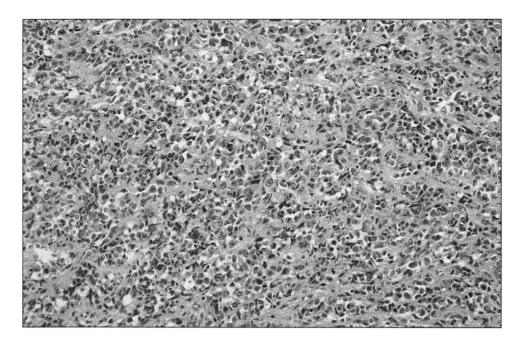

Figure 13.1 Small lymphocytic lymphoma involving the wall of the bladder.

monoclonality (Abraham et al, 1993), although rare T-cell lymphomas have been described (Mourad et al, 1998). The most common type of primary lymphoma is a low-grade lymphoma of the MALT type (Kempton et al, 1997). Primary Hodgkin's disease and immunoblastic sarcoma are extremely rare (Bocian et al, 1982; Forrest et al, 1983). Bladder outflow obstruction may result from lymphomatoid granulomatosis and Burkitt's lymphoma (Feinberg et al, 1987; Lewis et al, 1983).

The overall survival for bladder lymphoma is estimated to be 68%–73% at 1 year and 27%–34% at 5 years (Guthman et al, 1990; Kempton et al, 1997). Patients with nonlocalized bladder involvement without a prior history of lymphoma who present with symptoms attributable only to the bladder had a mean cancer-specific survival of 4 years. For primary bladder lymphoma, the type of treatment, including surgery, radiation, and chemotherapy, had no apparent effect on survival (Kempton et al, 1997).

The major differential diagnostic considerations are florid chronic cystitis, small cell carcinoma, lymphoepithelioma-like carcinoma, and lymphoma-like carcinoma.

13.1.2 Leukemia

At autopsy, fewer than 18% of patients who died of chronic lymphocytic leukemia and chronic myelogenous leukemia had bladder involvement (Gilver, 1971). The frequency is somewhat higher in patients with acute leukemia. Grossly, there are mucosal nodules or foci of hemorrhagic thickening. Granulocytic sarcoma rarely involves the urinary bladder.

13.1.3 Multiple Myeloma

The bladder is rarely involved with multiple myeloma or a solitary plasmacytoma (Gesme et al, 1994). There is no apparent sex predilection, and adult patients of all ages may be affected

(a)

(b)

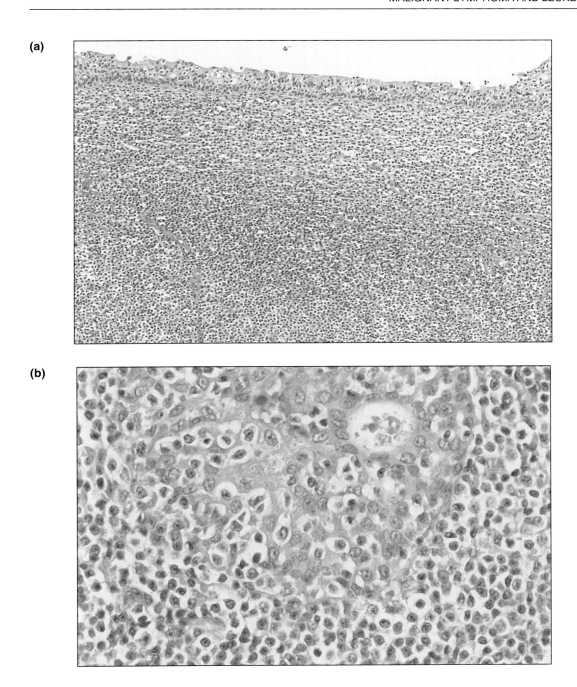

Figure 13.2 Mucosa-associated lymphoid tissue lymphoma of the bladder. **(a):** The infiltrate fills the submucosa; **(b):** lymphoepithelial lesion is typical.

(range: 28–89 years). Most patients present with hematuria, and urine cytology may reveal malignant plasma cells (Neal et al, 1985). The tumor forms solid polypoid or pedunculated masses composed of sheets of plasma cells with varying degrees of atypia (Yang et al, 1982). The mucosa is typically intact.

13.2 MELANOMA

Primary malignant melanoma is rare in the bladder, with fewer than 15 reported cases (Fig 13.3) (De Torres et al, 1995). It occurs with equal frequency in men and women, and the age ranges from 44 to 81 years. Most patients present with gross hematuria or metastases (Ironside et al, 1985). Macroscopically, melanoma is dark brown to black, polypoid or fungating, and solid or infiltrating. Some cases have a flat or "macular" appearance. It may arise anywhere in the bladder; histologically it resembles melanoma at other sites, with a variable amount of pigment. Occasionally, melanocytes may be present in the adjacent urothelium. All cases display immunoreactiviy for S-100 protein and HMB45. Two cases of spindle cell melanoma of the bladder were recently reported (De Torres et al, 1995).

The major differential diagnostic concern is metastatic melanoma to the bladder (Table 13.1). Metastasis is much more common than primary melanoma, and these patients invariably die of disease within 24 months. One case of melanoma metastasized to a urothelial carcinoma (Arapantoni-Dadioti et al, 1995).

13.3 GERM CELL TUMORS

13.3.1 Dermoid Cyst

Rarley, dermoid cyst arises in the bladder of women between 30 and 49 years old, all presenting with nonspecific symptoms (Cauffield,

1956). Typical pathologic features of a dermoid cyst are present, including hair, teeth, and calcifications (Sabnis et al, 1993). The possibility of direct extension from an ovarian teratoma should be considered (Valizadeh et al, 1991).

13.3.2 Choriocarcinoma

Fewer than 30 cases of choriocarcinoma arising in the bladder have been described (Fig 13.4) (Cho et al, 1992). At least 70% of these cases are mixed with a recognizable papillary or solid urothelial carcinoma component, although some apparently pure cases have been reported (Obe et al, 1983). Tumor giant cells and syncytiotrophoblastic giant cells may be seen without cytotrophoblasts (Fig 13.5), and such cases should be classified as urothelial carcinoma with trophoblastic differentiation rather than choriocarcinoma (Fowler et al, 1992). Some cases of urothelial carcinoma display human chorionic gonadotropin (HCG) immunoreactivity in mononuclear cells without evidence of trophoblastic differentiation (Seidal et al, 1993; Shah et al, 1986; Yokoyama et al, 1992). Patients usually have symptoms typical of other bladder cancers, including hematuria, dysuria, and frequency. Gynecomastia occurs in some men,

Table 13.1 Diagnostic criteria for distinction between primary and metastatic malignant melanoma of the urinary bladder

- No prior history of melanoma of the skin or other site
- Careful examination of the entire skin surface, including use of a Wood's light to exclude a depigmented area that may represent a regressed melanoma
- Clinical studies to exclude an ophthalmic or other visceral primary site
- Pattern of metastasis or recurrence should be consistent with a primary bladder tumor rather than metastatic melanoma
- Atypical melanocytes should be present in the mucosa adjacent to the tumor nodule

(a)

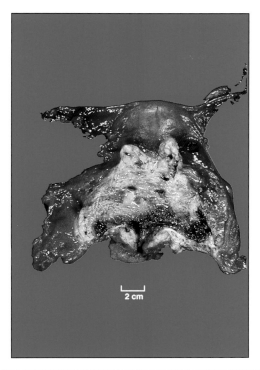

(b)

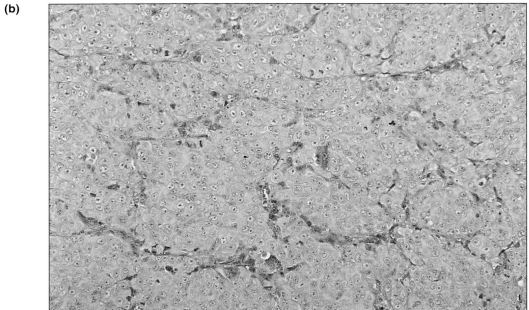

Figure 13.3 Primary malignant melanoma of the urethra and bladder neck. **(a):** Grossly, part of the tumor displays jet-black pigment; **(b):** typical features of melanoma, with a mixture of pigmented and non-pigmented cells. The tumor displayed intense cytoplasmic immunoreactivity for S-100 protein and HMB45 (not shown).

231

(a)

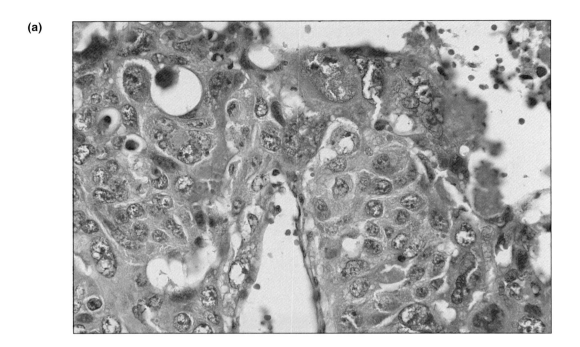

(b)

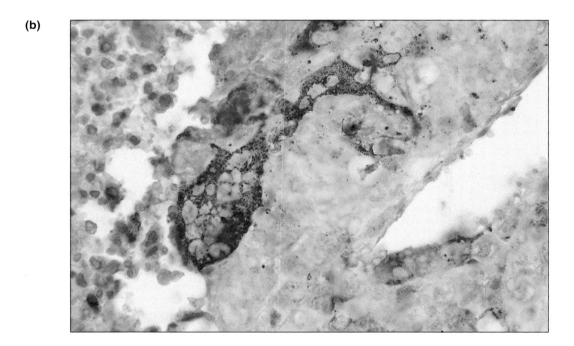

Figure 13.4 **(a):** Choriocarcinoma of the urinary bladder with classic findings of syncytiotrophoblasts forming an adherent covering over the cytotrophoblasts. **(b):** Immunoreactivity for human chorionic gonadotropin is limited to the syncytiotrophoblasts.

(a)

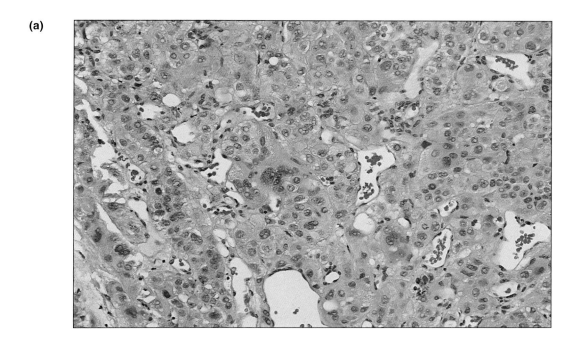

(b)

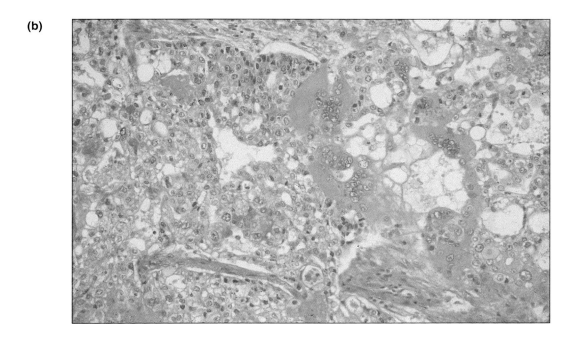

Figure 13.5 **(a):** Rare syncytiotrophoblasts in urothelial carcinoma; compare with **(b),** which contains an abundance of syncytiotrophoblasts. (Courtesy of Dr. Carlos Lopes, Oporto, Portugal.)

(a)

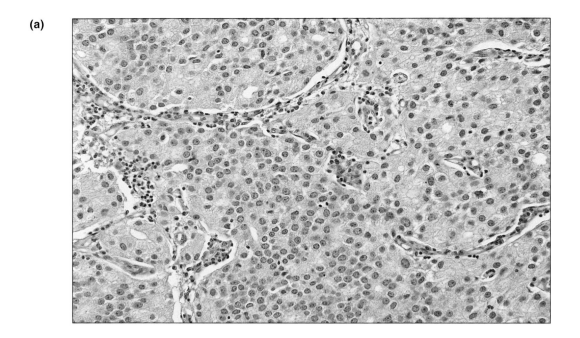

(b)

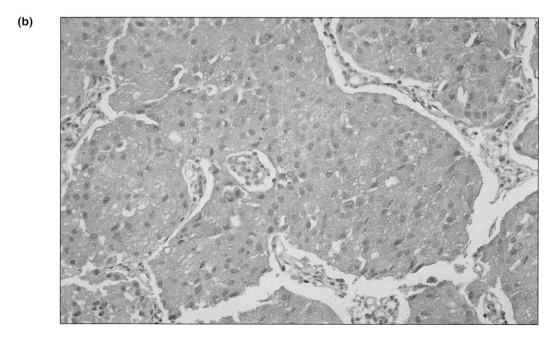

Figure 13.6 **(a):** High-grade prostatic adenocarcinoma mimicking urothelial carcinoma with contiguous spread to the bladder. **(b):** Prostatic origin was confirmed by diffuse immunoreactivity for prostate-specific antigen.

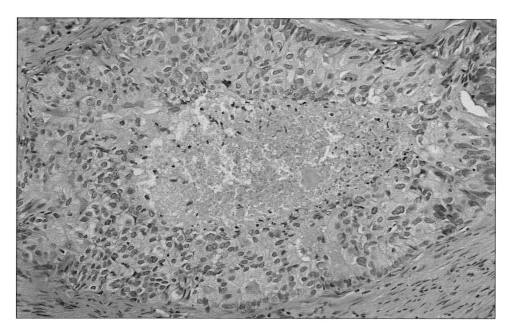

Figure 13.7 High-grade prostatic adenocarcinoma mimicking urothelial carcinoma with comedonecrosis that extensively involved the bladder neck.

and increased levels of serum or urinary gonadotropins may be present.

A pure choriocarcinoma is highly aggressive and usually associated with hemorrhage and necrosis. The significance of HCG production by a urothelial carcinoma with or without trophoblastic differentiation is uncertain, although in most cases with HCG immunoreactivity, there is concomitant elevation of the serum HCG (Martin et al, 1989). The presence of HCG immunoreactivity significantly correlated with the presence of squamous differentiation and a poor response to radiation therapy (Martin et al, 1989). Occasional HCG immunoreactivity has also been observed in squamous cell carcinoma of the bladder associated with schistosomiasis.

13.3.3 Other Germ Cell Tumors

Rare cases of teratoma have been described, including one arising in an 8-year-old, which was cured by complete excision (Misra et al, 1997). A case of seminoma involving the bladder was reported (Khandekar et al, 1993), and a yolk sac tumor has also been described (Taylor et al, 1983).

13.4 SECONDARY TUMORS

Secondary tumors represent up to 14% of bladder neoplasms. Most represent direct invasion from cancer arising in adjacent organs, including colonic cancer (Okaneya et al, 1991), prostatic cancer, and malignant lymphoma. Most cases of secondary involvement by prostatic adenocarcinoma are readily recognized by the distinctive histology of the tumor and the use of immunohistochemical stains for prostatic specific-antigen and prostatic acid phosphatase (Figs 13.6 and 13.7). The use of CEA, **OC125**, and vimentin may also be useful (Torenbeek et al, 1998).

Metastases to the bladder from distant organs are less common than contiguous spread. Overall, distant metastases account for up to

3.5% of secondary tumors. Malignant melanoma (38%) and carcinoma of the stomach (23%), breast (11%), kidney (10%), and lung (8%) are most common (Goldstein, 1967). Metastases should be suspected in any bladder tumor with an unusual histology and in cases of pure adenocarcinoma or squamous cell carcinoma. Occasional cases of pelvic lipomatosis can simulate a neoplasm extending to the bladder (Fogg & Smyth, 1968).

REFERENCES

Abraham NZ, Maher TJ, Hutchinson RE. Extra-nodal monocytoid B-cell lymphoma of the urinary bladder. *Mod Pathol.* 1993;6:145–149.

Arapantoni-Dadioti P, Panayiotides J, Kalkandi P, et al. Metastasis of malignant melanoma to a transitional cell carcinoma of the urinary bladder. *Eur J Surg Oncol.* 1995;21:92–93.

Biancari F, Lepidini G, D'Andrea V. Recurrent plasmacytoid lymphocytic lymphoma of the bladder secreting monoclonal and biclonal proteins. *J Urol.* 1998;159:985.

Bocian JJ, Elam MS, Mendoza CA. Hodgkin's disease involving the urinary bladder diagnosed by urinary cytology: a case report. *Cancer.* 1982;50: 2482–2485.

Cauffield EW. Dermoid cysts of the bladder. *J Urol.* 1956;75:801–803.

Cho JH, Yu E, Kim KH, et al. Primary choriocarcinoma of the urinary bladder: a case report. *J Korean Med Sci.* 1992;7:369–372.

Clarke NW, Maxwell AJ. Primary lymphoma of the urinary bladder. *Br J Urol.* 1991;64:761–762.

De Torres I, Fortuno MA, Raventos A, et al. Primary malignant melanoma of the bladder: immunohistochemical study of a new case and review of the literature. *J Urol.* 1995;154:525–527.

Feinberg SM, Leslie KO, Colby TV. Bladder outlet obstruction by so-called lymphomatoid granulomatosis (angicentric lymphoma). *J Urol.* 1987;137: 989–990.

Fogg LB, Smyth JW. Pelvic lipomatosis: a condition simulating pelvic neoplasm. *Radiology.* 1968;90: 558–559.

Forrest JB, Saypol DC, Mills SE, et al. Immunoblastic sarcoma of the bladder. *J Urol.* 1983;130:350–351.

Fowler AL, Hall E, Rees G. Choriocarcinoma arising in transitional cell carcinoma of the bladder. *Br J Urol.* 1992;70:333–334.

Freeman C, Berg JW, Cutler SJ. Occurrence and prognosis of extranodal lymphomas. *Cancer.* 1972;29: 253–260.

Gesme D Jr, Boatman D, Weinman G, et al. Extramedullary plasmacytoma of skin, bowel and bladder. *Iowa Med.* 1994;84:354–355.

Gilver RL. Involvement of the bladder in leukemia and lymphoma. *J Urol.* 1971;105:667–669.

Goldstein AG. Metastatic carcinoma to the bladder. *J Urol.* 1967;98:209–215.

Guthman DA, Malek RS, Chapman WR, et al. Primary malignant lymphoma of the bladder. *J Urol.* 1990;144:1367–1369.

Ironside JW, Timperley WR, Madden JW, et al. Primary melanoma of the urinary bladder presenting with intracerebral metastases. *Br J Urol.* 1985;57:593–594.

Kempton CL, Kurtin PJ, Inwards DJ, et al. Malignant lymphoma of the bladder: evidence from 36 cases that low-grade lymphoma of the MALT-type is the most common primary bladder lymphoma. *Am J Surg Pathol,* 1997;21:1324–1333.

Khandekar JD, Holland JM, Rochester D, Christ ML. Extragonadal seminoma involving urinary bladder and arising in the prostate. *Cancer.* 1993;71: 3972–3974.

Kuhara H, Tamura Z, Suchi T, et al. Primary malignant lymphoma of the urinary bladder. *Acta Pathol Jpn.* 1990;40:764–769.

Lewis RH, Mannarino FG, Worsham GF, et al. Burkitt's lymphoma presenting as urinary outflow obstruction. *J Urol.* 1983;130:120–124.

Martin JE, Jenkins BJ, Zuk RJ. Human chorionic gonadotropin expression and histological findings as predictor of response to radiotherapy in carcinoma of the bladder. *Virchows Arch A.* 1989;414: 273–277.

Misra S, Agarwal PK, Tandon RK, et al. Bladder teratoma: a case report and review of literature. *Indian J Cancer.* 1997;34:20–21.

Mourad WA, Khalil S, Radwi A, et al. Primary T-cell lymphoma of the urinary bladder. *Am J Surg Pathol.* 1998;22:373–377.

Neal MH, Swearingen ML, Gawronski L, et al. Myeloma cells in the urine. *Arch Pathol Lab Med.* 1985;109:870–872.

Obe JA, Rosen N, Koss LG. Primary choriocarcinoma of the urinary bladder. Report of a case with probable epithelial origin. *Cancer.* 1983;52:1405–1409.

Ohsawa M, Aozasa K, Horiuchi K, et al. Malignant lymphoma of bladder. Report of three cases and review of the literature. *Cancer.* 1993;72:1969–1974.

Okaneya T, Inoue Y, Ogawa A. Solitary urethral recurrence of sigmoid colon carcinoma. *Urol Int.* 1991;47:105–107.

Pawade J, Banerjee SS, Harris M, et al. Lymphomas of mucosa-associated lymphoid tissue arising in the urinary bladder. *Histopathology.* 1993;23:147–151.

Sabnis RB, Bradoo AM, Desai RM, et al. Primary benign vesical teratoma. A case report. *Arch Esp Urol.* 1993;46:444–445.

Seidal T, Breborowicz J, Malmstrom PU. Immunoreactivity to human chorionic gonadotropin in urothelial carcinoma: correlation with tumor grade, stage, and progression. *J Urol Pathol.* 1993;1:397–410.

Shah VM, Newman J, Crocker J, et al. Ectopic beta-human chorionic gonadotropin production by bladder urothelial neoplasia. *Arch Pathol Lab Med.* 1986;110:107–111.

Siegelbaum MH, Edmonds P, Seidmon EJ. Use of immunohistochemistry for identification of primary lymphoma of the bladder. *J Urol.* 1986;136:1074–1076.

Simpson RHW, Bridger JE, Anthony PP, et al. Malignant lymphoma of the lower urinary tract. A clinicopathological study with review of the literature. *Br J Urol.* 1990;65:254–260.

Taylor G, Jordan M, Churchill B, et al. Yolk sac tumor of the bladder. *J Urol.* 1983;129:591–594.

Torenbeek R, Lagendijk JH, Van Diest PJ, et al. Value of a panel of antibodies to identify the primary origin of adenocarcinomas presenting as bladder carcinoma. *Histopathology.* 1998;32:20–27.

Valizadeh A, Arend P, Diallo B, et al. Dermoid cyst of the bladder. Case report. *Acta Urol Belg.* 1991;59:79–83.

Yang C, Motteram R, Sandeman TF. Extramedullary plasmacytoma of the bladder: a case report and review of literature. *Cancer.* 1982;50:146–149.

Yokoyama S, Hayashida Y, Nagahama J, et al. Primary and metaplastic choriocarcinoma of the bladder. A report of two cases. *Acta Cytol.* 1992;36:176–182.

237

14

URINE CYTOLOGY

This chapter discusses the spectrum of cytologic abnormalities in voided urine samples and washings to allow comparison with the biopsy findings described elsewhere in the text. For a more complete description of urine cytology, the reader is referred to specialized texts in this field.

14.1 UTILITY OF URINE CYTOLOGY

14.1.1 Indications

Cytologic examination of the urine sediment may be of value in the diagnosis of a wide variety of benign and malignant diseases of the bladder, urethra, ureter, and renal pelvis (Koss, 1997; Ooms and Veldhuizen, 1993; Potts et al, 1997). This chapter focuses mainly on diagnostic cytology of the urothelium with special emphasis on bladder diseases. Urine cytology has important limitations; for example, this method is not fully reliable for the identification of low-grade papillary tumors despite recent improvements (Maier et al, 1995). However, cytology yields good to excellent results in the identification of urothelial dysplasia, carcinoma in situ, and high-grade cancer (Gamarra & Zeima, 1984). The principal indications for the use of cytology in disorders of the urinary tract are as follows:

- diagnosis of urothelial dysplasia, carcinoma in situ, and high-grade carcinoma.
- follow-up of patients with a urothelial tumor, regardless of grade.
- monitoring of patients with a urothelial tumor undergoing or after treatment (Badalament et al, 1987; Berlac & Holm, 1992; Chow et al, 1994; Koss, 1997; Koss et al., 1985; Schwalb et al, 1993).

The major diagnostic categories are presented in Table 14.1.

14.1.2 Types of Cytology Specimens

The source of most urine cytology specimens is voided or randomly voided urine (Matzkin et al, 1992), catheterized urine specimen, bladder washing (barbotage), brushing (Bian et al, 1995), or an ileal conduit urine specimen.

14.2 NORMAL COMPONENTS OF THE URINARY SEDIMENT

14.2.1 Superficial (Umbrella) Cells

Regardless of the type of sample and collection technique used, superficial urothelial cells are a common component of the urine sediment.

Table 14.1 Cytologic diagnostic categories in urine sediment

Non–tumor-associated cytology
  Normal cells/negative for malignant cells
  Inflammatory changes
    Specific type
    Nonspecific
Tumor-associated cytology
  Atypical cells present, favor reactive
    Specific type (eg, lithiasis, chemotherapy, other)
    Nonspecific
  Atypical cells present, favor malignancy
  Atypical cells present/malignant NOS
  Atypical cells present/papillary urothelial neoplasm of low malignant potential
  Atypical cells present/low-grade urothelial carcinoma (papillary, nonpapillary, mixed forms)
  Atypical cells present/high-grade urothelial carcinoma (papillary, nonpapillary, mixed forms)
  Atypical cells present/urothelial dysplasia
  Atypical cells present/carcinoma in situ
  Atypical cells present/other neoplastic categories (specify: squamous cell carcinoma, adenocarcinoma, prostatic adenocarcinoma, renal cell carcinoma, other).

NOS: not otherwise specified.

These cells have one or more nuclei that are large, measuring up to 3 μm in diameter, comparable to superficial squamous cells (Fig 14.1) (Koss, 1997). Binucleate cells are common. Such cells are often larger than the mononucleate superficial cells, and their nuclei are somewhat smaller. Large, multinucleate superficial cells are by far the most striking component of the urinary sediment, particularly in washings or brushings of the bladder or ureter. Multinucleate superficial cells are particularly large and may be mistaken for giant cells. A common error in diagnosis is misinterpreting large superficial cells as macrophages or tumor cells. The DNA content may be twice that of normal cells (tetraploid nuclei) (Amberson & Laino, 1993; Kline et al, 1995).

The chromatinic rim of the nucleus is thick and sharply demarcated. The chromatin is finely granular, often with a "salt and pepper" appearance, and may contain one or more prominent chromocenters. The structure of the nucleus is better preserved in bladder washings than in voided urine. In women, there may be a sex chromatin body attached to the nuclear membrane. The cytoplasm of these cells is usually eosinophilic, often finely granular, and sometimes vacuolated.

14.2.2 Cells Originating from the Deeper Layers of the Urothelium

Epithelial cells smaller than the superficial cells derived from the deeper layers of the urothelium often exfoliate in clusters, particularly if the specimen was obtained with an instrument. Single small urothelial cells are observed in voided urine, usually in the presence of inflammation and destruction of the superficial cell layer. The clusters of urothelial cells may be tightly packed and assume a spherical "papillary" configuration with sharp borders. Such clusters are often misinterpreted as low-grade papillary carcinoma (Highman & Wilson, 1982; Kannan & Bose, 1993). When the deep cells are removed by an instrument, they often appear in loose clusters. These cells are polygonal or elongate, sometimes columnar, and almost always display cytoplasmic extensions in contact with other cells. The amount of basophilic cy-

(a)

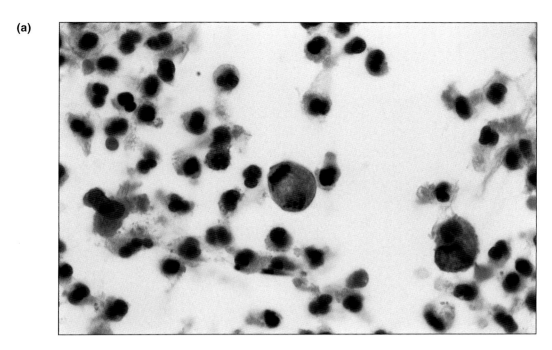

(b)

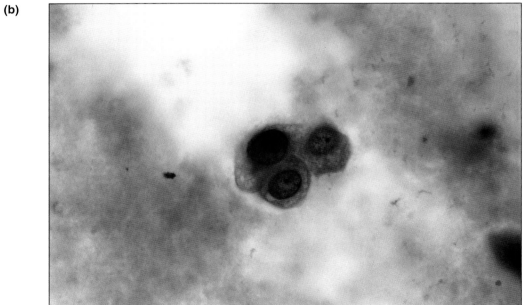

(c)

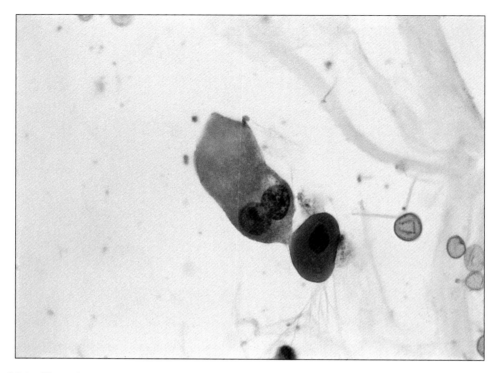

Figure 14.1 Normal components of voided urine and bladder washings. **(a, b)**: Superficial cells; **(c)**: superficial binucleate cell with nuclear enlargement in a catheterization specimen.

toplasm in such cells depends on the layer of origin and is more abundant in cells derived from superficial layers. Single cells resemble parabasal squamous cells in size and configuration. These cells are often spherical or round, particularly in voided urine, but may also show cytoplasmic extensions (Koss, 1997). The nuclei of the smaller urothelial cells are approximately the same size, measuring about 5 µm in diameter. They are usually finely granular and benign appearing, and contain one, or rarely, two small chromocenters. In voided urine, the nuclei may be pale or opaque and occasionally somewhat dark.

14.2.3 Mucus-Containing Epithelial Cells

Occasionally, urine cytology specimens contain mucus-secreting columnar epithelial cells with peripheral nuclei and distended clear cyto-

plasm. These cells may be ciliated. Such cells derive from cystitis cystica or cystitis glandularis.

14.2.4 Squamous Cells

Squamous cells of varying size and degree of maturation are common in urine sediment, particularly in voided specimens (Fig 14.2). Such cells are more abundant in female than in male patients (Koss, 1997). In women, these cells originate in the squamous epithelium and the trigone of the urinary bladder and are usually glycogenated. Voided urine sediment may also contain squamous cells derived from the vulva, vagina, or uterine cervix. In men, the origin of the squamous cells is the terminal portion of the urethra or, in rare cases, vaginal-type squamous metaplasia. Among the benign squamous cells, there may be superficial cells, intermedi-

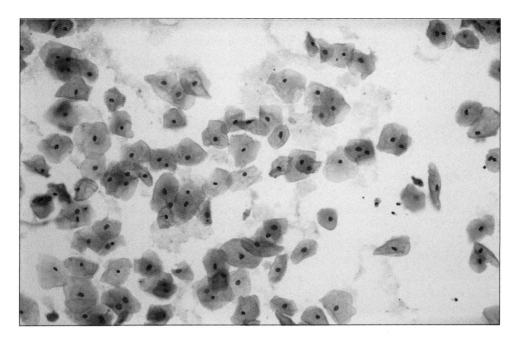

Figure 14.2 Squamous cells in the urine.

ate cells, and smaller parabasal cells. Navicular cells are intermediate squamous cells with abudant cytoplasmic glycogen content and peripheral nuclei; these cells stain yellow with Papanicolaou stain. Such cells may be observed during pregnancy, early menopause, and sometimes in women or men receiving hormonal therapy (estrogen therapy for prostate cancer in men). In women, the population of squamous cells in the urinary sediment may be used to determine the level of estrogenic activity (the so-called urocytogram). Squamous cells may also be anucleated and fully keratinized. The presence of such "ghost" cells may be of diagnostic significance, representing squamous cell carcinoma of the bladder.

14.2.5 Other Benign Cells

Cells derived from renal tubules may appear in the urine sediment. These cells are small and usually poorly preserved, with pyknotic, hyperchromatic, condensed, spherical nuclei and granular eosinophilic cytoplasm. Occasionally, the tubular cells form small clusters or casts. The significance of tubular cells in urine sediment remains uncertain. In patients who have undergone kidney transplant, the presence of renal tubular cells may indicate rejection of the allograft (Roberti et al, 1995). Occasionally, cells of prostatic and seminal vesicle origin may be present in the urinary sediment. Such cells accompany spermatozoa and are common after prostatic massage (Rupp et al, 1994).

Macrophages are often observed in inflammatory reactions of the urinary tract. The cells may be mononucleated or multinucleated and may contain fine cytoplasmic vacuoles, sometimes with phagocytic debris. Erythrocytes are a frequent component of the urinary sediment, particularly in patients with clinical evidence of hematuria (Fraccia et al, 1995). Normal urine sediment contains very few lymphocytes or neutrophils. The presence of large numbers of such cells may precede clinical evidence of inflammation.

14.2.6 Noncellular Components of the Urinary Sediment

Polygonal transparent crystalline precipitates of urates are common in voided urine. Their presence results from changes in the acidity of urine after collection but has no diagnostic significance. Crystals derived from true uric acid are exceedingly rare. Other crystals are very rarely of diagnostic value. Voided urine and occasional specimens obtained by instrumentation may contain contaminants and renal casts.

14.3 DIAGNOSTIC CRITERIA

14.3.1 Inflammatory Processes

14.3.1.1 Bacteria

A wide variety of bacteria may affect the epithelium of the urinary tract. Most are coliforms and other gram-negative rods. Cystitis may be acute or chronic. Acute cystitis is usually associated with symptoms that rarely require confirmatory tissue biopsy or cytologic examination. In those cases in which urine is studied, the sediment may contain numerous exfoliated urothelial cells, necrotic material, and inflammatory cells, with a predominance of neutrophils (Fig 14.3). Marked necrosis and inflammation may also occur in the presence of necrotic tumors, particularly high-grade urothelial carcinoma and squamous cell carcinoma.

The urinary sediment in chronic cystitis usually contains a background of chronic inflammation with macrophages and erythrocytes (Fraccia et al, 1995). Urothelial cells may be abundant and poorly preserved, occasionally forming small clusters. The cytoplasm in these cells tends to be granular and vacuolated; when

the cells are degenerate, the cytoplasm contains spherical eosinophilic inclusions of no significance (Fig 14.4). They may have slight nuclear enlargement and hyperchromasia, but the contours of the nuclei are usually regular and the chromatin texture is finely granular without the coarse granularity of urothelial cancer cells. There may be necrosis of urothelial cells, with nuclear pyknosis and marked cytoplasmic vacuolization. In ulcerative cystitis, large sheets of urothelial cells may be observed.

Interstitial cystitis, a form of chronic cystitis associated with chronic inflammation, displays nonspecific cytologic changes (Koss, 1997). Eosinophilic cystitis has a predominance of eosinophils, a pattern that may be seen in patients with allergic disorders, previous biopsies, or following mitomycin C treatment (Eltoum et al, 1992). Tuberculous cystitis may be observed in patients with acquired immune deficiency syndrome (AIDS) and those receiving treatment for urothelial carcinoma with bacillus Calmette-Guérin. In such patients, the sediment shows inflammatory cells and may contain fragments of tubercles in the form of clusters of elongate, carrot-shaped epithelioid cells, sometimes accompanied by multinucleated Langerhan's-type giant cells and reactive atypia of urothelial cells (Betz et al, 1993; Schwalb et al, 1994). Similar findings may occur in patients with tuberculosis of the bladder.

14.3.1.2 Fungi

Fungi occasionally affect the lower urinary tract, particularly the urinary bladder. *Candida albicans* is the most common, usually seen in pregnant women, patients with diabetes, and people with impaired immunity such as patients with AIDS, those undergoing chemotherapy for cancer, and bone marrow transplant recipients. In the urinary sediment, the fungi may appear as yeast forms, with small oval bodies, or pseudohyphae, with oblong branch-

(a)

(b)

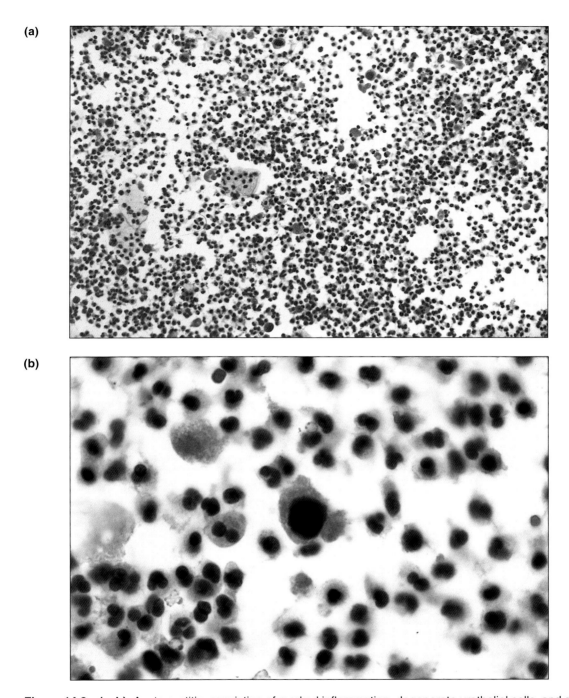

Figure 14.3 **(a, b):** Acute cystitis, consisting of marked inflammation, degenerate urothelial cells, and scattered superficial cells.

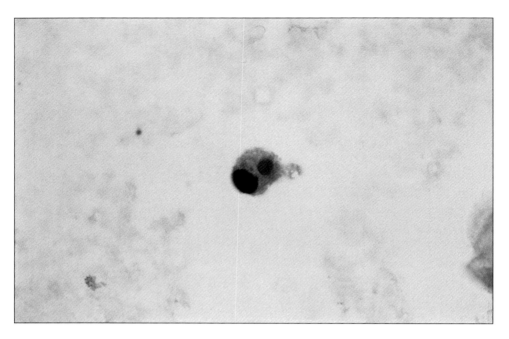

Figure 14.4 Degenerate urothelial cell with cytoplasmic inclusions.

ing non-encapsulated filaments (Fig 14.5). Other fungi are uncommon, including *Blastomyces dermatitidis*, *Aspergillus*, and mucormycosis. A fungus of the species *Alternaria* is a common laboratory contaminant (Koss, 1997).

14.3.1.3   Viruses

Several important viruses cause significant morphologic changes in the urothelial cells, many of which may be confused with malignancy. The dominant feature of viral infections is the formation of nuclear and cytoplasmic inclusions (Table 14.2).

Herpes simplex is an obligate intracellular virus, and florid infection with permissive replication of the virus causes abnormalities in urothelial cells that are readily recognized. In the early stages of viral replication, the nuclei of infected cells appear hazy with a ground glass appearance. Multinucleation is commonly observed in such cells. Multiple nuclei are often densely packed, with nuclear moulding and

tightly fitting contoured nuclei. In later stages of infection, the viral particles concentrate in the center of the nuclei, forming bright eosinophilic inclusions with a narrow clear zone or halo at the periphery. Infected cells may contain single or multiple nuclei (Koss, 1997).

Cytomegalovirus (CMV) is usually seen in newborn infants with impaired immunity. The infection is common in adults with AIDS. The characteristic changes are readily recognized in the urinary sediment, including large cells with large basophilic nuclear inclusions surrounded by a large peripheral clear zone (Fig 14.6). There is a distinct outer band of condensed nuclear chromatin.

Polyomavirus infection is widespread, according to serologic studies of adults. The occult virus can become activated and recognized in voided urine sediment. One form of polyomavirus, the BK virus, plays a major role in urine cytology because it produces cell abnormalities that may be readily confused with cancer; these cells are also known as "decoy cells" (Fig 14.7). In permissive

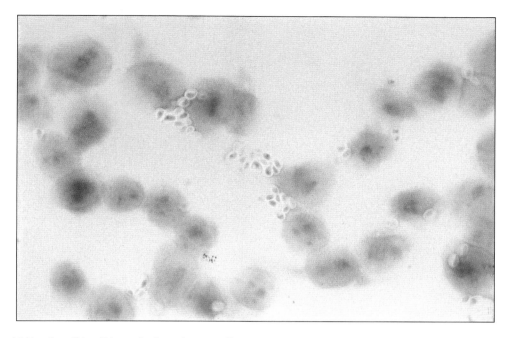

Figure 14.5 *Candida albicans* in the urinary sediment. Note the small oval bodies that stand in contrast with the urothelial cells.

Table 14.2 Characteristic cytologic changes associated with specific types of viruses

CMV
    Enlarged cells
    High nucleus-to-cytoplasm (N/C) ratio
    Basophilic intranuclear inclusion with "owl's-eye" appearance; occasionally small, dark intracytoplas-
    mic inclusions
Herpes virus
    Enlarged, multinucleated cells with "ground-glass" chromatin
    High N/C ratio
    Opaque, structureless chromatin
    Eosinophilic intranuclear inclusion
Polyomavirus
    Enlarged cells
    High N/C ratio
    Opaque, structureless chromatin, chromatinic membrane is common
    Nuclei stain with a magenta hue
    Intranuclear inclusion fills almost the entire nuclear area
Papillomavirus
    Perinuclear clear cytoplasmic zones (koilocytosis)
    Nuclear enlargement and homogeneous hyperchromasia

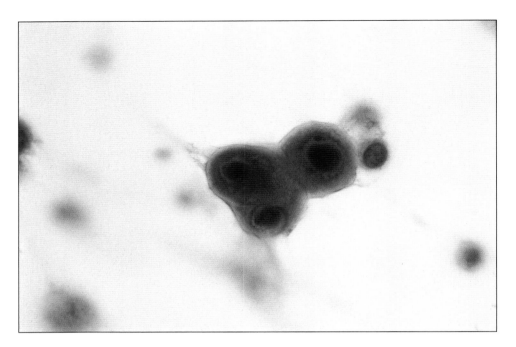

Figure 14.6 CMV infection.

infections, the BK virus produces large, homogeneous, basophilic nuclear inclusions that occupy almost the entire volume of the nuclei. Occasionally, a narrow rim of clearing separates the inclusion from the chromatinic rim. The infected cells are often enlarged and usually contain a single nucleus, but binucleation and occasional large multinucleated cells may be seen (Koss et al, 1984). The cytologic picture in some cases may be quite dramatic and has led to the misdiagnosis of carcinoma (Seftel et al, 1996). Another rare form of polyomavirus infection of the urine is caused by the JC virus, which is associated with progressive multifocal leucoencephalopathy

More than 70 types of human papillomavirus are recognized, and types 6 and 11 are associated with condyloma acuminata. Condyloma may also appear in the urethra and invariably induces koilocytosis. Urothelial carcinoma exhibits a low incidence of concomitant human papillomavirus types 16 and 18 infection (Lopez-Beltran et al, 1996).

14.3.1.4 *Trematodes and Other Parasites*

The most important of these parasites is *Schistosoma haematobium* (Bilharzia) (see Chapter 3). There are two important cytologic manifestations of infection with *Schistosoma haematobium*: recognition of the ova and the malignant tumors that may be associated with infection (Eltoum et al, 1992). The ova are elongate structures with a thick transparent capsule and a sword-shaped protrusion known as the "terminal spine" located at the narrow end of the ova. Fresh or calcified ova may be readily recognized in the urinary sediment. The embryonal form of the parasite, known as miracidium, is released in human stool and urine, retaining the shape of the ovum with its terminal spine.

Other common intestinal parasites that affect the bladder include *Ascaris lumbricoides, Enterobius vermicularis,* and filariasis.

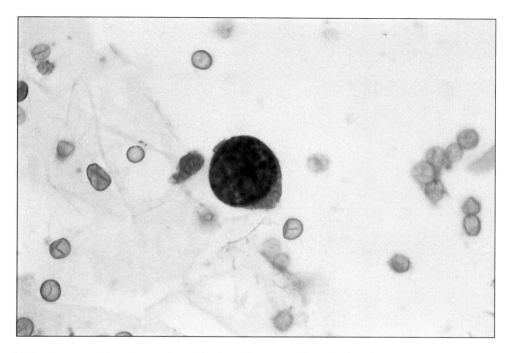

Figure 14.7 Decoy cell in polyomavirus infection. These may be mistaken for malignant cells.

14.3.2 Reactive Cytologic Changes

Numerous reactive and atypical changes involving the urothelium may be mistaken for malignancy (Tables 14.3 and 14.4).

14.3.2.1 *Lithiasis*

About 40% of patients with calculi have abnormal cytologic findings in voided urine (Highman & Wilson, 1982). These patients have numerous large smooth-bordered clusters of benign urothelium with an abundance of superficial cells (Fig 14.8). These changes may overlap with the spectrum of findings of low-grade urothelial carcinoma, but the cells tend to cluster, with fewer single cells (Highman & Wilson, 1982). Calculi are abrasive to the mucosa when present in the renal pelvis, ureter, or urinary bladder, and the resultant cytologic specimens closely resemble the effects of instrumentation. Significant atypia of urothelial cells

caused by lithiasis is uncommon (Koss, 1996a). Nonetheless, lithiasis remains a major diagnostic pitfall in urinary cytology interpretation.

14.3.2.2 *Drug Effects*

Intravesically administered drugs such as mitomycin C and thiotepa are commonly used for the treatment of bladder tumors and their recurrence (Figs 14.9 and 14.10) (Ross, 1996). They may induce cell enlargement or cytoplasmic vacuolization. Intravesical chemotherapy contributes to a high rate of false–positive results in urine cytology (Maier et al, 1995).

Systemically administered drugs such as the alkylating agents cyclophosphamide and busulfan have a marked effect on the urothelium, with significant cytologic abnormalities (Fig 14.11). These drugs may induce changes that include bizarre abnormal urothelial cells with marked nuclear and nucleolar enlargement mimicking poorly differentiated carcinoma (Forni et al, 1964;

Table 14.3 Differential diagnosis of urothelial atypia found in urinary sediment

Urinary tract conditions
  Urethral catheterization
  Urinary calculi
  Chronic cystitis and cystitis glandularis
  Cellular changes as a result of radiation therapy and chemotherapy
  Atypical and/or hyperplastic urothelium
  Papillary urothelial tumor of low malignant potential and low-grade urothelial carcinoma
Renal parenchymal conditions
  Acute tubular necrosis
  Papillary necrosis
  Renal infarction
  Acute allograft rejection with ischemic necrosis

Table 14.4 Cellular features of reactive urothelium versus urothelial neoplasia

Cells	Atypia	CIS	Papillary urothelial neoplasm of low malignant potential	Urothelial carcinoma
Arrangement	Papillary aggregates	Numerous single cells	Papillary and loose clusters	Isolated and loose clusters
Size	Increased	Increased	Increased, uniform	Increased, pleomorphic
Number	Variable	Variable	Often numerous	Variable
Cytoplasm	Vacuolated	Variable maturation	Homogeneous	Variable
Nucleus-to-cytoplasm ratio	Normal/increased	Increased	Increased	Increased
Nuclei				
Position	Non-eccentric	Non-eccentric	Eccentric	Eccentric
Size	Enlarged	Enlarged	Enlarged	Variable
Morphology	Uniform within aggregates	Syncytia, cannibalism	Variable within aggregates	Variable
Borders	Smooth	Marked membrane irregularity	Irregular (notches, creases)	Irregular
Chromatin	Dusty, peripheral concentration	Increased coarsely granular, evenly distributed	Fine, even	Coarse, uneven
Nucleoli	Often large	Rare nucleoli	Small/absent	Variable
Background	Variable	Clean	Clean	Dirty, tumor diathesis

Murphy, 1990). Large doses of cyclophosphamide have been shown to induce urothelial carcinoma, leiomyosarcoma, and carcinosarcoma (Lopez-Beltran et al, 1998; Travis et al, 1989; Wall & Kalusen, 1995).

14.3.2.3 Effects of Radiation Therapy

Radiation therapy typically induces marked cell enlargement, with bizarre cell shapes and vacuolated nuclei and cytoplasm (Fig 14.12). These findings may persist for years after treatment (Ross, 1996).

14.3.2.4 Urine Cytology in Renal Transplant Recipients

The epithelial cells of collecting tubules are well preserved in patients following renal transplantation. The cells that appear in urine specimens have scant vacuolated cytoplasm with spherical and somewhat opaque nuclei. A feature of

(a)

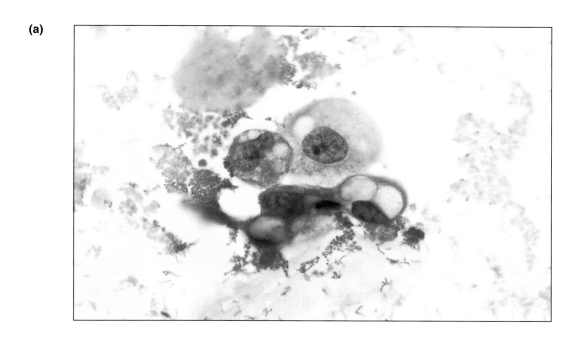

(b)

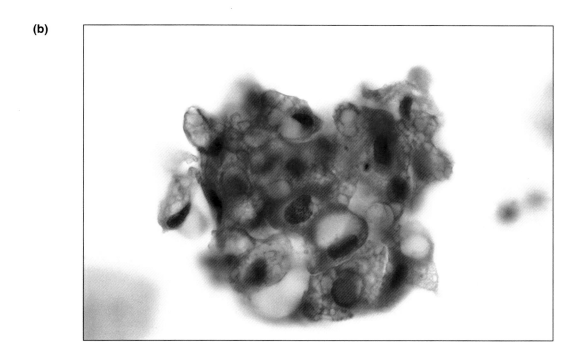

(c)

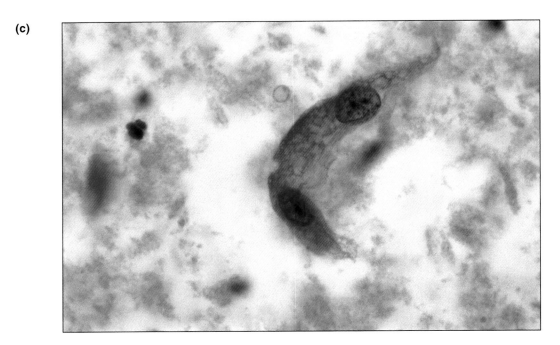

Figure 14.8 Renal lithiasis, with findings that may be mistaken for malignancy. **(a):** Cluster of benign urothelial cells; **(b):** tissue fragment resembling the effects of instrumentation; **(c):** superficial cells with mild nuclear atypia.

(a)

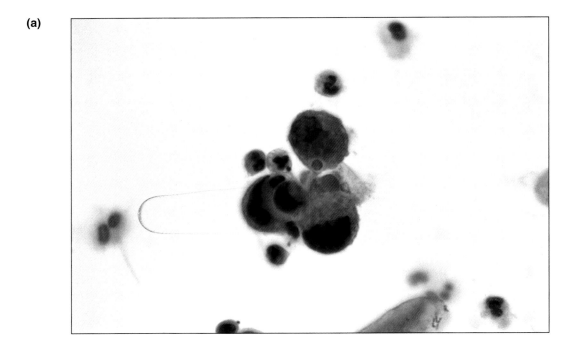

(b)

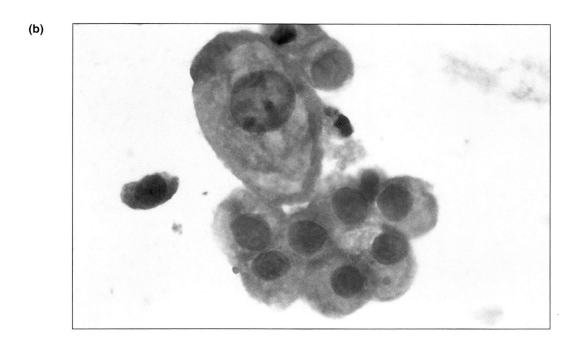

(c)

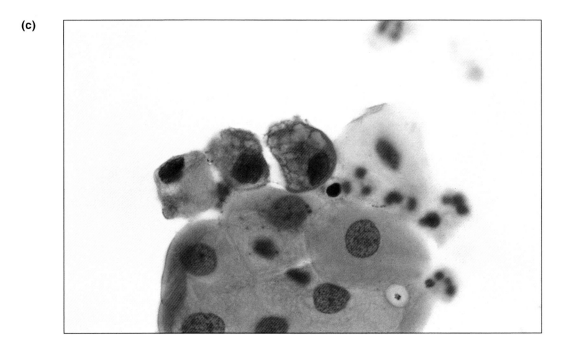

Figure 14.9   (a, b, c): Mitomycin C changes in the urine mimicking malignancy.

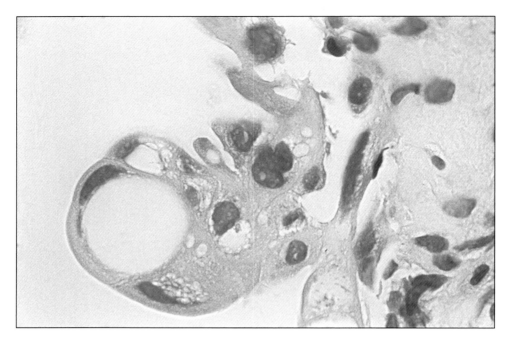

Figure 14.10 Thiotepa-induced changes, including urothelial detachment with nuclear atypia and cytoplasmic vacuolization.

(a)

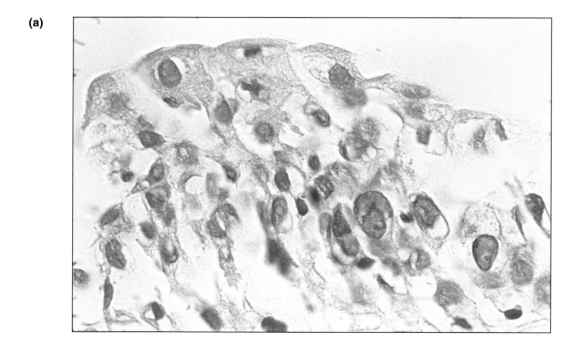

(b)

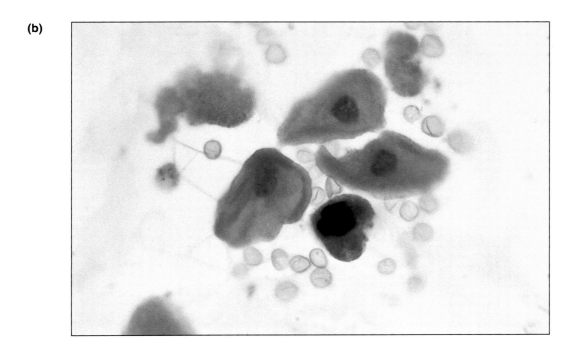

(c)

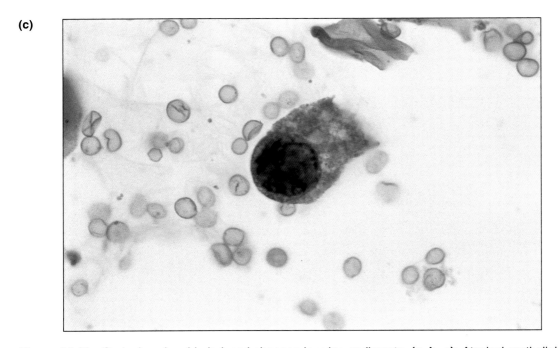

Figure 14.11 Cyclophosphamide-induced changes in urine sediments. **(a, b, c):** Atypical urothelial cells with large hyperchromatic nuclei that may be misinterpreted as malignant.

(a)

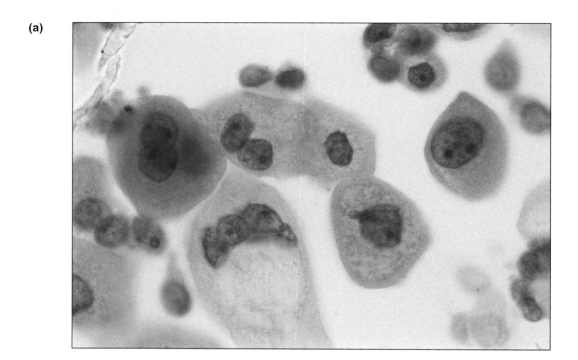

(b)

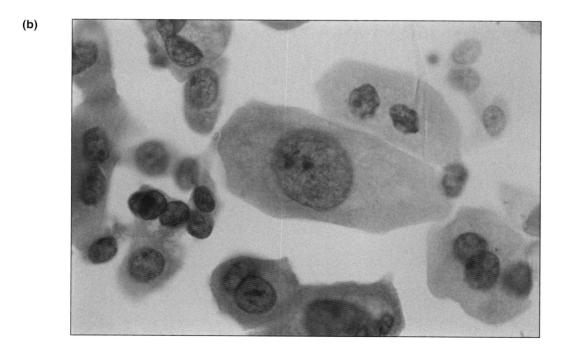

Figure 14.12   (a, b): Radiation-induced changes in urine sediments. Note bizarre enlarged urothelial cells with abundant vacuolation.

impending rejection is the presence of numerous T lymphocytes and erythrocytes in the urine. The erythrocytes have a thick outer border and clear center suggestive of renal origin. In rejection, tissue fragments may be present, including necrotic renal tubules and hyaline casts (Roberti et al, 1995).

14.3.3 Other Benign Conditions

Partial or complete keratinization of the squamous epithelium, referred to clinically as "leukoplakia," often replaces the urothelium, resulting in a cystoscopic gray-white appearance of the mucosa. In the urinary sediment, anucleated keratinized cells, so-called "ghost cells," may be present. When such cells are identified, the possibility of squamous cell carcinoma should be excluded (Koss 1996a; Schumann et al, 1995). Cystitis glandularis may shed ciliated mucus-containing epithelial cells that contain peripheral nuclei and clear cytoplasm. Such cells may be mistaken for adenocarcinoma. Large numbers of macrophages may be present in urine samples in patients with malakoplakia, but the release of such inflammatory cells usually occurs after biopsy and is detected in the urine stream. The spherical, intracytoplasmic, eosinophilic, or calcified Michaelis-Gutmann bodies in the cytoplasm of the macrophages are usually readily identified.

14.3.4 Benign Tumors and Tumor-Like Processes

There are no cellular changes that are characteristic of an inverted papilloma or nephrogenic metaplasia, and cytologic findings from these tumors may be difficult to interpret (Stilmant et al, 1986).

Condyloma acuminata of the urinary bladder is uncommon and may be associated with condyloma of the urethra or external genitalia. The typical finding, koilocytosis, is characterized by squamous cells containing large hyperchromatic nuclei with perinuclear clear zones or halos. These changes result from infection by human papillomavirus types 6 and 11. The presence of koilocytes in voided urine sediment in men often indicates a lesion in the bladder or urethra. In women, such cells may also indicate contamination from the lower genital tract. Occasionally, koilocytes may mimic squamous cell carcinoma. Endometrial-type glandular cells in urine sediment have been reported in women with endometriosis (Schneider et al, 1980).

14.3.5 Cytologic Diagnosis of Urothelial Tumors

14.3.5.1 Dysplasia

In cases of dysplasia, the only cytologic finding is the presence of atypical urothelial cells (Fig 14.13) (Murphy & Soloway, 1982). It is difficult, if not impossible, to specifically recognize cell changes corresponding to dysplasia (Koss, 1996a). Severe dysplasia and carcinoma in situ are considered to be synonymous (see below).

14.3.5.2 Carcinoma in Situ

Urothelial carcinoma in situ (CIS) is characterized by the presence of malignant cells that are often uniform in size and may be small or large (Fig 14.14; Table 14.5) (Gamarra & Zeima, 1984; Murphy, 1990). The background of the smears is often clean and free of necrotic debris and lacks inflammation. Occasionally, the cells may be heterogeneous and large, particularly after biopsies. When prominent inflammation is present, it is often prudent not to attempt to separate CIS from invasive carcinoma. Microinvasive carcinoma may not be recognizable in cytologic samples, particularly when CIS is

(a)

(b)

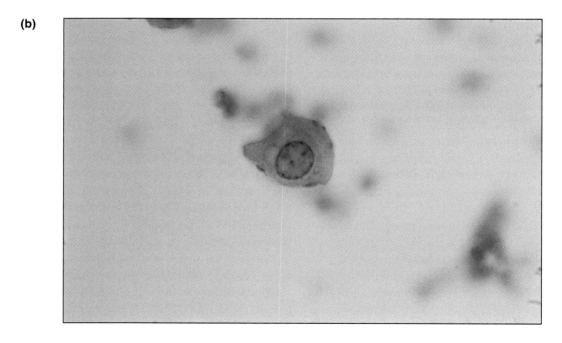

Figure 14.13   (a, b): Atypical urothelial cells consistent with dysplasia. Multiple biopsies of the bladder revealed dysplasia but no evidence of carcinoma in situ.

(a)

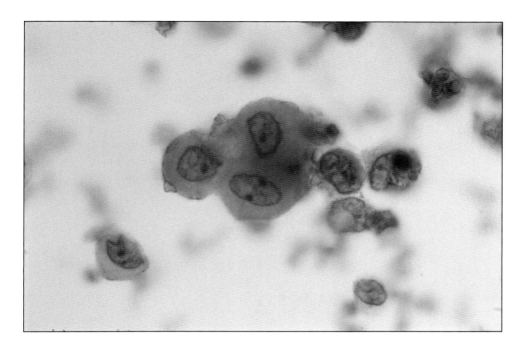

(b)

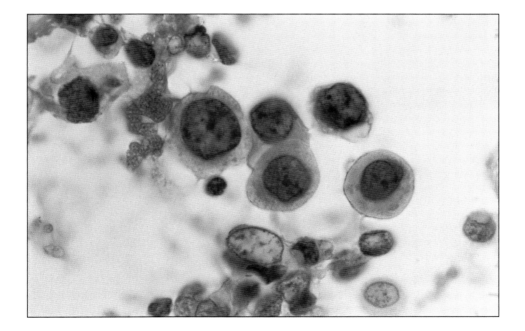

(c)

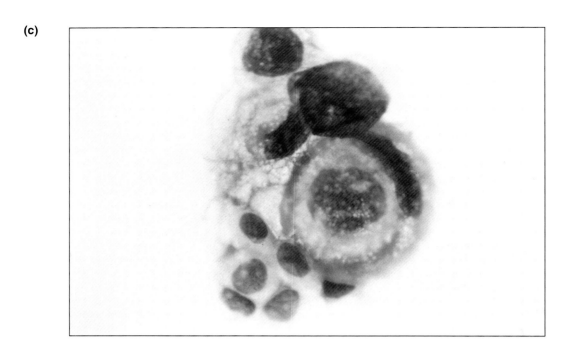

(d)

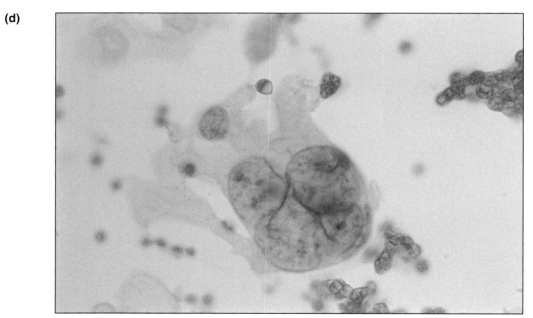

(e)

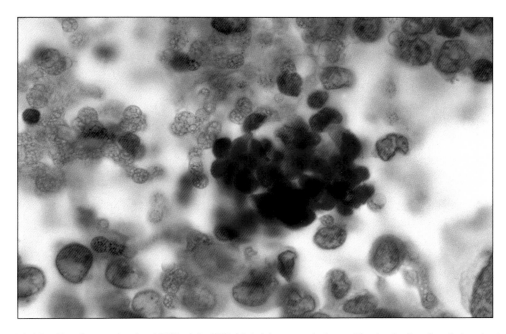

Figure 14.14 Carcinoma in situ (CIS). **(a):** CIS (right) in association with atypical cells of dysplasia (left); **(b, c):** cluster of CIS cells; **(d):** multinucleated CIS cell; **(e):** small cell variant of CIS.

Table 14.5 Criteria for cytologic grading of urothelial cancer

Morphologic features	CIS	Papillary neoplasm of low malignant potential	Low-grade urothelial carcinoma	High-grade urothelial carcinoma
Background	Clean	Clean	Clean	Dirty, tumor diathesis
Cellular arrangement	Numerous single cells, rare fragments	Large fragments of urothelium	Large fragments of urothelium and single cells	Large fragments and numerous single cells
Nuclear features	Syncytia,* cannibalism	Slightly enlarged	Nuclear crowding and overlap	Syncytia,* cannibalism
Nuclear membrane	Marked membrane irregularity	Regular, round or oval	Minimal membrane irregularity	Marked membrane irregularity
Chromatin	Increased coarsely granular, evenly distributed	Finely granular (vesicular)	Finely granular, evenly distributed	Increased chromatin, coarsely granular, unevenly distributed
Nucleolus	Rare nucleoli	Occasional micronucleoli	Variable micronucleoli	Macronucleoli
Cytoplasmic features	Variable maturation	Cell maturation present	Moderate degree of maturation	Maturation absent, squamoid and/or glandular features

*Loss of cell borders.

261

present. CIS may persist after intravesical therapy such as treatment with bacillus Calmette-Guérin (Fig 14.15).

14.3.5.3 *Papilloma, Papillary Neoplasm of Low Malignant Potential, and Low-Grade Papillary Carcinoma*

It may be difficult in cytology specimens to separate papillary urothelial tumor of low malignant potential from papilloma (Renshaw et al, 1996; Wolinska et al, 1985). The urothelial cell clusters often show a papillary configuration and are difficult to distinguish from those shed from the normal benign urothelium after palpation, instrumentation, or irritation by calculi or inflammation (Figs 14.16 and 14.17) (Highman & Wilson, 1982; Kannan & Bose, 1993). In voided urine, spontaneously shed complex clusters of morphologically benign urothelial cells may be suggestive of a papillary tumor, provided that trauma can be excluded clinically. Diagnostic features of papillary tumor of low malignant potential include the presence of tumor fragments with connective tissue stalks or central capillary vessels (Table 14.5) (Green & Meistrich, 1995).

Numerous attempts to define the precise microscopic features of neoplasm fragments that separate benign urothelial cell clusters from papillary urothelial tumor of low malignant potential have met with limited success (Weiner et al, 1993). Some authors claim that papillary urothelial neoplasm sheds recognizable cells in the urinary sediment (Sack et al, 1995); characteristic features (present in 70% of such tumors) include an increased ratio of nucleus to cytoplasm, enlarged and eccentric nuclei, but the absence of nucleoli (Murphy et al, 1984). Others report a correct cytologic diagnosis in 33% of cases (Wiener et al, 1993).

Differentiation between papillary urothelial neoplasm of low malignant potential and instrumentation artifacts is based on the presence of cell clusters with ragged borders, unlike the smooth borders lined by densely stained cytoplasm at the edge of benign cell clusters (Kannan & Bose, 1993). Papillary urothelial neoplasm of low malignant potential can be identified with 45% sensitivity and 98% specificity based on the cytologic criteria of increased nucleus-to-cytoplasm ratio, irregular nuclear borders, and cytoplasmic homogeneity (Raab et al, 1994). Overall observer accuracy was 76%, with a sensitivity of 82% for a definitive negative diagnosis and a specificity for a definitive positive diagnosis of 96% (Raab et al, 1996). In another study, the sensitivity of 90% and specificity of 65% for papillary urothelial neoplasm of low malignant potential was based on the absence of inflammation, the presence of single and overlapping groups of cells with high nucleus-to-cytoplasm ratio, hypochromasia, nuclear grooves and notches, and small nucleoli (Maier et al, 1995). Despite these findings, papillary urothelial neoplasm of low malignant potential is a major source of false–negative results in urine cytology (Maier et al, 1995).

Ancillary techniques may be valuable for separating benign and neoplastic urothelial cells, including DNA ploidy analysis (Sack et al, 1995), immunohistochemical markers (Panosian et al, 1989), and numeric chromosomal abnormalities detected by fluorescence in situ hybridization (FISH) (Cajulis et al, 1994). Digital image analysis is superior to bladder wash cytology for prediction of tumor recurrence (van der Poel et al, 1997).

14.3.5.4 *Low-Grade and High-Grade Urothelial Carcinoma*

It may be difficult to separate low-grade and high-grade urothelial carcinomas from urothelial carcinoma in situ (Table 14.5). Unlike benign urothelial cells, these cells have substantial nuclear and cytoplasmic abnormalities (Fig 14.18). The principal value of urine cytology is

(a)

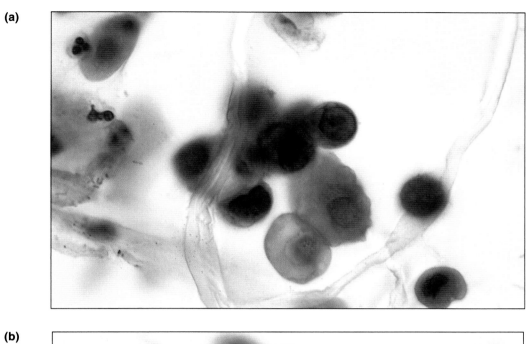

(b)

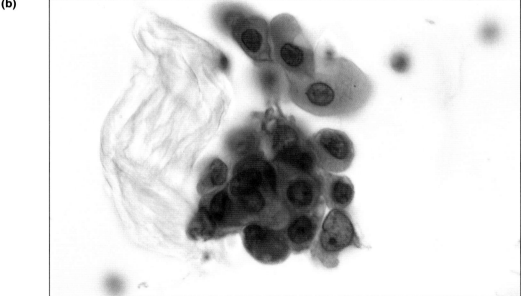

Figure 14.15 (a, b): Carcinoma in situ resistant to therapy with bacillus Calmette-Guérin, with clusters of hyperchromatic neoplastic cells.

(a)

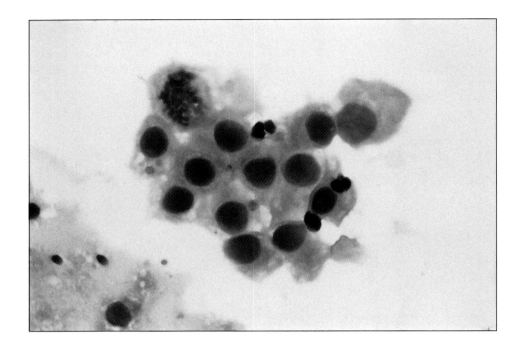

(b)

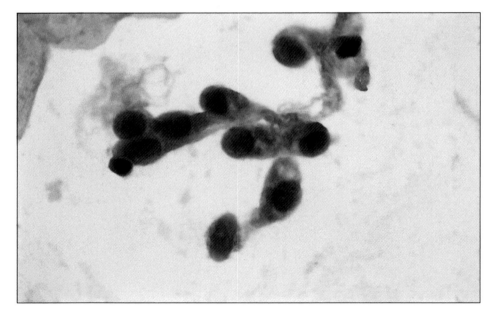

(c)

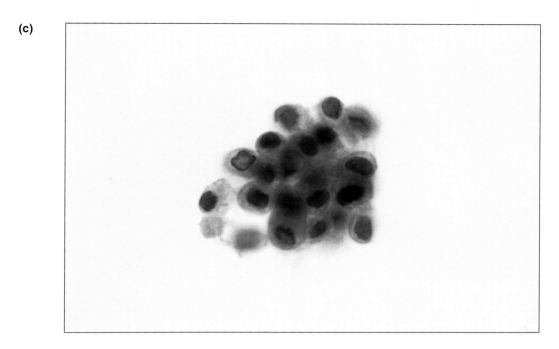

(d)

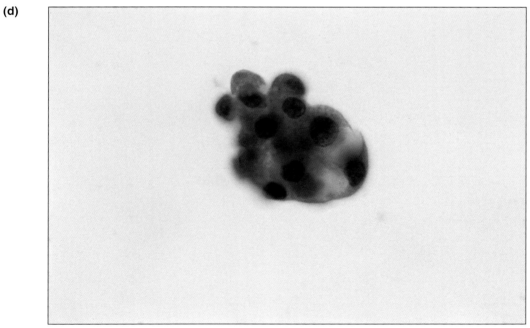

Figure 14.16 (a, b, c, d): Examples of papillary urothelial neoplasm of low malignant potential. In each case, the diagnosis was confirmed by a biopsy.

(a)

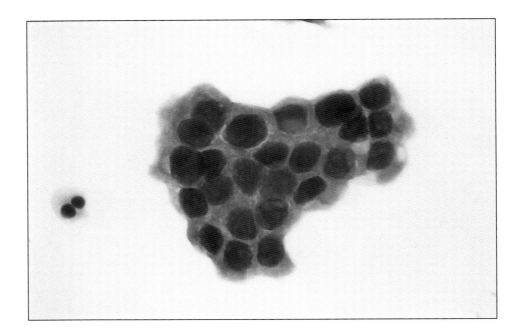

(b)

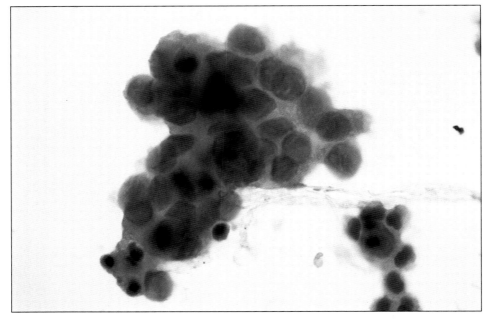

(c)

(d)

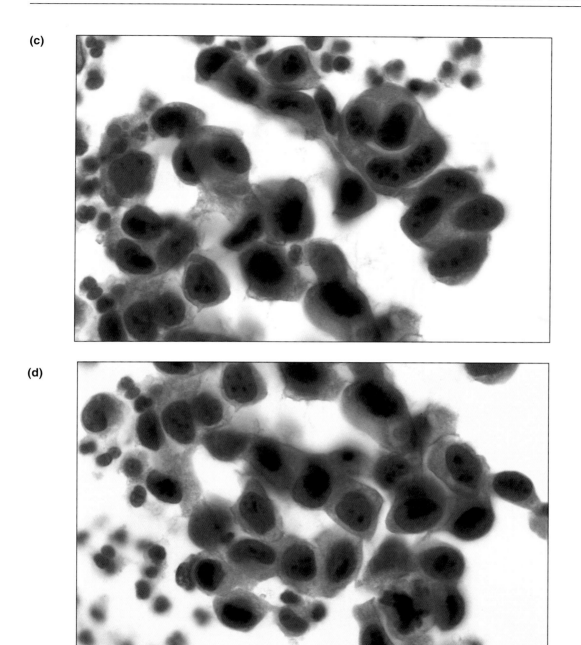

Figure 14.17 (a, b, c, d): Examples of low-grade papillary urothelial carcinoma. In each case, the diagnosis was confirmed by a biopsy.

267

(a)

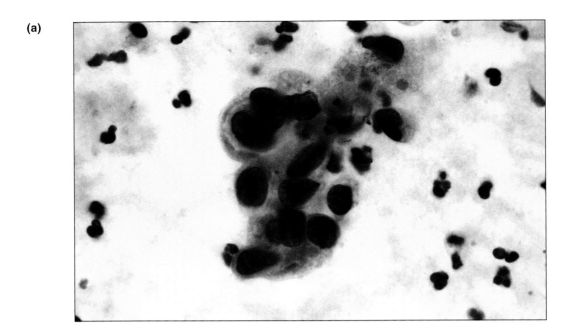

(b)

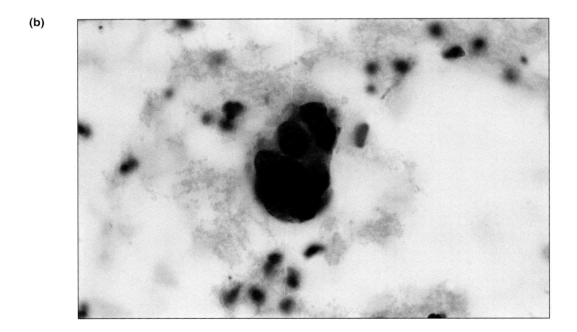

(c)

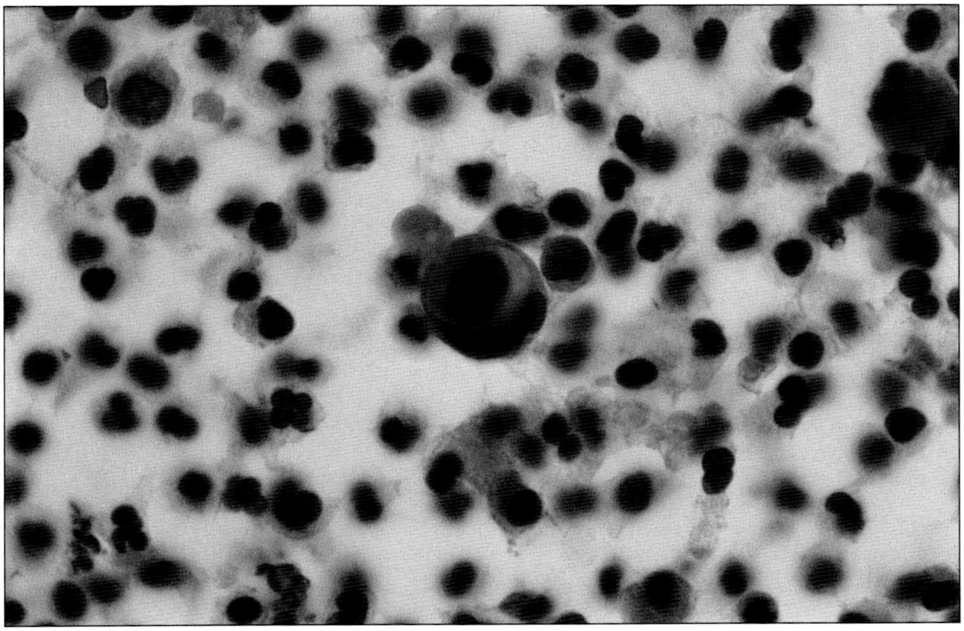

Figure 14.18 **(a, b):** High-grade papillary urothelial carcinoma, with marked cytologic abnormalities. **(c):** Note cell cannibalism.

in the diagnosis and monitoring of high-grade tumors that may not be evident cystoscopically, including CIS and occult invasive carcinoma (Gamarra & Zeima, 1984; Potts et al, 1997; Rife et al, 1979).

In voided urine, low-grade and high-grade urothelial carcinoma cells vary in size and shape and may be small or large. The nuclei are enlarged, with coarsely granular chromatin, hyperchromasia, abnormal nuclear contours, and prominent nucleoli. Multinucleate cancer cells and mitotic figures are often readily identified (Shenoy et al, 1985).

In bladder washings, urothelial carcinoma may demonstrate a lower degree of nuclear hyperchromasia, perhaps resulting in more prominent large nucleoli. The cells may be poorly preserved, particularly when there is inflammation or necrosis, and a variety of changes may be seen, including frayed or vacuolated cytoplasm, nonspecific eosinophilic cytoplasmic inclusions, and pyknotic nuclei. In some high-grade papillary tumors, the dominant cytologic finding may be the presence of isolated cancer cells, either singly or in groups of two or three. Papillary tumors of low grade often present a diagnostic challenge (Koss, 1997; Rife et al, 1979; Segura et al, 1995). In some cases, the cells are similar to those in a papillary urothelial tumor of low malignant potential. Unfortunately, in most cases, atypical urothelial cells are observed, and these alert the clinician to the need for cystoscopic examination. For high-grade urothelial carcinoma, digital image analysis and bladder wash cytology are equally predictive (van der Poel et al, 1997).

14.3.6 Other Carcinomas

14.3.6.1 *Squamous Cell Carcinoma*

Invasive squamous cell carcinoma is common in Africa and the Middle East, particularly in

269

patients infected with *Schistosoma haematobium*, but it is relatively uncommon in developed countries, accounting for no more than 3% of bladder tumors (Eltoum et al, 1992). Squamous cell carcinoma has been observed with increasing frequency in long-term survivors with severe spinal cord injury and a neurogenic bladder.

Squamous cell carcinoma may display varying degrees of differentiation (Fig 14.19). In well-differentiated invasive cell carcinoma, the cytologic findings in voided urine are somewhat characteristic. The presence of markedly keratinized cells with thick yellow or orange cytoplasm and large, irregular, often dark pyknotic nuclei are useful. Squamous pearls, characterized by cell aggregates concentrically arranged around a core of keratin, may be observed (Koss, 1997). The background of the smear often shows evidence of marked necrosis, and ghost cells may be present. A mixture of cancer cells is observed in the urine of patients with poorly differentiated squamous cell carcinoma, including sharply demarcated cells

with eosinophilic cytoplasm and large nuclei (Koss, 1997). Most cases are aneuploid (Shaaban et al, 1990).

14.3.6.2   *Adenocarcinoma*

In colonic-type adenocarcinoma of the bladder, the urinary sediment contains columnar cancer cells with large hyperchromatic nuclei and a large nucleoli, sometimes in clusters. In poorly differentiated mucus-producing carcinoma, the cancer cells are small, more spherical or cuboidal in shape, and contain large hyperchromatic nuclei, often with prominent nucleoli. The cytoplasm is usually basophilic, often scant, and sometimes poorly preserved. When there are large cytoplasmic vacuoles containing mucus, the nuclei may be pushed to the periphery of the cell, a feature diagnostic of signet-ring cell carcinoma.

In clear cell adenocarcinoma, the cancer cells are large, with abundant finely vacuolated or granular cytoplasm, open vesicular nuclei, and

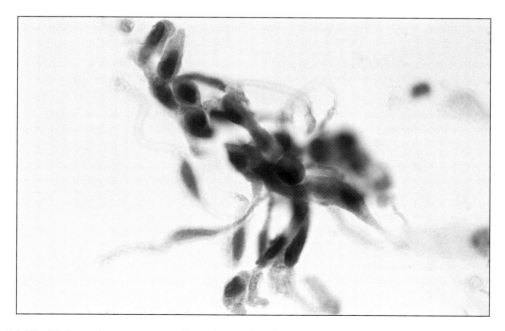

Figure 14.19   High-grade squamous cell carcinoma in urine.

prominent nucleoli. Such cells usually form round "papillary" clusters. Most cases are DNA aneuploid (Tribukait, 1984).

14.3.6.3 *Small Cell Undifferentiated Carcinoma (Oat Cell Carcinoma)*

In small cell carcinoma, the cancer cells are small and contain compact, often pyknotic nuclei and scant basophilic cytoplasm (Rollins & Schumann, 1991). Nucleoli are not visible. The presence of small clusters of tightly packed tumor cells with nuclear moulding may be diagnostically useful (Koss, 1996a). The presence of cell clusters without prominent nucleoli is helpful in differentiating these cells from malignant lymphoma. In lymphoma, the cells do not cluster and usually contain at least a small nucleolus. The demonstration of neuroendocrine differentiation in small cell carcinoma may require immunohistochemical or ultrastructural studies.

14.3.6.4 *Mixed Carcinoma*

Urothelial cancer may contain foci with more than one histologic type, including squamous cell carcinoma, adenocarcinoma, and small cell carcinoma. The cytologic findings in such tumors rarely allow the diagnosis of mixed carcinoma. Usually, one cytologic pattern is dominant, although, rarely, a mixed population of cancer cells may be observed.

14.3.6.5 *Other Malignant Tumors*

Rare cases of carcinoid (low-grade neuroendocrine carcinoma) have been diagnosed by urine cytology (Rudrick et al, 1995). Other rare cancers that may be diagnosed by cytology include sarcoma, carcinoma, primary and secondary lymphoma (Tanaka et al, 1993), and choriocarcinoma. In many cases, urine cytology may not be diagnostic.

14.3.7 **Major Diagnostic Pitfalls**

Most errors in urine cytology are overdiagnosis of benign cellular changes as malignant (Table 14.6). Knowledge of these changes is fundamental to the practice of urine cytology. Listed below is a summary of some of the most vexing problems, which are also described and illustrated elsewhere in this chapter and the remaining text.

14.3.7.1 *Trauma or Instrumentation*

The normal urothelium tends to exfoliate in the form of tissue fragments that are round or oval, commonly called "papillary clusters." Vigorous palpation, catheterization, or any form of instrumentation may result in the formation of such epithelial clusters. When present in large numbers, these clusters may be misinterpreted as papillary carcinoma (Kannan & Bose, 1993). Another important source of error is the pres-

Table 14.6 Major diagnostic pitfalls in lower urinary tract cytology

Underdiagnosis
  Low-grade urothelial carcinoma as benign
Overdiagnosis
  Normal and degenerated urothelium as malignant
  Human polyomavirus infection as malignant
  Effects of cyclophosphamide as malignant

ence of numerous superficial urothelial cells that may be mistaken for cancer cells because of their variable nuclear features (Murphy, 1990).

14.3.7.2 Cell Preservation

Cells in voided urine sediment, particularly in the first morning voiding, are often poorly preserved, compounding the diagnostic difficulty. The diagnosis of cancer in voided urine should be avoided unless the findings are unequivocal (Koss, 1997).

14.3.7.3 Human Polyomavirus

Polyomavirus forms large intranuclear inclusions that may mimic cancer cell nuclei. However, the inclusions are homogeneous and lack the coarse granularity of chromatin seen in cancer (Koss et al, 1984). Polyomavirus is an important source of diagnostic errors that can contribute to costly and lengthy investigations.

14.3.7.4 Lithiasis

Calculi originating anywhere in the lower urinary tract may act as an abrasive instrument, dislodging epithelial fragments that be may be quite large and display papillary appearance mimicking low-grade papillary carcinoma (Highman & Wilson, 1982). The presence of numerous superficial cells may also create diagnostic difficulty as a result of nuclear abnormalities (Koss, 1997; Maier et al, 1995; Murphy, 1990).

14.3.7.5 Medications and Other Therapeutic Procedures

Urine cell changes may result from a wide variety of inciting agents, including chemotherapeutic agents, radiotherapy, and other interventions. Intravesical chemotherapy is responsible for a high rate of false–positive results (Maier et al, 1995). A further source of diagnostic difficulty may be synchronous infection with polyomavirus in patients who are immunocompromised (Koss, 1997). It should be remembered that urothelial carcinoma or sarcoma may develop in patients receiving cyclophosphamide for the treatment of malignant lymphoma (Lopez-Beltran et al, 1998; Travis et al, 1989; Wall & Kalusen, 1995).

14.3.7.6 Special Aspects of Anatomic Sites Other Than Urinary Bladder

Primary cancer of the urethra that is not associated with a bladder tumor is rare. The most common cancers are squamous cell carcinoma, adenocarcinoma, and urothelial carcinoma, although all are rare. Other rare cancers include malignant melanoma and clear cell adenocarcinoma.

A common cytologic examination of the urethra occurs after cystectomy for bladder cancer. Frequently, these examinations may reveal carcinoma in situ or early invasive carcinoma (Gamarra & Zeima, 1984).

Urine cytology is usually diagnostic in urothelial carcinoma of the renal pelvis and ureter, particularly when the cancers are high grade. In low-grade malignancies, the same diagnostic problems are encountered as in the bladder (Gourlay et al, 1995).

Urine cytology is unsatisfactory for the detection of renal cell carcinoma. When malignant cells are present, they are large with clear or vacuolated cytoplasm and distinct nucleoli.

Prostatic adenocarcinoma may produce cells in voided urine spontaneously or after prostatic massage, particularly if the carcinoma is of high grade. The cancer cells in the urine sediment are usually small, often spherical, and columnar. Small cell clusters may be observed. The cytoplasm is usually basophilic with open vesicular nuclei and prominent nucleoli. This procedure is not considered useful for the early detection of prostatic carcinoma.

14.3.7.7 Secondary Tumors

Numerous metastatic malignant tumors may be observed in the urinary sediment. The most common metastases arise from adjacent or contiguous organs, including the uterine cervix and endometrium or ovary in women, the prostate in men, and the colon in both sexes. Urine cytology often shows a cellular background of squamous cell carcinoma or adenocarcinoma. Clinical–pathologic correlation is usually required for diagnosis. Rare cases of lymphoma, leukemia, and melanoma may be diagnosed from urine samples.

14.3.8 Ancillary Studies

Numerous auxillary studies are emerging to assist in detection of malignant cells or associated cell products. Described below are many typical cytology-based studies; the reader is referred to Chapter 15 for additional information.

14.3.8.1 Flow Cytometry

Voided urine is generally not adequate for flow cytometry, and the cell samples must be obtained by vigorous flushing of the bladder through a soft rubber catheter 5 to 10 times with saline solution or during cystoscopy by lavage. Subpopulations of bladder epithelial cells can be identified by interactive digital image analysis. The diagnosis of cancer is strongly suspected in cases with an aneuploid stemline or 16% or more of measured cells with hyperdiploid DNA (greater than 2xDNA content). A specimen is less likely to be cancerous if no aneuploid stemline is detected and fewer than 11% of the cells are hyperdiploid. If 11% to 15.9% of the measured cells are hyperdiploid and no aneuploid stemline is detected, the samples are considered suspicious. Recurrent cancer can be detected by using combined urine cytology and image analysis (Delaroza et al, 1996; Giella et al, 1992; Gourlay et al, 1995; Mellon et al, 1991; Mora et al, 1996).

14.3.8.2 Digital Image Analysis

Digital image analysis was found to be superior to flow cytometry for DNA ploidy analysis, with sensitivities of 91% and 71%, respectively (Cajulis et al, 1994). Furthermore, image analysis was superior to cytologic examination for the prediction of tumor recurrence after normal findings at cystoscopic examination and was equivalent to cytology for the detection of high-grade lesions (Richman et al, 1998; van der Poel et al, 1997).

14.3.8.3 Blood Group Antigens and Other Tumor Markers Detected by Immunohistochemistry

Deletion of A,B, and H blood group antigens is associated with biochemical and structural changes of glycoprotein components of the cell surface during neoplastic transformation. Blood group reactivity is decreased in high-grade and aggressive tumors (Golijanin et al, 1995; Sheinfeld et al, 1990). Carcinoembryonic antigen has been used in the evaluation of exfoliated urothelial cancer cells. The URO series of monoclonal antibodies and the proliferation marker Ki67 has been detected (Panosian et al, 1989).

14.3.8.4 Molecular Cytogenetics

FISH is useful for investigating numeric chromosomal abnormalities (Cajulis et al, 1994). FISH revealed abnormalities for chromosomes 8 and 12 in 83% of 26 bladder tumors of all grades.

14.4 CORRELATION OF URINE CYTOLOGY AND BIOPSY FINDINGS (DIAGNOSTIC ACCURACY)

The diagnostic accuracy of urine cytology is high in patients who are symptomatic or are being followed after diagnosis and treatment for bladder cancer. The reported results vary considerably. In general, all reports of series of bladder tumors indicate that papilloma and papillary urothelial tumor of low malignant potential cannot be reliably diagnosed by urine cytology despite the several key cytologic findings investigated. Approximately two-thirds of cases of papillary urothelial tumor of low malignant potential are diagnosed as suspicious or malignant. The sensitivity increases to 80% for low-grade carcinoma and 95% for high-grade urothelial carcinoma. Urothelial carcinoma in situ can be diagnosed as suspicious or positive in virtually all instances. The overall sensitivity of urine cytology for primary carcinoma of the bladder ranges from 45% to 97%. In a recent report, urine cytology predicted 82% of all recurrent tumors in the bladder (Loh et al, 1996). Two major drawbacks of urinary cytology are the high rate of false–positive results in patients on intravesical chemotherapy and the high rate of false–negative results in those with papillary urothelial tumor of low malignant potential.

REFERENCES

Amberson JB, Laino J. Image cytometric deoxyribonucleic acid analysis of urine specimens as an adjunct to visual cytology in the detection of urothelial cell carcinoma. *J Urol.* 1993;149:42–45.

Badalament RA, Gay H, Cibas ES, et al. Monitoring endoscopic treatment of superficial bladder carcinoma by postoperative urinary cytology. *J Urol.* 1987;138:760–762.

Berlac PA, Holm HH. Bladder tumor control by abdominal ultrasound and urine cytology. *J Urol.* 1992;147:1510–1512.

Betz SA, See WA, Cohen NB. Granulomatous inflammation in bladder washed specimens after intravesical bacillus Calmette-Guerin therapy for transitional cell carcinoma of the bladder. *Am J Clin Pathol.* 1993;99:244–248.

Bian Y, Ehya H, Bagley DH. Cytologic diagnosis of upper urinary tract neoplasms by ureteroscopic sampling. *Acta Cytol.* 1995;39:733–740.

Cajulis RS, Haines GK III, Frias-Hidregi D, et al. Cytology, flow cytometry, image analysis, and interphase cytogenetics by fluorescence in situ hybridization in the diagnosis of transitional cell carcinoma in bladder washes: a comparative study. *Diag Cytopathol.* 1995;13:214–223.

Chow NH, Tzai TS, Cheng HL, et al. Urinary cytodiagnosis: can it have a different prognostic implication than a diagnostic test. *Urol Int.* 1994; 53:18–23.

Delaroza GL, Hopkovitz A, Caraway NP, et al. DNA image analysis of urinary cytology. Prediction of recurrent transitional cell carcinoma. *Mod Pathol.* 1996;9:571–578.

Eltoum IA, Suliaman SM, Ismail BM, et al. Evaluation of eosinophiluria in the diagnosis of schistosomiasis hematobium: a field-based study. *Am J Trop Med Hyg.* 1992;46:732–736.

Forni AM, Koss LG, Geller W. Cytological study of the effect of cyclophosphamide on the epithelium of the urinary bladder in man. *Cancer.* 1964; 17:1348–1355.

Fraccia JA, Motta J, Miller LS, et al. Evaluation of asymptomatic microhematuria. *Urology.* 1995; 46:484–489.

Gamarra MC, Zeima T. Cytologic spectrum of bladder cancer. *Urology.* 1984;23:23–36.

Giella JG, Ring K, Olsson CA, et al. The predictive value of flow cytometry in urinary cytology in the follow up of patients with transitional cell carcinoma of the bladder. *J Urol.* 1992;148:293–296.

Golijanin D, Sherman Y, Shapiro A, et al. Detection of bladder tumors by immunostaining of the Lewis X antigen in cells from voided urine. *Urology.* 1995; 46:173–177.

Gourlay W, Chan V, Gilks CB. Screening for urothelial malignancies by cytologic analysis and flow cytometry in a community urologic practice. *Mod Pathol.* 1995;8:394–397.

Green LK, Meistrich H. Dramatically increased specificity and sensitivity in detecting low grade papillary TCC in urologic cytology via a combination of cytospin and cell blocking techniques (Abstract). *Mod Pathol.* 1995;8:40A.

Highman W, Wilson E. Urine cytology in patients with calculi. *J Clin Pathol.* 1982;35:25–48.

Kannan V, Bose S. Low grade transitional cell carcinoma and instrument artifact. A challenge in urinary cytology. *Acta Cytol.* 1993;37:899–902.

Kline MJ, Wikinson EJ, Askeland R, et al. DNA tetraploidy in Feulgen-stained bladder washings assessed by image cytometry. *Anal Quant Cytol Histol.* 1995;17:129–134.

Koss LG. Errors and pitfalls in cytology of the lower urinary tract. *Monogr Pathol.* 1997;39:60–74.

Koss LG, Sherman AB, Eppich E. Image analysis and DNA content of urothelial cells infected with human polyomavirus. *Analyt Quant Cytol.* 1984;6:89–94.

Koss LG, Deitch D, Ramanathan R, et al. Diagnostic value of cytology of voided urine. *Acta Cytol.* 1985; 29:810–816.

Loh CS, Spedding AV, Ashworth MT, et al. The value of exfoliative urine cytology in combination with flexible cystoscopy in the diagnosis of recurrent transitional cell carcinoma of the urinary bladder. *Br J Urol.* 1996;77:655–658.

Lopez-Beltran A, Escudero AL, Carrasco-Aznar JC, et al. Human papillomavirus infection and transitional cell carcinoma of the bladder. Immunohistochemistry and in situ hybridization. *Pathol Res Pract.* 1996;192:154–159.

Lopez-Beltran A, Pacelli A, Rothenberg HJ, et al. Carcinosarcoma and sarcomatoid carcinoma of the bladder: clinicopathologic study of 41 cases. *J Urol.* 1998;159:1497–1503.

Maier U, Simak R, Neuhold N. The clinical value of urinary cytology: 12 years of experience with 615 patients. *J Clin Pathol.* 1995;48:314–317.

Matzkin H, Moinuddin SM, Soloway MS. Value of urine cytology versus bladder washing in bladder cancer. *Urology.* 1992;39:201–203.

Mellon K, Shenton BK, Neal DE. Is voided urine suitable for flow cytometric DNA analysis? *Br J Urol.* 1991;67:48–53.

Mora LB, Nicosia SV, Powsang JM, et al. Ancillary techniques in the follow up of transitional cell carcinoma. A comparison of cytology, histology, and deoxyribonucleic acid image analysis cytometry in 91 patients. *J Urol.* 1996;156:49–54.

Murphy WM. Current status of urinary cytology in the evaluation of bladder neoplasms. *Hum Pathol.* 1990;21:886–896.

Murphy WM, Soloway MS. Urothelial dysplasia. *J Urol.* 1982;127:849–854.

Murphy WM, Soloway MS, Jukkola AF, et al. Urinary cytology and bladder cancer: the cellular features of transitional cell neoplasms. *Cancer.* 1984; 53:1555–1565.

Ooms EC, Veldhuizen RW. Cytological criteria and diagnostic terminology in urinary cytology. *Cytopathology.* 1993;4:51–54.

Panosian KJM, Lopez-Beltran A, Croghan G, et al. An immunohistochemical evaluation of urinary bladder cytology utilizing monoclonal antibodies. *World J Urol.* 1989;7:73–79.

Potts SA, Thomas PA, Cohen MB, et al. Diagnostic accuracy and key cytologic features of high-grade

transitional cell carcinoma in the upper urinary tract. *Mod Pathol.* 1997;10:657–662.

Raab SS, Lenel JC, Cohen MB. Low-grade transitional cell carcinoma of the bladder: cytologic diagnosis by key features as identified by logistic regression analysis. *Cancer.* 1994;74:1621–1626.

Raab SS, Slagel DD, Jensen CS, et al. Transitional cell carcinoma: cytologic criteria to improve diagnostic accuracy. *Mod Pathol.* 1996;9:225–232.

Renshaw AA, Nappi D, Weinberg DS. Cytology of grade 1 papillary transitional cell carcinoma. A comparison of cytologic, architectural and morphometric criteria in cytoscopically obtained urine. *Acta Cytol.* 1996;40:676–682.

Richman AM, Mayne ST, Jekel JF, et al. Image analysis combined with visual cytology in the early detection of recurrent bladder carcinoma. *Cancer.* 1998;82:1738–1748.

Rife CC, Farrow GM, Utz DC. Urine cytology of transitional cell neoplasms. *Urol Clin North Am.* 1979; 6:599–612.

Roberti I, Reisman L, Burrows L, et al. Urine cytology and urine flow cytometry in renal transplantation—a prospective double blind study. *Transplantation.* 1995;59:495–500.

Rollins S, Schumann GB. Primary urinary cytodiagnosis of a bladder small cell carcinoma. *Diagn Cytopathol.* 1991;7:79–82.

Ross JS. Therapy associated atypia in urothelial cytology. Genitourinary pathology case 5. United States and Canadian Academy of Pathology Meeting, Washington, DC, March 26, 1996: 26–35. [conference handout]

Rudrick B, Nguyen GK, Lakey WH. Carcinoid tumor of the renal pelvis: report of a case with positive urine cytology. *Diagn Cytopathol.* 1995;12:360–363.

Rupp M, O'Hara B, McCullough L, et al. Prostatic carcinoma cells in urine specimens. *Cytopathology.* 1994;5:164–170.

Sack MJ, Artymyshyn RL, Tomaszewski JE, et al. Diagnostic value of bladder wash cytology, with special reference to low-grade urothelial neoplasms. *Acta Cytol.* 1995;39:187–194.

Schneider V, Smith MJ, Frable WJ. Urinary cytology in endometriosis of the bladder. *Acta Cytol.* 1980;24:30–33.

Schwalb DM, Herr HW, Fair WR. The management of clinically unconfirmed positive urinary cytology. *J Urol.* 1993;150:1751–1756.

Schwalb MD, Herr HW, Sogany PC, et al. Positive urinary cytology following a complete response to intravesical balillus Calmette-Guerin therapy: pattern of recurrence. *J Urol.* 1994;152: 382–387.

Seftel AD, Matthews LA, Smith MC, et al. Polyomavirus mimicking high grade transitional cell carcinoma. *J Urol.* 1996;156:1764–1766.

Segura A, Upton M, Duren L, et al. Cytologic diagnosis of low grade transitional cell carcinoma of the bladder. New cytologic criteria (Abstract). *Mod Pathol.* 1995;8:43A.

Shaaban AA, Tribukait B, el-Bedeiwy AF, et al. Characterization of squamous cell carcinoma bladder tumors by flow cytometric deoxyribonucleic acid analysis: a report of 100 cases. *J Urol.* 1990;144:879–883.

Sheinfeld J, Reuter VE, Melamed MR, et al. Enhanced bladder cancer detection with the Lewis-X antigen as a marker of neoplastic transformation. *J Urol.* 1990;143:285–288.

Shenoy UA, Colby TV, Schumann GB. Reliability of urinary cytodiagnosis in urothelial neoplasms. *Cancer.* 1985;56:2041–2045.

Stilmant M, Murphy JL, Merriam JC. Cytology of nephrogenic adenoma of the urinary bladder. *Acta Cytol.* 1986;30:35–40.

Tanaka T, Yoshimi N, Sawada K, et al. Ki-1-positive large cell anaplastic lymphoma diagnosed by urinary cytology. A case report. *Acta Cytol.* 1993;37: 520–524.

Travis LB, Curtis RE, Boice JD, et al. Bladder cancer after chemotherapy for non-Hodgkin's lymphoma. *N Engl J Med.* 1989;321:544–545.

Tribukait B. Clinical DNA flow cytometry. *Med Oncol Tumor Pharmacother.* 1984;1:211–218.

van der Poel HG, Boon ME, van Stratum P, et al. Conventional bladder wash cytology performed by four experts versus quantitative image analysis. *Mod Pathol.* 1997;10:976–982.

Wall RL, Kalusen KP. Carcinoma of the urinary bladder in patients receiving cyclophosphamide. *N Engl J Med.* 1995;295:271–273.

Wiener HG, Vooijs GP, van Hof-Grootenboer B. Accuracy of urinary cytology in the diagnosis of primary and recurrent bladder cancer. *Acta Cytol.* 1993;37:163–169.

Wolinska W, Melamed MR, Klein FA. Cytology of bladder papilloma. *Acta Cytol.* 1985;29:817–822.

15

MOLECULAR BIOLOGY OF THE BLADDER

Our understanding of the molecular and genetic alterations underlying urothelial carcinoma has expanded significantly over the past decade. Many new biomarkers are now available commercially and are often touted as superior to urine cytology in select patient cohorts. A recent large comparative study defined the predictive value of many of these markers (Ramakumar S, Bhuiyan J, Roberts SG, *J Urol*, 1999, in press). This chapter is an introduction to many of the promising new markers and is not meant to be all-inclusive (Tables 15.1 and 15.2).

15.1 PROPRIETARY COMMERCIAL MARKERS

15.1.1 Bladder Tumor Antigen

The Bard Bladder Tumor Antigen (BTA) stat™ test (Bard Diagnostics, Redmond, WA) is a latex agglutination assay that detects high molecular weight basement membrane complexes in urine produced when cancer cells become invasive and induce proteolytic degradation. It is rapid, easily performed, and readily interpretable in a clinician's office. Recent modifications of the test (BTA TRAK™ test) allow quantitation of immunoenzymatic results and superior sensitivity and specificity (Ellis et al, 1997; Leyh et al, 1998).

The specificity of the BTA™ test in monitoring patients with a history of urothelial carcinoma varies from 40% to 70%, significantly greater than 17%–32% for cytology; sensitivity results were 90%–96% and 100%, respectively (Ishak & Ellis, 1998; Raitanen et al, 1998; reviewed in Ianari et al, 1997). Interestingly, cytology was more predictive than the BTA™ test in patients with carcinoma in situ (Landman et al, 1998; Leyh et al, 1998), so the utility of the BTA™ test appears to be greatest in follow-up of patients with low-grade papillary tumors

Table 15.2   Prospective comparison of urine-based detection methods in bladder cancer

	Telomerase	Cytology	BTA Stat™	NMP22
Sensitivity	75%	42%	75%	24%
Specificity	92%	93%	68%	93%

Data from Ramakumar S, Bhuiyan J, Roberts SG, *J Urol*, 1999, in press.

Table 15.1 Select molecular markers in urothelial cancer

Proprietary commercial markers
    BTA™
    NMP22
    Immunocyt™
DNA ploidy
Fluorescence in situ hybridization (FISH)
Proliferation markers
    Proliferating cell nuclear antigen (PCNA)
    Ki-67
    MIB-1
Oncogenes, tumor suppressor genes, and mutator genes
    p53
    Retinoblastoma gene (Rb)
    Her-2/*neu*
    ras
    bcl-2
Loss of heterozygosity
Growth factors and receptors
    Epidermal growth factor receptor
    Acidic fibroblast growth factor
    Basic fibroblast growth factor
Cell adhesion markers
    E-cadherin
    Integrins
    Cyclin D1
    CD44
    F- and G-actin
Telomerase
Microvessel density and vascular endothelial growth factor
    Microvessel density
    Vascular endothelial growth factor
Miscellaneous markers
    Autocrine motility factor
    Luminal epithelial antigen (LEA.135)
    Androgen receptor
    Urokinase-type plasminogen activator factor
    FHIT gene
    Cytokeratin 20
    T138
    Hyaluronic acid

(Van der Poel et al, 1998). This test is now commonly used as an adjunct to cystoscopy and is being investigated as a possible screening test in high-risk patients (Leyh et al, 1998).

15.1.2 Nuclear Matrix Protein 22

The Matritech Nuclear Matrix Protein 22 (NMP22) immunoassay (Matritech, Newton, MA) detects a skeletal protein of the cell nucleus generated by cell lysis in the urine. It is rapid, easily performed, readily interpretable, and available in many clinical laboratories. NMP22 had a sensitivity of 88%–91% and specificity of 70%–76% for urothelial carcinoma in patients with microscopic hematuria, greater than respective values of 54%–55% and 90%–100% for urine cytology (Carpinito et al, 1998; Miyanaga et al, 1998). The sensitivity of NMP22 in patients with a history of bladder cancer was 59%–100% (Ludecke et al, 1998; Stampfer et al, 1998). The optimal reference range for recurrent cancer was 6.4 units/mL in one study, with higher results indicating a greater likelihood of recurrence (Stampfer et al, 1998). NMP22 may allow lengthening of the interval between follow-up cystoscopies in patients with low-risk cancer. Urinary tract infections and calculi must be excluded owing to interference with the test.

15.1.3 Immunocyt™ (M344 and 19A211 Antigens)

The use of fluorescently labeled antibodies directed against two superficial antigens, M344 and 19A211, is the basis of the Immunocyt™ diagnostic test (DiagnoCure, Inc., Quebec, Canada). This urine test has 90% specificity and 90% sensitivity in cancer detection and invariably identified all high-grade cancers in one study (Fradet, 1998).

15.2 DNA PLOIDY ANALYSIS OF UROTHELIAL CANCER

DNA ploidy analysis correlates with cancer grade and stage in urothelial carcinoma of the bladder and upper urinary tract, squamous cell carcinoma, and adenocarcinoma. At present, it remains a research tool in most laboratories. Most cases of papillary neoplasm of low malignant potential (formerly WHO grade 1 carcinoma) are diploid, whereas high-grade carcinoma (formerly WHO grade 3 carcinoma), including carcinoma in situ, is usually aneuploid (Al-Abadi & Nagel, 1994; Lee et al, 1996; Pantazopoulos et al, 1997; Shiina et al, 1996b; Velthoven et al, 1996). Low-grade carcinoma (formerly WHO grade 2 carcinoma) is equally likely to be diploid or nondiploid (Nakopoulou et al, 1995).

Ploidy results are strongly correlated with cancer invasion. Diploid cancer is usually confined to the lamina propria, whereas muscle-invasive cancer tends to be aneuploid (Lee & Park, 1996; Lopez-Beltran et al, 1992b, 1994). About half of aneuploid low-grade carcinomas are tetraploid, and very few tetraploid cancers are deeply invasive, suggesting that tetraploid low-grade carcinoma is less likely to invade into the wall of the bladder than aneuploid cancer. Tetraploidy may be an intermediate stage in the development of invasive aneuploid cancer (Bucci et al, 1995). Carcinoma in situ with two aneuploid peaks is more likely to progress to invasive cancer than CIS with a single peak (Norming et al, 1992). Adjacent urothelium often shares the same DNA ploidy abnormality as cancer (Norming et al, 1989), suggesting that aneuploid cancer arises from aneuploid epithelial abnormalities (Lee & Park, 1996). The significance of the S-phase fraction in the prognosis of bladder cancers is uncertain, although a recent report found that it was better than DNA ploidy as a predictor of progression in patients with cancer treated by intravesical chemotherapy (deVere White et al, 1998).

DNA ploidy as assessed by flow cytometry increases the predictive value of urine cytology for cancer in untreated patients, those with low- and high-stage cancer, and after treatment with intravesical or systemic chemotherapy. DNA content according to computer-based image analysis is at least as sensitive as flow cytometry for detecting malignant cells and is superior in hypocellular specimens (Slaton et al, 1997). DNA content is predictive of recurrence in papillary urothelial carcinoma after controlling for grade and stage (Pantazopoulos et al, 1997; Slaton et al, 1997).

DNA ploidy patterns of urothelial carcinoma of the renal pelvis and ureter are similar to those in the bladder (Al-Abadi & Nagel, 1994). Patients with an aneuploid cancer have a poorer prognosis than those with a diploid cancer (Al-Abadi & Nagel, 1994; Lopez-Beltran et al, 1992b, 1994, 1996a).

Well-differentiated squamous cell carcinoma is usually diploid, whereas moderately and poorly differentiated carcinoma is usually aneuploid (Shaaban et al, 1990). Most cases of primary adenocarcinoma of the urinary bladder are aneuploid.

15.3 FLUORESCENCE IN SITU HYBRIDIZATION

Diploid cells of urothelial carcinoma display numeric abnormalities of individual chromosomes according to fluorescence in situ hybridization (FISH) studies (Nemoto et al, 1995). Diploid histograms in cancer vary less with time than aneuploid histograms (Cajulis et al, 1994). Chromosomes involved nonrandomly and frequently in bladder cancer include 1, 6, 11, and 13 (Hopman et al, 1991; Sandberg & Berger, 1994; Yokogi et al, 1996). In some cancers, trisomy 7 or 5q deletion was the only chromosomal change. Trisomy 7, when present as the sole abnormality, may be associated with noninvasive growth and may represent a primary event in low-grade papillary cancers (Cajulis et al, 1994). Deletion of chromosomes 3p and 18q correlates with high-grade and cancer invasion (Brewster et al, 1994). Allelic loss of chromosome 9q is frequent in low-grade low-stage cancer (Gonzalez-Zulueta et al, 1995;

Sauter et al, 1995), whereas loss of chromosomes 11p and 17p is seen predominantly in high-grade invasive cancer (Olumi et al, 1990; Matsuyama et al, 1994; Shaw & Knowles, 1995). Deletion of chromosome 8p is common in invasive urothelial cancer, suggesting the possibility of a tumor suppressor gene (Wagner et al, 1997). FISH has also shown that there is frequent deletion of cyclin-dependent kinase inhibitor 2 (CDKN2, MTS1, INK4, or p16) at 9p21 in bladder cancer (Balazs et al, 1997).

15.4 PROLIFERATION MARKERS

Cell proliferation measures include counting mitotic figures; immunohistochemical analysis of proliferating cell nuclear antigen, Ki-67, and MIB-1; quantitation of tritiated thymidine uptake or bromodeoxyuridine uptake, and measurement of S phase fraction.

Proliferating cell nuclear antigen (PCNA, or cyclin) is a nonhistone nuclear protein that acts as an accessory of DNA polymerase. Its expression is maximal during the S phase and is closely linked to the cell cycle. The PCNA labeling index in bladder cancer varies from 5% to 92% and was predictive of cancer recurrence (Blasco-Olaetxea et al, 1996; Chen et al, 1997; Cheng et al, 1997), response to radiation therapy (Ogura et al, 1995), and survival (Shiina et al, 1996a). Diploid urothelial cancer with PCNA labeling index below 30% of cells did not recur, whereas aneuploid cancer with PCNA index greater than 30% usually recurred (Pantazopoulos et al, 1997). PCNA expression correlated with nuclear morphometric findings in bladder cancer cells (Ogura et al, 1997).

Ki-67 is a monoclonal antibody that recognizes a human nuclear antigen expressed in the S, G1, G2, and M phases of the cell cycle. Ki-67 expression, measured as the number of immunoreactive cells in frozen tissue specimens, correlated with cancer grade and stage (Busch et al, 1991; Mulder et al, 1992; Nakopoulou et al,

1998; Okamura et al, 1990). Also, it was predictive of recurrence of urothelial carcinoma (Asakura et al, 1997; Fontana et al, 1992; Stavropoulos et al, 1993) but not always by multivariate analysis (Nakopoulou et al, 1998).

MIB-1 is a monoclonal antibody that is the equivalent of Ki-67 and that displays immunoreactivity in formalin-fixed paraffin-embedded sections. Its expression is significantly associated with p53 expression (Liukkonen et al, 1997).

15.5 ONCOGENES, TUMOR SUPPRESSOR GENES, AND MUTATOR GENES

Some oncogenes and tumor suppressor genes appear to play a significant role in urothelial carcinogenesis (Theodorescu, 1996). The most likely factors include p53, retinoblastoma, Her-2/*neu*, and the *ras* family of genes.

15.5.1 p53 Gene

p53 is a 53-kd DNA-binding phosphoprotein that is coded for by a tumor suppressor gene located on the short arm of chromosome 17 (17p13.1). This transcription factor regulates cell growth and inhibits cells from entering the S phase. Mutations of p53 or functional inactivation with intact p53 genes are common in many human cancers, reflecting loss of normal growth regulation (Dalbagni et al, 1995). Mutations result in prolonged half-life and accumulation of the p53 protein to a level that makes it detectable immunohistochemically in cancer cell nuclei (Underwood et al, 1996). Overexpression of p53 protein is associated with a poor prognosis in a variety of cancers (Cordon-Cardo et al, 1994, 1997a,b).

Most antibodies for p53 require antigen retrieval procedures when used with deparaffinized formalin-fixed sections. Staining results may vary because of differences in fixation, specimen pretreatment, and antibody binding sites. Immunohistochemical methods rely on the accumulation of p53 protein in cells with p53 missense mutations. The cause of this is unknown, and recent studies indicate that immunoreactivity is not always indicative of p53 mutations. Wild-type p53 protein may accumulate in the setting of p53 activation, including hypoxia and DNA damage. In addition, not all p53 missense mutations result in protein accumulation, and they may cause false–negative immunohistochemical results. Finally, there may be a gradient of p53 inactivation that varies according to the site and extent of the mutation. Nonetheless, there is a strong positive correlation of immunoreactivity and p53 mutations (Cordon-Cardo et al, 1994). Benign urothelium rarely if ever displays staining, whereas expression in carcinoma is observed in 18% to 78% of cases (Burkhard et al, 1997; Caliskan et al, 1997; Esrig et al, 1994; Sinik et al, 1997). Different cut points have been used for positive and negative staining, most commonly being 0% of cells (Casetta et al, 1997; Vatne et al, 1995), 10% of cells (Gardiner et al, 1994; Grossman et al, 1998; Nakopoulou et al, 1998; Sinik et al, 1997), and 20% of cells (Caliskan et al, 1997; Cordon-Cardo et al, 1997b; Esrig et al, 1994; Liukkonen et al, 1997; Raitanen et al, 1997). Intratumoral heterogeneity is reflected in the heterogeneous expression of staining. The cellular urine sediment may be used for genetic analysis of p53 mutations (Friedrich et al, 1998; Sachs et al, 1998a).

In urothelial carcinoma, nuclear p53 protein immunoreactivity correlates with high grade (Dalbagni et al, 1993; Inagaki et al, 1997; Lipponen, 1993; Miyamoto et al, 1993; Nakopoulou et al, 1998; Oyasu et al, 1995), high stage (Al-Abadi et al, 1998; Dalbagni et al, 1993; Inagaki et al, 1997; Miyamoto et al, 1993; Nakopoulou et al, 1995, 1998; Pfister et al, 1998), vascular invasion (Dalbagni et al, 1993), cancer recurrence and progression (Cordon-Cardo et al, 1997b; Schmitz-Drager et al, 1997; Grossman et al, 1998; Lerner et al, 1998; Lipponen, 1993), survival (Cordon-Cardo et al, 1997b; Esrig et al, 1994; Lerner et al, 1998; Llopis et al, 1998; Sarkis et al, 1995; Tsuji et al, 1997; Uchida et al, 1995), and p53 mutations, including 17p deletion and 17 polysomy (Esrig et al, 1994; Fujimoto et al, 1992; Liukkonen et al, 1997; Nakopoulou et al, 1998; Oyasu et al, 1995; Raitanen et al, 1997; Vet et al, 1994, 1995; Vollmer et al, 1998). Immunoreactivity may have independent prognostic significance (Casetta et al, 1997; Cordon-Cardo et al, 1997b; Esrig et al, 1994; Sarkis et al, 1993, 1994, 1995), but this has been refuted (Al-Abadi et al, 1998; Burkhard et al, 1997; Inagaki et al, 1997; Lipponen, 1993; Nakopoulou et al, 1995, 1998; Vatne et al, 1995). Stage T1 bladder carcinoma with more than 20% p53-immunoreactive cells had a higher progression rate than cancer with fewer stained cells (21% vs 3% progression per year, respectively) (Sarkis et al, 1993). Similarly, carcinoma in situ with more than 20% p53-immunoreactive cells had a higher progression rate than cases with fewer stained cells (86% vs 16% per year, respectively) (Sarkis et al, 1994). These results have been confirmed by other authors (Esrig et al, 1994; Glick et al, 1996; Grossman et al, 1998; Terrel et al, 1995; Watanabe et al, 1994). Conversely, a recent study showed that cancer grade and stage were the only independent predictive factors for patient survival when p53 and bcl-2 were included in the analysis (Nakopoulou et al, 1998). p53 status is not predictive of initial clinical response to bacillus Calmette-Guerin therapy in T1 cancer treated by transurethral resection, regardless of grade (Lebret et al, 1998; Pages et al, 1998).

The predictive value of p53 may be increased when combined with other factors. p53 immunoreactivity and DNA aneuploidy are closely associated and, when found in combination, predict a very poor outcome for patients with invasive cancer (Nakopoulou et al, 1995); conversely, another study found no correlation of p53 expression and DNA ploidy status (Al-Abadi et al, 1998).

p53 alterations in urothelial carcinoma may result in increased sensitivity to chemotherapeutic agents that damage DNA, including doxorubicin and ciplatin (Cote et al, 1997). In patients with p53 mutations, adjuvant chemotherapy resulted in a threefold decreased risk of recurrence and a 2.6-fold increased chance of survival with median follow-up of about 9 years (Cote et al, 1997). Patients without p53 mutations derived no survival advantage with chemotherapy. These results suggest that patients at greatest risk of progression and death (those with p53 mutations) may also derive the maximum benefit from adjuvant chemotherapy and that p53 status may identify such patients.

Wild-type p53 leads to apoptotic cell death, whereas mutant p53 inhibits apoptotic death, similar to *bcl*-2. Thus, it is interesting to note that *bcl*-2 is expressed more frequently in low-grade and low-stage urothelial cancer, whereas mutant p53 is more frequent in high-grade and high-stage cancer. One possible explanation is that mutant p53 prolongs survival of cells with established genetic defects, allowing them to become more unstable and clinically aggressive; conversely, *bcl*-2 may be an early event that prolongs survival of cells, allowing them to acquire initial genetic defects (Nakopoulou et al, 1998).

p53 protein can be inactivated by viral proteins such as the E6 protein of human papillomavirus (HPV) 16. HPV is detected in occasional cases of papillary noninvasive and invasive cancer, and the presence of HPV correlates with higher stage and grade (Lopez-Beltran & Escudero, 1997; Lopez-Beltran & Munoz, 1995; Lopez-Beltran et al, 1992a, 1996b). p53 mutations are rarely observed in patients with HPV-positive cancer, suggesting separate etiologic pathways (LaRue et al, 1995). Also, p53 can activate the proto-oncogene nuclear protein MDM2 (Lianes et al, 1994; Schmitz-Drager et al, 1997). This protein is increased in 67% of cases of noninvasive and early invasive bladder cancer but is present in only 27% of cases of muscle-invasive carcinoma. The p16 gene, present on chromosome 9, is abnormal in up to 60% of cases of squamous cell carcinoma associated with *Schistosomiasis* but only 18% of cases of urothelial carcinoma (Gonzalez-Zulueta et al, 1995; Orlow et al, 1995; Warren et al, 1995). Moreover, anomalies of p16 and p53 are mutually exclusive, suggesting a complementary role in the pathogenesis of bladder cancer (Orlow et al, 1995). Synchronous p53 and nm23-H-1 detection showed significant correlation with poor patient survival (Nakopoulou et al, 1996).

p53 induces p53-dependent genes. A prototype of this class of genes, Cip-1 (WAF-1), encodes a 21-kd protein that inhibits cyclin-dependent kinases responsible for initiation of the G1 phase of the cell cycle. Mutations in the p53 gene result in failure to stimulate Cip-1, with subsequent loss of inhibition of cyclin-dependent kinase complexes and initiation of G1 (Miyamoto et al, 1996). The discovery of p53-dependent cyclin-dependent kinase inhibitors linked this gene to the basic enzyme mechanisms operative in cell cycle regulation. Mutations in p53 are usually missense substitutions that cluster in one particular region of the gene product between amino acids 130 and 290, involving residues 117–142, 171–181, 239–258, and 270–286. These regions are highly conserved among species and are probably necessary for normal p53 function. The regions encompassing codons 280 and 285 are a hot spot for p53 mutations (Xu et al, 1997).

Loss of heterozygosity of the p53 locus occurs in many human cancers (Miyamoto et al, 1996). Therefore, p53 most likely contributes to human carcinogenesis when its normal allele is deleted or inactivated. Transforming activity in the heterozygous state may be a result of formation of an oligomeric complex between mutant and wild-type p53. In cells transformed with mutant p53 gene, the altered protein complex remains in the cytoplasm.

Mutated p53 genes can cooperate with *ras* genes to transform primary cultured fibroblasts in the presence of endogenous wild-type p53 protein (Cordon-Cardo et al, 1994). In some cancers, deletion of chromosome 17 loci occurs simultaneously with other chromosomal abnormalities, suggesting that p53 mutation is a late event in carcinogenesis. Cancer cell aneuploidy, reflecting chromosomal instability, may play a role in selection of cancer cells with p53 gene mutations. This process could lead to loss of the remaining wild-type allele and inactivation of growth control function of the normal p53 protein (Dalbagni et al, 1995).

About 65% of cases of carcinoma in situ contain p53 mutations (Schmitz-Drager et al, 1994; Spruck et al, 1994), considerably greater than the 28%–33% of cases of atypia and dysplasia (Sinik et al, 1997). This high frequency of mutations is similar to that found in invasive urothelial carcinoma and may explain on a genetic basis the great propensity of carcinoma in situ to progress (Schmitz-Drager et al, 1994). Moreover, germ-line transmission of p53 mutations occurs in cancer-prone families, including those with Li-Fraumeni syndrome (Schulte, 1988). p53 gene mutations were present in 11 of 18 invasive bladder cancers, and the most common mutation was single base-pair substitution (Sidransky et al, 1991). Missense mutations were present in 7 of 11, cases and nonsense mutations in three. Mutations of p53 are also detectable in urine sediment (Sidransky et al, 1991) and may be predictive of progression (Vet et al, 1996). In a study of 25 bladder cancers from 23 patients, the incidence of p53 mutations was significantly higher in muscle-invasive than non–muscle-invasive cancer (58% vs 8%, respectively) (Fujimoto et al, 1992). High-grade bladder cancer contains diverse p53 mutations in 36% of cases, according to one study (Cordon-Cardo et al, 1994). These molecular studies confirm the immunohistochemical observations of p53 protein expression in bladder carcinoma. The identification of mutations of Cip-1 and MTS1 genes in urothelial carcinoma and other human cancers indicates that similar biologic effects can be the result of alterations of different genes in the p53 regulatory pathway (Kinzler & Vogelstein, 1996; Patard et al, 1995). Importantly, p53 immunoreactivity correlates with detection of p53 mutated protein (Zhang et al, 1994).

15.5.2 Retinoblastoma Gene

The retinoblastoma (Rb) gene on chromosome 13p14 encodes a 105-kd protein that regulates transcription in all adult cells. The normal gene product suppresses expression of genes required for cell cycle progression. Cyclin and cyclin-dependent kinases inactivate the Rb gene product by phosphorylation. pRb can be inactivated by the protein corresponding to the open reading frames E6 of HPV 16 without mutation of the Rb gene (Cordon-Cardo et al, 1992; Lopez-Beltran & Escudero, 1997). Loss of function of the MTS-1 gene, which encodes the p16 protein, is an upstream regulator of Rb maintaining the Rb in its active or hypophosphorylated state. Absence of p16 correlates with functional inactivation of the Rb protein, perhaps accounting for the equal prognosis in patients with Rb absence or overexpression in some studies (Benedict et al, 1998).

pRb is expressed in all human tissues. Mutational inactivation of Rb gene and reduction of pRb expression occurs in retinoblastoma and other cancers (Ishikawa et al, 1991). The two main types of alteration of Rb in human cancer are deletion and mutation. Major deletions of large segments of the gene result in the absence of a properly functioning gene product (Ishikawa et al, 1991). Mutations, including nucleotide substitutions that alter gene function, create improperly located initiation signals, splicing sites, stop codons, amino acid substitutions, and other changes that destabilize transcription, producing a truncated gene product or otherwise modifying the messenger RNA. These changes cause absence of a functional Rb protein (Kubota et al, 1995). Rb alterations in bladder cancer appear to be subtle point mutations rather than major deletions. Rb gene is one of the major genetic factors responsible for development and progression of high-grade muscle-invasive bladder cancer (Cordon-Cardo et al, 1992, 1997b). Loss of Rb function occurs in 30% of high-grade papillary and nonpapillary urothelial carcinomas. Loss of Rb correlates with loss of heterozygosity at the Rb gene locus, as well as high grade and muscle invasion.

Altered expression of pRb is associated with decreased survival of patients with urothelial carcinoma (Grossman et al, 1998; Kubota et al, 1995). Benign urothelial mucosa and noninvasive urothelial carcinoma have pRb immunoreactivity in most cells (Goodrich et al, 1992). Immunohistochemical detection of pRb appears to be a useful marker of cancer progression but is not routinely used (Cordon-Cardo et al, 1992; Geradts et al, 1996; Lipponen & Liukkonen, 1995; Wright et al, 1995).

15.5.3   Her-2/*neu*; p185 (c-*erb*B2)

The Her-2/*neu* proto-oncogene is present as a single copy gene in normal cells, present on chromosome 17q12-21.32. It encodes a protein in the cytoplasmic membrane that has an external (Her-1) component, a transmembrane component, and an internal (Her-2/*neu*) 185-kd cytoplasmic component (Mellon et al, 1996). Her-2/*neu* has tyrosine kinase activity and is 85% homologous with epidermal growth factor receptor protein (EGFr) (Mellon et al, 1996). The transmembrane segment is not closely related to EGFr, as the extracellular domain shares 40% homology.

Her-2/*neu* immunoreactivity in urothelial carcinoma is usually present on the cell membrane (Gorgoulis et al, 1995), although cytoplasmic reactivity has also been reported (Tetu et

al, 1996). Stained cells are distributed diffusely, with no preference for superficial or basal cells. The frequency of Her-2/*neu* protein expression varies from 2% to 65% in the normal and inflamed urothelium and is present in 19% of cases of dysplasia and 64% of cases of carcinoma in situ (Underwood et al, 1995). Immunoreactivity increases with urothelial cancer stage and recurrence (Mellon et al, 1996; Ravery et al, 1997), although some reports found no correlation of Her-2/*neu* staining and outcome (Moch et al, 1994).

15.5.4   *ras* Genes

The human *ras* gene family, including Ha-*ras*, Ki-*ras*, and N-*ras*, is a prototype of cellular genes whose mutations or overexpression can lead to malignant transformation (Barbacid, 1987). These genes encode a group of closely related 21-kd proteins (p21). *ras* p21 binds guanine nucleotides with high affinity and has guanosine triphosphate activity. The protein is anchored to the cytoplasmic surface of the cell membrane and is a transducer molecule for signals affecting cell proliferation (Barbacid, 1987).

Two mechanisms may explain how *ras* genes transform cells. One involves a single nucleotide mutation in the coding sequence that occurs most frequently at codons 12, 13, 159, and 61, resulting in an amino acid substitution of the gene product p21 that affects the GTP binding domain and reduces its enzyme activity. The second mechanism involves overexpression of the *ras* gene product.

Mutations of the coding sequence of *ras* genes are the most frequent genetic alterations in urothelial cancer (Barbacid, 1987). These mutations usually involve codon 12 and, less frequently, codon 13 or 61 of Ha-*ras*. Sporadically, the Ki-*ras* gene is also affected. The elimination of functional Ha-*ras* gene in human bladder cancer cell line T24 by an antisense oligonucleotide inhibited cell proliferation. Ha-*ras* mutations occur in about 50% of bladder cancers (Knowles

& Williamson, 1993). G-T substitution in the second nucleotide of codon 12 of the Ha-*ras* gene results in replacement of glycine for valine in the gene product p21 and is a dominant mutation in human bladder cancer (Cerutti et al, 1994; Czerniak et al, 1992). Ha-*ras* gene codon 12 mutations occur more frequently in high-grade aneuploid bladder carcinoma than in low-grade diploid papillary carcinoma, but there is no definitive correlation with cancer grade or stage. Similar results have been obtained with p21 by immunohistochemistry; p21 expression correlates with DNA ploidy status but not with grade and stage (Lopez-Beltran et al, 1992b). c-Ha-*ras*-1 gene polymorphisms have been found in bladder cancer, but c-Ha-*ras*-1 genotyping appears to be of limited value in the clinical management of patients (Bittard et al, 1996).

15.5.5 *bcl*-2

The proto-oncogene *bcl*-2 encodes a mitochondrial membrane protein that blocks apoptosis without influencing cell proliferation. *bcl*-2 immunoreactivity was observed in benign and dysplastic urothelium and in about half of cases of urothelial carcinoma but was negative in carcinoma in situ (Furihata et al, 1996; Lipponen et al, 1996; Liukkonen et al, 1997; Nakopoulou et al, 1998). There was decreased expression with higher stage and higher grade cancer (Liukkonen et al, 1997; Nakopoulou et al, 1998; Posch et al, 1998).

15.6   LOSS OF HETEROZYGOSITY

Loss of heterozygosity (LOH) in bladder cancer can be detected by cytogenetics, restriction fragment length polymorphisms, and microsatellite polymorphism analysis (Knowles, 1995). Some chromosomal deletions are common in urothelial carcinoma (Sandberg & Berger, 1994), and the most common is loss of chromosome 9p, present in more than 50% of cases of well to moderately differentiated T1

and T2 cancer (Miyao et al, 1993). Both 9p and 9q probably harbor tumor suppressor genes involved in the initiation of bladder carcinogenesis (Simoneau et al, 1996). The total number of alterations is higher in pT1 tumors than in pTa tumors (Richter et al, 1997).

LOH of chromosomes 11p and 17p13 (the p53 locus) usually occurs in high-grade invasive cancer (Olumi et al, 1990), whereas allelic loss of chromosome 3 is seen in only 26% of high-stage urothelial cancers (Li et al, 1996). Loss of the Y chromosome is common in urothelial carcinoma and is associated with advanced stage, coexistent carcinoma in situ, and poor prognosis (Sidransky & Messing, 1992). LOH of the short arm of chromosome 3 is not present in superficial papillary cancer, whereas it is present in 54% of cases of muscle-invasive cancer. LOH has also been observed on chromosomes 4p, 4q, 5q, 8p, and 10q (Cappellen et al, 1997). Loss of 14q is common in invasive bladder cancer and suggests that there are potential tumor suppressor loci on 14q12 and 14q32.1-32.2 (Chang et al, 1995). LOH of chromosome 18q is associated with muscle-invasive bladder cancer (Brewster et al, 1994). LOH at the DEL-27 locus on 5p13-12 predicted progression in bladder cancer (Bohm et al, 1997).

Other chromosomal imbalances in bladder carcinoma have been found by comparative genomic hybridization (Kallioniemi et al, 1995; Richter et al, 1997; Voorter et al, 1995). A recent report described a novel method of detecting polymorphic microsatellite markers in urine sample with a high sensitivity for bladder cancer recurrence (Steiner et al, 1997).

15.7   GROWTH FACTORS AND RECEPTORS

15.7.1   Epidermal Growth Factor Receptor

The epidermal growth factor receptor (EGFr), encoded by a proto-oncogene located on chromosome 7p13, is a transmembrane, growth-regulating 170-kd glycoprotein. The extracellular domain represents the ligand binding site and is a receptor for epidermal growth factor (EGF) and transforming growth factor alpha (TGF-a). Binding of EGF to its receptor results in downregulation of the receptor and stimulation of tyrosine kinase (Nakanishi et al, 1996). EGFr is present in many cells, including the basal cell layer of normal urothelium (Gorgoulis et al, 1995). Staining is predominantly membranous. EGFr immunoreactivity is present in about 50% of bladder cancers, with increased expression in stage T2-4 cancers (71% of cases) (Sauter et al, 1994). Staining is most common at the advancing edge of the invasive cancer (Sauter et al, 1994).

EGFr immunoreactivity correlates with bladder cancer recurrence, time to recurrence, and survival (Sauter et al, 1994; Turkeri et al, 1998), although there are some conflicting results (Ravery et al, 1997). The strong association between EGFr immunoreactivity and the proliferation index (using bromodeoxyuridine staining) in bladder cancer suggests that it may be involved in cancer promotion and proliferation (Sauter et al, 1994). Furthermore, the combination of increased EGFr immunoreactivity and loss of blood group antigen and spontaneous expression of the T antigen suggests that defective glycosylation is involved in urothelial carcinogenesis and increasing stage (Pinnock et al, 1995). EGFr immunoreactivity may be related to expression of c-*jun* oncoprotein (Tiniakos et al, 1994). At present, immunoreactivity for growth factors provides no practical prognostic value in urothelial carcinoma of the upper urinary tract (Nakanishi et al, 1996).

15.7.2 Acidic Fibroblast Growth Factor

Acidic fibroblast growth factor is a monomeric 16-kd protein originally purified from normal brain and widely distributed in normal human tissues (Sauter et al, 1994). It is present in most cases of urothelial carcinoma, and the intensity and frequency of immunoreactivity correlates with grade and stage.

15.7.3 Basic Fibroblast Growth Factor

Basic fibroblast growth factor (bFGF) is one of a family of nine fibroblast growth factors, all of which have a strong affinity for heparin and are functional ligands for FGF receptors that have intrinsic tyrosine kinase activity. bFGF is present in the basal lamina of the normal urothelium, normal muscle, and blood vessels but in only 13% of cases of urothelial carcinoma (O'Brien et al, 1997). bFGF is a potent angiogenic factor.

15.8 CELL ADHESION MARKERS

15.8.1 E-cadherin

E-cadherin is the epithelial member of the cadherin molecule family, a group of glycoproteins of the cell membranes of 80- to 120-kd molecular weight and 723–748 amino acids. They have an extracellular, membranous, and cytoplasmic domain, and the extracellular domain contains the binding site for calcium, which protects the molecule from proteolysis (Lipponen & Eskelinen, 1995). The cytoplasmic domain forms complexes with catenins and cytoplasmic elements.

The normal human urothelium displays homogeneous immunohistochemical expression of E-cadherin, with membranous staining at cell borders (Ross et al, 1995, 1996). The luminal membrane of superficial cells was devoid of staining, as was the part of the cells in contact with the basement membrane. Abnormal staining is present in 21% of low-stage cancers and 76% of invasive cancers (Lipponen & Eskelinen, 1995). The strong correlation of E-cadherin expression with cancer stage indicates that it plays a role in invasion (Wakatsuki et al, 1996). There is also a strong correlation between E-cadherin expression and survival; conversely, the presence of normal E-cadherin staining appears to indicate a good prognosis, even if the cancer is high stage (Otto et al, 1997; Ross et al, 1995). Serum concentration of E-cadherin correlated with cancer grade, number of cancers at presentation, and cancer recurrence but not with immunoreactivity in tissue sections (Griffiths et al, 1996).

15.8.2 Integrins

The integrins are a family of adhesion molecules that are transmembrane heterodimers of noncovalently linked alpha and beta subunits. There are at least eight different subfamilies of integrins, each with a common beta subunit capable of combining with various alpha subunits. Integrins function as receptors for extracellular molecules and can be segregated broadly into those that bind primarily to major constitutents of the basement membrane (collagens, and laminin), those that bind primarily to the extracellular matrix proteins (fibrinogen, fibronectin, and thrombospondin), and those that function as cell adhesion molecules (found primarily on lymphocytes) (Liebert et al, 1994). Normal urothelium does not express alpha 1, alpha 4, and alpha 5 subunits but shows cell membrane staining for alpha 2 and alpha 3 that is stronger in the basal cell layer than in luminal cells (Saito et al, 1996). There is progressive loss of alpha 2 beta 1 expression and, to a lesser extent, alpha 3 beta 1 in progression from Ta and T1 cancer to T2–3 cancer (Liebert et al, 1994). In normal urothelium, the alpha 6 beta 4 integrin colocalizes with type VII collagen at the junction of the basal cell and the lamina propria (Liebert et al, 1994). In 83% of noninvasive bladder cancers, integrin expression is present on the suprabasal and basal cells, whereas type VII collagen remains at the

hemidesmosomal anchoring complex. This finding suggests that the anchoring complex in low-stage cancer is normal or only slightly altered, whereas in 83% of invasive cancers, loss of integrin or type VII collagen or both indicate abnormalities (Liebert et al, 1994).

15.8.3 Cyclin D1

Cyclin D1 is a nuclear protein encoded by the CCND1 gene on chromosome 11q13 that has been identified as the PRAD1 proto-oncogene and the most likely candidate for the *bcl*-1 proto-oncogene. Cyclin D1 binds to cyclin-dependent kinases and displays specific and periodic expression during cell cycle progression, suggesting an important role in growth regulation. It interacts with pRB and other cell cycle–related proteins such as PCNA and p21. Benign and dysplastic urothelium, including inverted papilloma, do not express cyclin D1 (Lee et al, 1997).

Conflicting results have been obtained with immunohistochemical studies of cyclin D1 expression. One study identified nuclear cyclin D1 only in stage Ta and T1 papillary urothelial cancer but not in invasive cancer or non-papillary cancer, and a marked decline with cancer grade (Lee et al, 1997; Tut et al, 1998). There was an inverse correlation of cyclin D1 expression and PCNA and p53 expression, suggesting that cyclin D1 plays a role in negatively controlling cellular proliferation and allowing cancer differentiation. Conversely, other studies found no correlation of cyclin D1 expression with grade and stage, although cyclin D1–immunoreactive cancers recurred more rapidly than unreactive cancer (Proctor et al, 1991; Shin et al, 1997). Overexpression of cyclin D1 mRNA was found in 81% of non–muscle-invasive cancer and 38% of muscle-invasive cancer (Bringuier et al, 1996). For comparison, about 10%–15% of bladder cancers have amplification of the 11q13 region (Bringuier et al, 1996). The cumulative results indicate that genetic alterations in cyclin D1 are probably early events in urothelial carcinogenesis.

15.8.4   CD44

CD44 (PgP-1, ECM III, Hermes antigen) designates a family of cell surface glycoproteins present chiefly in epithelial cells that are involved in cell–cell and cell–matrix interactions (reviewed in Cohen et al, 1997). The normal urothelium expresses CD44, but the greatest expression is present in early noninvasive papillary urothelial carcinoma, with progressive loss with invasion (Iczkowski et al, 1998; Ross et al, 1996; Sugino et al, 1996). CD44 protein isoforms and mRNA species are also detectable in exfoliated cancer cells in urine specimens (Muller et al, 1996; Sugiyama et al, 1995). Soluble CD44 proteins are detectable in serum, with lower levels in men with bladder cancer than in matched healthy controls (Lein et al, 1997). CD44v6 immunostaining discriminates small cell carcinoma of the bladder (negative) from poorly differentiated urothelial carcinoma (usually positive) (Iszkowski et al, 1998).

15.8.5   F- and G-Actin

The amounts of the cytoskeletal protein, F-actin, or its precursor, G-actin, are markers for decreased differentiation that identify patients at risk for bladder cancer (Hemstreet et al, 1996; Rao et al, 1991). The differentiation-related changes occur early in carcinogenesis and can be reversed by in vitro treatment with retinoids or other differentiation-promoting agents (Rao et al, 1990).

15.9   TELOMERASE

The chromosome ends, referred to as telomeres, progressively shorten with each cell division, ultimately resulting in destruction of the chromosome. Telomere shortening acts as a biologic clock to induce cell senescence and death and is reversed by telomerase, a DNA polymerase that repairs the ends of chromosomes, thereby prolonging cell life and replicative potential. The presence or increased expression of telomerase has been implicated in the immortality and growth advantage of cancer cells in a variety of organs.

Benign urothelium displays little or no telomerase activity, whereas virtually every cancer expressed high levels, according to studies of tissue extracts (Kamata et al, 1996; Kyo et al, 1997; Lin et al, 1996). An in situ hybridization assay revealed comparable results recently in formalin-fixed paraffin-embedded tissues (Fagelson et al, 1998).

The majority of urine samples with cancer cells contain telomerase activity, whereas most benign samples do not (Heine et al, 1998; Kinoshita et al, 1997; Landman et al, 1997; Lee et al, 1998; Muller et al, 1996; Yoshida et al, 1997). Analysis of telomerase activity in urine samples using PCR-based amplification in the Telomeric Repeat Amplification Protocol (TRAP) assay revealed an optimal combination of sensitivity and specificity (75% and 92%, respectively) when compared with cytology, the BTA stat™ test, and NMP22 (Table 15.2) (Landman et al, 1998; Ramakumar S, Bhuiyan J, Roberts SG, unpublished observations, 1998). Telomerase activity did not correlate with cancer stage, grade, multifocality, or cancer recurrence (Fagelson et al, 1998; Kyo et al, 1997).

15.10   MICROVESSEL DENSITY AND VASCULAR ENDOTHELIAL GROWTH FACTOR

15.10.1   Microvessel Density

Angiogenesis is an essential component of cancer growth, and it is indirectly measured by counting the number of small blood vessels to create the microvessel density score (number of blood vessels per unit area). All studies of microvessel density in bladder cancer to date have been retrospective, and comparison is often difficult owing to differences in methods of microvessel density measurement, patient populations, and outcome variables. Standards have recently been proposed for analysis of microvessel density to facilitate confirmation of the suggested predictive value of this factor in bladder cancer and other cancers (Vermeulen et al, 1996; Weidner, 1996).

Increased microvessel density in urothelial carcinoma is predictive of lymph node metastases (Jaeger et al, 1995), recurrence, and survival (Bochner et al, 1995; Dickinson et al, 1994) and appears to be an independent prognostic factor (Bochner et al, 1995; Dickinson et al, 1994).

15.10.2 Vascular Endothelial Growth Factor

Vascular endothelial growth factor (VEGF) and, to a lesser extent, basic fibroblast growth factor, are the primary inducers of angiogenesis in bladder cancer cells (Campbell et al, 1998). VEGF mRNA and protein levels are higher in cancer than benign urothelium (Brown et al, 1993), and high VEGF predicts a poor prognosis (Crew et al, 1997). An inhibitor of VEGF, thrombospondin-1, appears to play a key role in angiogenesis; its downregulation is associated with the switch from an antiangiogenic to an angiogenic phenotype that occurs early in urothelial carcinoma (Campbell et al, 1998).

15.11 MISCELLANEOUS MARKERS

A variety of other markers have been evaluated in limited series. Autocrine motility factor (AMF-R, or gp78) was not expressed by benign urothelium, whereas its expression in urothelial carcinoma was an independent predictor of outcome in patients treated surgically (Otto et al, 1997). Expression of the surface gly-coprotein luminal epithelial antigen (LEA.135) in immunohistochemical assays showed progressive loss with high-grade and higher stage cancer (Jones et al, 1997). Androgen receptor, a member of the steroid hormone nuclear receptor superfamily, is expressed in the majority of cases of urothelial carcinoma (Zhuang et al, 1997) but not in benign urothelium (Ruizeveld de Winter et al, 1991). Urokinase-type plasminogen activator is a serine protease whose expression was an independent predictor of survival in node-negative muscle-invasive bladder cancer (Hofmann et al, 1998) but not in upper urinary tract carcinoma (Nakanishi et al, 1998). The fragile histidine triad (FHIT) gene on chromosome 3p14.2 is aberrantly expressed in most primary urothelial cancers (Baffa et al, 1998). Cytokeratin 20 is expressing in neoplastic urothelial cells but apparently not in normal urothelium, and mRNA extraction from urine samples of patients with bladder cancer revealed a sensitivity of 91% and specificity of 67% (Klein et al, 1998). Progression marker T138 detected a surface antigen that, together with cancer stage, was an independent predictor of metastases (Fradet, 1998). The glycosaminoglycan hyaluronic acid promotes cell migration and adhesion, and levels in the urine, when measured by enzyme-linked immunoabsorption assay, are elevated three- to fivefold in patients with urothelial carcinoma (Lokeshwar et al, 1997). Expression of the nm 23-H1 gene product in musele-invasive urothelial carcinoma was predictive of poor patient survival in multivariate analysis (Nakopoulou et al, 1996).

15.12 CLONAL ORIGIN OF UROTHELIAL CARCINOMA

Bladder cancer is often multifocal and may recur at another site following excision. Synchronous multiple bladder cancers appear to be monoclonal according to molecular genetic studies based on analysis of X chromosome inactivation pattern in female patients (Sidransky & Messing, 1992). Clonal origin is also likely according to analysis of p53 gene mutations in patients whose cancers were resected at different times (Habuchi et al, 1993; Sachs et al, 1998b); each patient's cancers contained identical p53 mutations, suggesting that the cancers arose from the same transformed cell and were monoclonal. LOH studies of chromosome 9, 17p, and p53 gene in synchronous and asynchronous bladder cancers revealed identical gene lesions in most, indicating that the cancers were probably monoclonal (Miyao et al, 1993). The cumulative findings suggest that intravesical metastases are common.

15.13 GENETIC PATHWAYS IN UROTHELIAL CARCINOMA

Molecular abnormalities vary according to the histologic type and stage of bladder cancer (Reznikoff et al, 1993, 1996). Low-grade noninvasive papillary cancer (pTa) frequently shows only loss of heterozygosity of chromosome 9, suggesting that inactivation of one or more putative tumor suppressor genes on this chromosome is an initiating event in carcinogenesis (Gonzalez-Zulueta et al, 1993; Miyao et al, 1993; Gonzalez-Zulueta et al, 1995). In contrast, carcinoma in situ frequently contains p53 gene mutations but only infrequently shows loss of heterozygosity of chromosome 9. These observations suggest that there are two separate pathways in bladder carcinogenesis with different initiating events, including chromosome 9 deletion or p53 gene alteration (Simoneau & Jones, 1994; Spruck et al, 1994). After transformation, urothelial cells may acquire additional genetic abnormalities that determine transition from noninvasive to invasive cancer. Subsequent changes may involve deletions in chromosomes 3p, 4p, 8p, 11p, 13q, 18q, and others.

REFERENCES

Al-Abadi H, Nagel R. Deoxyribonucleic acid content and survival rates of patients with transitional cell carcinoma of the bladder. *J Urol.* 1994;151:37–42.

Al-Abadi H, Nagel R, Neuhaus P. Immunohistochemical detection of p53 protein in transitional cell carcinoma of the bladder in correlation to DNA ploidy and pathohistological stage and grade. *Cancer Detect Prev.* 1998;22:43–50.

Asakura T, Takano Y, Iki M, et al. Prognostic value of Ki-67 for recurrence and progression of superficial bladder cancer. *J Urol.* 1997;158:385–388.

Baffa R, Gomella LG, Strup SE, et al. Pathologic role of the FHIT gene in transitional cell carcinoma of the bladder (Abstract). *J Urol.* 1998;1159 (Suppl 5):278.

Balazs M, Carroll P, Kerschmann R, et al. Frequent homozygous deletion of cyclin-dependent kinase inhibitor 2 (MTS1, p16) in superficial bladder cancer detected by fluorescence in situ hybridization. *Genes Chromosomes Cancer.* 1997;19:84–89.

Barbacid M. *ras* genes. *Ann Rev Biochem.* 1987;56:779–827.

Benedict WF, Lerner SP, Czerniak BA, et al. Level of retinoblastoma protein expression correlates with P16 status in bladder cancer (Abstract). *J Urol.* 1998;159 (Suppl 5):281.

Bittard H, Descotes F, Billerey C, et al. A genotype study of the C-Ha-ras-1 locus in human bladder tumors. *J Urol.* 1996;155:1083–1088.

Blasco-Olaetxea E, Belloso L, Gracia-Tamayo J. Superficial bladder cancer: study of the proliferative nuclear fraction as a prognostic factor. *Eur J Cancer.* 1996;32A:444–446.

Bochner BP, Cote RJ, Weidner N, et al. Angiogenesis in bladder cancer: relationship between microvessel density and tumor prognosis. *J Natl Cancer Inst.* 1995;87:1603–1612.

Bohm M, Kirch H, Otto T, et al. Deletion analysis at the DEL-27, APC and MTS1 loci in bladder cancer: LOH at the DEL-27 locus on 5p13-12 is a prognostic marker of tumor progression. *Int J Cancer.* 1997;74:291–295.

Brewster SF, Gingell JC, Browne S, et al. Loss of heterozygosity on chromosome 18q is associated with muscle-invasive transitional cell carcinoma of the bladder. *Br J Cancer.* 1994;70:697–700.

Bringuier PP, Tamimi E, Schuuring E, et al. Expression of cyclin D1 and EMS1 in bladder tumours: relationship with chromosome 11q13 amplification. *Oncogene.* 1996;12:1747–1753.

Brown LF, Berse B, Jackman RW, et al. Increased expression of vascular permeability factor (vascular endothelial growth factor) and its receptors in kidney and bladder carcinoma. *Am J Pathol.* 1993; 143:1255–1262.

Bucci B, Pansadoro V, De Paula F, et al. Biologic characteristics of T1 papillary bladder cancer. Flow cytometric study of paraffin-embedded material. *Analyt Quant Cytol Histol.* 1995;17:121–128.

Burkhard FC, Markwalder R, Thalmann GN, et al. Immunohistochemical determination of p53 expression. *Urol Res.* 1997;25 (Suppl 1):S31–S35.

Busch C, Price P, Norton J, et al. Proliferation in human bladder carcinoma measured by Ki-67 antibody labeling: its potential clinical importance. *Br J Cancer.* 1991;64:357–363.

Cajulis RS, Haines GK III, Frias-Hidvegi D, et al. Interphase cytogenetics as an adjunct in the cytodiagnosis of urinary bladder carcinoma. A comparative study of cytology, flow cytometry and interphase cytogenetics in bladder washes. *Analyt Quant Cytol Histol.* 1994;16:1–10.

Caliskan M, Turkeri LN, Mansuroglu B, et al. Nuclear accumulation of mutant p53 protein: a possible predictor of failure of intravesical therapy in bladder cancer. *Br J Urol.* 1997;79:373–377.

Campbell SC, Volpert OV, Ivanovich M, et al. Molecular mediators of angiogenesis in bladder cancer. *Cancer Res.* 1998;58:1298–1304.

Cappellen D, de Medina SGD, Chopin D, et al. Frequent loss of heterozygosity on chromosome 19q in muscle-invasive transitional cell carcinomas of the bladder. *Oncogene.* 1997;14:3059–3066.

Carpinito GA, Rukstalis DB, Pandrangi LV, et al. Prospective multi-center study of NMP22 and cytology in patients with hematuria (Abstract). *J Urol.* 1998;159 (Suppl 5):245.

Casetta G, Gontero P, Russo R, et al. p53 expression compared with other prognostic factors in OMS grade-1 stage-Ta transitional cell carcinoma of the bladder. *Eur Urol.* 1997;32:229–236.

Cerutti P, Hussain P, Pourzand C, et al. Mutagenesis of the H-ras proto-oncogene and p53 tumor suppressor gene. *Cancer Res.* 1994;54:1934s–1938s.

Chang WY-H, Cairns P, Schoenberg MP, et al. Novel suppressor loci on chromosome 14q in primary bladder cancer. *Cancer Res.* 1995;55: 3246–3249.

Chen G, Lin MS, Li RC. Expression and prognostic value of proliferating cell nuclear antigen in transitional cell carcinoma of the urinary bladder. *Urol Res.* 1997;25:25–30.

Cheng H-I, Chow N-H, Tzai T-S, et al. Prognostic significance of proliferating cell nuclear antigen expression in transitional cell carcinoma of the upper urinary tract. *Anticancer Res.* 1997;17:2789–2794.

Cohen MB, Griebling TL, Ahaghotu CA, et al. Cellular adhesion molecules in urologic malignancies. *Am J Clin Pathol.* 1997;107:56–63.

Cordon-Cardo C, Wartinger D, Petrylak D, et al. Altered expressions of the retinoblastoma gene product: prognostic indicator of bladder cancer. *J Natl Cancer Inst.* 1992;84:1251–1256.

Cordon-Cardo C, Dalbagni G, Saez GT, et al. p53 mutations in human bladder cancer: genotypic versus phenotypic patterns. *Int J Cancer.* 1994; 56:347–353.

Cordon-Cardo C, Sheinfeld J, Dalbagni G. Genetic studies and molecular markers of bladder cancer. *Sem Surg Oncol.* 1997a;13:319–327.

Cordon-Cardo C, Zhang Z-F, Dalbagni G, et al. Cooperative effects of p53 and pRB alterations in primary superficial bladder tumors. *Cancer Res.* 1997b;57:1217–1221.

Cote RJ, Esrig D, Groshen S, et al. p53 and treatment of bladder cancer. *Nature.* 1997;385:123–124.

Crew JP, O'Brien T, Bradburn M, et al. Vascular endothelial growth factor is a predictor of relapse and stage progression in superficial bladder cancer. *Cancer Res.* 1997;57:5281–5285.

Czerniak B, Cohen GL, Etkind P, et al. Concurrent mutations of coding and regulatory sequences of the Ha-ras gene in urinary bladder carcinomas. *Hum Pathol.* 1992;23:1199–1203.

Dalbagni G, Presti JC Jr, Reuter VE, et al. Molecular genetic alterations of chromosome 17 and p53 nuclear overexpression in human bladder cancer. *Diag Mol Pathol.* 1993;2:4–13.

Dalbagni G, Cordon-Cardo C, Reuter V, et al. Tumor suppressor gene alterations in bladder carcinoma. Translational correlates to clinical practice. *Surg Oncol Clin North Am.* 1995;4:231–240.

deVere White R, Deitch AD, Daneshmand S, et al. Predictors of outcome in bladder transitional cell carcinoma (TCC) treated by intravesical chemotherapy (Abstract). *J Urol.* 1998;159 (Suppl 5):145.

Dickinson AJ, Fox SB, Persad RA, et al. Quantification of angiogenesis as an independent predictor in invasive bladder carcinoma. *Br J Urol.* 1994;74: 762–766.

Ellis WJ, Blumenstein BA, Ishak LM, et al. Clinical evaluation of the BTA TRAK assay and comparison to voided urine cytology and the Bard BTA test in patients with recurrent bladder tumors. The Multi Center Study Group. *Urology.* 1997;50:882–887.

Esrig D, Elmajian D, Groshen S, et al. Accumulation of nuclear p53 and tumor progression in bladder cancer. *New Engl J Med.* 1994;331:1259–1264.

Fagelson JE, Rathi A, Miura N, et al. Detection of telomerase expression by in situ hybridization: a promising new technique in the evaluation of bladder cancer (Abstract). *J Urol.* 1998;159 (Suppl 5):283.

Fontana D, Bellina M, Gubetta L, et al. Monoclonal antibody Ki-67 in the study of the proliferative activity of bladder carcinoma. *J Urol.* 1992; 148:1149–1152.

Fradet Y. Phenotypic characterization of bladder cancer. *Eur Urol.* 1998;33 (Suppl 4):5–6.

Friedrich M, Erbersdobler A, Schwalbold H, et al. Detection of loss of heterozygosity (LOH) in the P53-gene among bladder cancer patients in tumor and urinary sediment using a simple polymerase chain reaction (PCR) technique (Abstract). *J Urol.* 1998;159 (Suppl 5):280.

Fujimoto K, Yamada Y, Okajima E, et al. Frequent association of p53 gene mutation in invasive bladder cancer. *Cancer Res.* 1992;52:1393–1398.

Furihata M, Sonobe H, Ohtsuki Y, et al. Detection of p53 and bcl-2 protein in carcinoma of the renal pelvis and ureter including dysplasia. *J Pathol.* 1996;178:133–139.

Gardiner RA, Walsh MD, Allen V, et al. Immunohistological expression of p53 in primary pT1 transitional cell bladder cancer in relation to tumour progression. *Br J Urol.* 1994;73:526–532.

Geradts J, Kratzke RA, Crush-Stanton S, et al. Wild-type and mutant retinoblastoma protein in paraffin sections. *Mod Pathol.* 1996;9:339–347.

Glick S, Howell LP, Devere White RW. Relationship of p53 and bcl-2 to prognosis in muscle invasive transitional cell carcinoma of the bladder. *J Urol.* 1996;155:1754–1757.

Gonzalez-Zulueta M, Ruppert JM, Tokino K, et al. Microsatellite instability in bladder cancer. *Cancer Res.* 1993;53:5620–5623.

Gonzalez-Zulueta M, Shibata A, Ohneseit PF, et al. High frequency of chromosome 9p allelic loss and CDKN2 tumor suppressor gene alterations in squamous cell carcinoma of the bladder. *J Natl Cancer Inst.* 1995;87:1383–1393.

Goodrich DW, Chen Y, Scully P, et al. Expression of retinoblastoma gene product in bladder carcinoma cells associates with a low frequency of tumor formation. *Cancer Res.* 1992;52:1968–1973.

Gorgoulis VG, Barbatis C, Poulias I, et al. Molecular and immunohistochemical evaluation of epidermal growth factor receptor and c-erb-B-2 gene product in transitional cell carcinomas of the urinary bladder: a study in Greek patients. *Mod Pathol.* 1995;8:758–764.

Griffiths TRL, Brotherick I, Bishop RI, et al. Cell adhesion molecules in bladder cancer: soluble serum E-cadherin correlates with predictors of recurrence. *Br J Cancer.* 1996;74:579–584.

Grossman HB, Liebert M, Antelo M, et al. p53 and RB expression predict progression in T1 bladder cancer. *Clin Cancer Res.* 1998;4:829–834.

Habuchi T, Takahashi R, Yamada H, et al. Metachronous multifocal development of urothelial cancers by intraluminal seeding. *Lancet.* 1993; 342:1087–1088.

Heine B, Hummel M, Muller M, et al. Non-radioactive measurement of telomerase activity in human bladder cancer, bladder washings, and in urine. *J Pathol.* 1998;184:71–76.

Hemstreet GP III, Rao J, Hurst RE, et al. G-actin as a risk factor and modulatable endpoint for cancer chemoprevention trials. *J Cell Biochem.* 1996;25 (suppl):197–204.

Hofmann R, Krusmann G, Lehmer S, et al. Prognostic factors for muscle invasive bladder cancer (Abstract). *J Urol.* 1998;159 (Suppl 5):246.

Hopman AHN, Hooren EV, van de Kaa CA, et al. Detection of numerical chromosome aberrations using in situ hybridization in paraffin sections of routinely processed bladder cancers. *Mod Pathol.* 1991;4:503–513.

Ianari A, Sternberg CN, Rossetti A, et al. Results of Bard BTA test in monitoring patients with a history of transitional cell cancer of the bladder. *Urology.* 1997;49:786–789.

Iczkowski KA, Shanks JH, Bostwick DG. Loss of CD 44 variant 6 expression differentiates small cell carcinoma of urinary bladder from urothelial (transitional cell) carcinoma. *Histopathology.* 1998;32:322–327.

Inagaki T, Ebisuno S, Uekado Y, et al. PCNA and p53 in urinary bladder cancer: correlation with histological findings and prognosis. *Int J Urol.* 1997; 4:172–177.

Ishak L, Ellis WJ. A comparison of the BTA stat and the BTA TRAK assays: two new tests for the detection of recurrent bladder cancer (BC) in urine (Abstract). *J Urol.* 1998;159 (Suppl 5):245.

Ishikawa J, Xu HJ, Hu SX, et al. Inactivation of the retinoblastoma gene in human bladder and renal cell carcinomas. *Cancer Res.* 1991;51:5736–5743.

Jaeger TM, Weidner N, Chew K, et al. Tumor angiogenesis correlates with lymph node metastases in invasive bladder cancer. *J Urol.* 1995;154:69–71.

Jones HL, Delahunt B, Bethwaite PB, et al. Luminal epithelial antigen (LEA.135) expression correlates with tumor progression for transitional carcinoma of the bladder. *Anticancer Res.* 1997;17:685–688.

Kallioniemi A, Kallioniemi OP, Citro G, et al. Identification of gains and losses of DNA sequences in primary bladder cancer by comparative genomic hybridization. *Genes Chromosom Cancer.* 1995;12:213–219.

Kamata S, Kageyama Y, Yonese J, et al. Significant telomere reduction in human superficial transitional cell carcinoma. *Br J Urol.* 1996;78:704–708.

Kinoshita H, Ogawa O, Kakehi Y, et al. Detection of telomerase activity in exfoliated cells in urine from patients with bladder cancer. *J Natl Cancer Inst.* 1997;89:724–730.

Kinzler KW, Vogelstein B. Life (and death) in a malignant tumour. *Nature.* 1996;379:19-20.

Klein A, Zemer R, Buchumensky V, et al. Expression of cytokeratin 20 in urinary cytology of patients with bladder carcinoma. *Cancer.* 1998;82:349–354.

Knowles MA. Molecular genetics of bladder cancer. *Br J Urol.* 1995;75:57–66.

Knowles MA, Williamson M. Mutation of Ha-ras is infrequent in bladder cancer: confirmation by single strand conformation polymorphism analysis, designed fragment length polymorphism and direct sequencing. *Cancer Res.* 1993;53:133–139.

Kubota Y, Miyamoto H, Noguchi S, et al. The loss of retinoblastoma gene in association with c-myc and transforming growth factor-ß1 gene expression in human bladder cancer. *J Urol.* 1995;154:371–374.

Kyo S, Kunimi K, Uchibayashi T, et al. Telomerase activity in human urothelial tumors. *Am J Clin Pathol.* 1997;107:555–560.

Landman J, Kavaler E, Droller MJ, et al. Applications of telomerase in urologic oncology. *World J Urol.* 1997;15:120–124.

Landman J, Kavaler E, Chang Y, et al. Sensitivity and specificity of NMP-22, telomerase, and BTA in the detection of human bladder cancer (Abstract). *J Urol.* 1998;159 (Suppl 5):245.

LaRue H, Simoneau M, Fradet Y. Human papillomavirus in transitional cell carcinoma of the urinary bladder. *Clin Cancer Res.* 1995;1:435–440.

Lebret T, Becette V, Barbagelatta M, et al. Correlation between p53 overexpression and response to bacillus Calmette-Guerin therapy in a high risk select population of patients with T1G3 bladder cancer. *J Urol.* 1998;159:788–791.

Lee CCR, Yamamoto S, Morimura K, et al. Significance of cyclin D1 overexpression in transitional cell carcinomas of the urinary bladder and its correlation with histopathologic features. *Cancer.* 1997;79:780–789.

Lee D-H, Yang S-C, Hong S-J, et al. Telomerase: a potential marker of bladder transitional cell carcinoma in bladder washes. *Clin Cancer Res.* 1998;4:535–538.

Lee SH, Lin JSN, Tzai TS, et al. Prognostic factors of primary transitional cell carcinoma of the upper urinary tract. *Eur Urol.* 1996;29:266–270.

Lee SE, Park MS. Prognostic factor for survival in patients with transitional cell carcinoma of the bladder: evaluation by histopathologic grade, pathologic stage and flow-cytometric analysis. *Eur Urol.* 1996;29:193–198.

Lein M, Jung K, Weiss S, et al. Soluble CD44 variants in the serum of patients with urological malignancies. *Oncology.* 1997;54:226–230.

Lerner SP, Benedict WF, Green A, et al. Molecular staging and prognosis following radical cystectomy using p53 and retinoblastoma protein expression (Abstract). *J Urol.* 1998;159 (Suppl 5):165.

Leyh H, Treiber U, Thomas L, et al. Results of a European multicenter trial comparing the BTA TRAK test to urine cytology in patients suspected of having bladder cancer (Abstract). *J Urol.* 1998;159 (Suppl 5):244.

Li MM, Zhang ZF, Reuter VE, et al. Chromosome 3 allelic losses and microsatellite alterations in transitional cell carcinoma of the urinary bladder. *Am J Pathol.* 1996;149:229–235.

Lianes P, Orlow I, Zhang ZF, et al. Altered patterns of MDM2 and TP53 expression in human bladder cancer. *J Natl Cancer Inst.* 1994;86:1325–1330.

Liebert M, Washington R, Wedemeyer G, et al. Loss of co-localization of alpha 6 beta 4 integrin and collagen VII in bladder cancer. *Am J Pathol.* 1994;144:787–795.

Lin Y, Miyamoto H, Fujinami K, et al. Telomerase activity in human bladder cancer. *Cancer Res.* 1996;2:929–932.

Lipponen PK. Overexpression of p53 nuclear oncoprotein in transitional-cell bladder cancer and its prognostic value. *Int J Cancer.* 1993;53:365–370.

Lipponen PK, Eskelinen MJ. Reduced expression of E-cadherin is related to invasive disease and frequent recurrence in bladder cancer. *J Cancer Res Clin Oncol.* 1995;121:303–308.

Lipponen PK, Liukkonen TJ. Reduced expression of retinoblastoma (Rb) gene protein is related to cell proliferation and prognosis in transitional-cell bladder cancer. *J Cancer Res Clin Oncol.* 1995; 121:44–50.

Lipponen PK, Aaltomaa S, Eskelinen M. Expression of the apoptosis suppressing bcl-2 protein in transitional cell bladder tumours. *Histopathology.* 1996;28:135–140.

Liukkonen TJO, Lipponen PK, Helle M, et al. Immunoreactivity of bcl-2, p53 and EGFr is associated with tumor stage, grade and cell proliferation in superficial bladder cancer. *Urol Res.* 1997;25:1–8.

Llopis J, Alcaraz A, Ribal MJ, et al. p53 expression predicts progression and poor survival in T1 bladder tumors (Abstract). *J Urol.* 1998;159 (Suppl 5):144.

Lokeshwar VB, Obek C, Soloway MS, et al. Tumor-associated hyaluronic acid: a new sensitive and specific urine marker for bladder cancer. *Cancer Res.* 1997;57:773–777.

Lopez-Beltran A, Escudero AL. Human papillomavirus and bladder cancer (review). *Biomed Pharmacother.* 1997;51:252–257.

Lopez-Beltran A, Munoz E. Low incidence of human papillomavirus DNA in transitional cell carcinoma. *Histopathology.* 1995;26:565–570.

Lopez-Beltran A, Carrasco-Aznar JC, Reymundo C, et al. Bladder cancer survival in human papillomavirus infection. Immunohistochemistry and in-situ hybridization. In: CA Olsson, ed. *Oncogenes and molecular genetics of urological tumours.* London: Churchill Livingstone; 1992a.

Lopez-Beltran A, Croghan GA, Croghan I, et al. Prognostic factors in survival of bladder cancer. *Cancer.* 1992b;70:799–807.

Lopez-Beltran A, Croghan GA, Croghan I, et al. Prognostic factors in bladder cancer. A pathologic, immunohistochemical, and DNA flow-cytometric study. *Am J Clin Pathol.* 1994;102:109–114.

Lopez-Beltran A, Escudero AL, Cavazzana AO, et al. Sarcomatoid transitional cell carcinoma of the renal pelvis: a report of five cases with clinical, pathological, immunohistochemical and DNA ploidy analysis. *Path Res Pract.* 1996a;192:1181–1296.

Lopez-Beltran A, Lopez Escudero A, Vicioso L, et al. Prognostic implication of human papillomavirus DNA in transitional cell carcinoma. *Br J Cancer.* 1996b;73:124–127.

Ludecke G, Farkas P, Edler M, et al. Nuclear matrix protein 22 (NMP22): A tumor marker in primary diagnosis and follow up of bladder cancer (Abstract). *J Urol.* 1998;159 (Suppl 5):244.

Matsuyama H, Pan Y, Mahdy EA, et al. p53 deletion as a genetic marker in urothelial tumor by fluo-rescence in situ hybridization. *Cancer Res.* 1994;54: 6057–6060.

Mellon JK, Lunec J, Wright C, et al. C-erbB-2 in bladder cancer: molecular biology, correlation with epidermal growth factor receptors and prognostic value. *J Urol.* 1996;155:321–326.

Miyamoto H, Kubota Y, Shuin T, et al. Analyses of p53 gene mutations in primary human bladder cancer. *Oncol Res.* 1993;5:245–249.

Miyamoto H, Shuin T, Ikeda I, et al. Loss of heterozygosity at the p53, RB, DCC, and APC tumor suppressor gene loci in human bladder cancer. *J Urol.* 1996;155:1444–1447.

Miyanaga N, Akaza H, Tsukamoto T, et al. Urinary nuclear matrix protein 22 (NMP22) as a marker for screening urothelial cancer patient with microscopic hematuria (Abstract). *J Urol.* 1998;159 (Suppl 5):243.

Miyao N, Tsai YC, Lerner SP, et al. Role of chromosome 9 in human bladder cancer. *Cancer Res.* 1993;53:4066–4070.

Moch H, Sauter G, Mihatsch MJ, et al. p53 but not erbB-2 expression is associated with rapid tumor proliferation in urinary bladder cancer. *Hum Pathol.* 1994;25:1346–1351.

Mulder AH, Van Hootegem JC, Sylvester R, et al. Prognostic factors in bladder carcinoma: histologic parameters and expression of a cell cycle-related nuclear antigen (Ki-67). *J Pathol.* 1992;166:37–43.

Muller M, Heine B, Heicappell R, et al. Telomerase activity in bladder cancer, bladder washings and in urine. *Int J Oncol.* 1996;9:1169–1173.

Nakanishi K, Kawai T, Suzuki M, et al. Growth factors and oncogene products in transitional cell carcinoma. *Mod Pathol.* 1996;9:292–297.

Nakanishi K, Kawai T, Torikata C, et al. Urokinase-type plasminogen activator, its inhibitor, and its receptor in patients with upper urinary tract carcinoma. *Cancer.* 1998;82:724–732.

Nakopoulou L, Constantinides C, Papandropoulos J, et al. Evaluation of overexpression of p53 tumor suppressor protein in superficial and invasive transitional cell bladder cancer: comparison with DNA ploidy. *Urology.* 1995;46:334–340.

Nakopoulou LL, Constantinides CA, Tzonou A, et al. Immunohistochemical evaluation of nm23H1 gene product in transitional cell carcinoma of the bladder. *Histopathology.* 1996;28:429–435.

Nakopoulou L, Vourlakou C, Zervas A, et al. The prevalence of bcl-2, p53, and Ki-67 immunoreactivity in transitional cell bladder carcinomas and their clinicopathologic correlates. *Hum Pathol.* 1998;29:146–154.

Nemoto R, Nakamura I, Uchida K, et al. Numerical chromosome aberrations in bladder cancer detected by in situ hybridization. *Br J Urol.* 1995; 75:470–476.

Norming U, Nyman CR, Tribukait B. Comparative flow cytometric deoxyribonucleic acid studies on exophytic tumors and random mucosal biopsies in untreated carcinoma of the bladder. *J Urol.* 1989;142:1442–1447.

Norming U, Tribukait B, Gustafson H, et al. Deoxyribonucleic acid profile and tumor progression in primary carcinoma in situ of the bladder: a study of 63 patients with grade 3 lesions. *J Urol.* 1992;147:11–15.

O'Brien T, Cranston D, Fuggle S, et al. Two mechanisms of basic fibroblast growth factor induced angiogenesis in bladder cancer. *Cancer Res.* 1997;57:136–140.

Ogura K, Habuchi T, Yamada H, et al. Immunohistochemical analysis of p53 and proliferating cell nuclear antigen (PCNA) in bladder cancer: positive immunostaining and radiosensitivity. *Int J Urol.* 1995;2:302–308.

Ogura K, Fukazawa S, Habuchi T, et al. Correlation of nuclear morphometry and immunostaining for p53 and proliferating cell nuclear antigen in transitional cell carcinoma of the bladder. *Int J Urol.* 1997;4:561–566.

Okamura K, Miyake K, Koshikawa T, et al. Growth fractions of transitional cell carcinomas of the bladder defined by the monoclonal antibody Ki-67. *J Urol.* 1990;144:875–879.

Olumi AF, Tsai YS, Nichols PW, et al. Allelic loss of chromosome 17p distinguishes high grade from low grade transitional cell carcinomas of the bladder. *Cancer Res.* 1990;50:7081–7083.

Orlow I, Lacombe L, Hannon GJ, et al. Deletions of p16 and p15 genes in human bladder tumors. *J Natl Cancer Inst.* 1995;87:1524–1529.

Otto T, Bex A, Schmidt U, et al. Improved prognosis assessment for patients with bladder carcinoma. *Am J Pathol.* 1997;150:1919–1923.

Oyasu R, Nan L, Szumel R, et al. p53 gene mutations in human urothelial carcinomas: analysis by immunohistochemistry and single-strand conformation polymorphism. *Mod Pathol.* 1995;8:170–176.

Pages F, Flam TA, Vieillefond A, et al. p53 status does not predict initial clinical response to bacillus Calmette-Guerin intravesical therapy in T1 bladder tumors. *J Urol.* 1998;159:1079–1084.

Pantazopoulos D, Ioakim-Liossi A, Karakitsos P, et al. DNA content and proliferation activity in superficial transitional cell carcinoma of the bladder. *Anticancer Res.* 1997;17:781–786.

Patard JJ, Brasseur F, Gil-Diez S, et al. Expression of MAGE genes in transitional cell carcinomas of the urinary bladder. *Int J Cancer.* 1995;64:60–64.

Pfister C, Flaman JM, Dunet F, et al. Preliminary results in detection of p53 mutations in bladder tumors with a functional assay (Abstract). *J Urol.* 1998;159 (Suppl 5):277.

Pinnock CB, Roxby DJ, Ross JM, et al. Ploidy and Tn-antigen expression in the detection of transitional cell neoplasia in non-tumor-bearing patients. *Br J Urol.* 1995;75:461–469.

Posch B, Haitel A, Pycha A, et al. Bcl-2 is a prognostic factor in advanced bladder cancer (Abstract). *J Urol.* 1998;159 (Suppl 5):246.

Proctor AJ, Coombs LM, Cairns JP, et al. Amplification at chromosome 11q13 in transitional cell tumors of the bladder. *Oncogene.* 1991;6:789–795.

Raitanen M-P, Tammela TLJ, Kallioinen M, et al. p53 accumulation, deoxyribonucleic acid ploidy and expression of bladder cancer. *J Urol.* 1997;157:1250–1253.

Raitanen M-P, Marttila T, Tammela TIJ, et al. The Bard BTA stat test in monitoring of bladder cancer (Abstract). *J Urol.* 1998;159 (Suppl 5):244.

Rao JY, Hurst RE, Bales WD, et al. Cellular F-actin levels as a marker for cellular transformation: relationship to cell division and differentiation. *Cancer Res.* 1990;50:2215–2220.

Rao JY, Hemstreet GP, Hurst RE, et al. Cellular F-actin levels as a marker for cellular transformation: correlation with bladder cancer risk. *Cancer Res.* 1991;51:2762–2767.

Ravery V, Grignon D, Angulo J, et al. Evaluation of epidermal growth factor receptor, transforming growth factor alpha, epidermal growth factor and c-erbB2 in the progression of invasive bladder cancer. *Urol Res.* 1997;25:9–17.

Reznikoff CA, Kao C, Messing EM, et al. A molecular genetic model of human bladder carcinogenesis. *Sem Cancer Biol.* 1993;4:143–152.

Reznikoff CA, Belair CD, Yeager TR, et al. A molecular genetic model of human bladder cancer pathogenesis. *Sem Oncol.* 1996;23:571–584.

Richter J, Jiang F, Gorog J-P, et al. Marker genetic differences between stage pTa and stage pT1 papillary cancer detected by comparative genomic hybridization. *Cancer Res.* 1997;57:2860–2864.

Ross JS, Del Rosario AD, Figge HL, et al. E-cadherin expression in papillary transitional cell carcinoma of the urinary bladder. *Hum Pathol.* 1995;26:940–944.

Ross JS, Delrosario AD, Bui HX, et al. Expression of the CD44 cell adhesion molecule in urinary bladder transitional cell carcinoma. *Mod Pathol.* 1996;9:854–860.

Ruizeveld de Winter JA, Trapman J, Vermay M, et al. Androgen receptor expression in human tissues: an immunohistochemical study. *J Histochem Cytochem.* 1991;39:927–936.

Sachs M, Schlecgte H, Lenk SV. Genetic analysis of TP 53 in the urine sediment for diagnosing recurrences of bladder cancer (Abstract). *J Urol.* 1998a;159 (Suppl 5):279.

Sachs M, Schlechte HH, Lenk SV, et al. TP 53—Genetic analysis shows monoclonality of primary and recurrent tumor of the urinary bladder (Abstract). *J Urol.* 1998b;159 (Suppl 5):279.

Saito T, Kimura M, Kawasaki T, et al. Correlation between integrin alpha 5 expression and the malignant phenotype of transitional cell carcinoma. *Br J Cancer.* 1996;73:327–331.

Sandberg A, Berger CS. Review of chromosome studies in urological tumors. II. Cytogenetics and molecular genetics of bladder cancer. *J Urol.* 1994; 155:545–560.

Sarkis AS, Dalbagni G, Cordon-Cardo C, et al. Nuclear overexpression of p53 protein in transitional cell carcinoma: a marker for disease progression. *J Natl Cancer Inst.* 1993;85:53–59.

Sarkis AS, Dalbagni G, Cordon-Cardo C, et al. Association of p53 nuclear overexpression and tumor progression in carcinoma in situ of the bladder. *J Urol.* 1994;152:388–392.

Sarkis AS, Bajorin DF, Reuter VE, et al. The prognostic value of p53 nuclear overexpression in patients with invasive bladder cancer treated with neoadjuvant MVAC. *J Clin Oncol.* 1995;13:1384–1390.

Sauter G, Haley J, Chew K, et al. Epidermal-growth-factor-receptor expression is associated with rapid tumor proliferation in bladder cancer. *Int J Cancer.* 1994;57:508–514.

Sauter G, Moch H, Carroll P, et al. Chromosome-9 loss detected by fluorescence in situ hybridization in bladder cancer. *Int J Cancer.* 1995;64:99–103.

Schmitz-Drager BJ, van Roeyen CRC, Grimm MO, et al. p53 accumulation in precursor lesions and early stages of bladder cancer. *World J Urol.* 1994;12:79–83.

Schmitz-Drager BJ, KushimaM, Goebell P, et al. p53 and MDM2 in the development and progression of bladder cancer. *Eur Urol.* 1997;32:487–493.

Schulte PA. The role of genetic factors in bladder cancer. *Cancer Det Prev.* 1988;11:379–388.

Shaaban AA, Tribukait B, Abdel-Fattah AEB, et al. Characterization of squamous cell bladder tumors by flow cytometric deoxyribonucleic acid analysis: a report of 100 cases. *J Urol.* 1990;144:879–883.

Shaw ME, Knowles MA. Deletion mapping of chromosome 11 in carcinoma of the bladder. *Genes Chromosomes Cancer.* 1995;13:1–8.

Shiina H, Igawa M, Nagami H, et al. Immunohistochemical analysis of proliferating cell nuclear antigen, p53 protein and nm23 protein, and nuclear DNA content in transitional cell carcinoma of the bladder. *Cancer.* 1996a;78:1762–1774.

Shiina H, Urakami S, Shirakawa H, et al. Evaluation of the argyrophilic nucleolar organizer region, nuclear DNA content and mean nuclear area in transitional cell carcinoma of bladder using a quantitative image analyzer. *Eur Urol.* 1996b;29:99–105.

Shin KY, Kong G, Kim WS, et al. Overexpression of cyclin D1 correlates with early recurrence in superficial bladder cancers. *Br J Cancer.* 1997;75:1788–1792.

Sidransky D, Messing E. Molecular genetics and biochemical mechanisms in bladder cancer. Oncogenes, tumor suppressor genes, and growth factors. *Urol Clin North Am.* 1992;19:629–639.

Sidransky D, von Eschenbach A, Tsai YC, et al. Identification of p53 mutations in bladder cancer and urine samples. *Science.* 1991;252:706–709.

Simoneau AR, Jones PA. Bladder cancer: the molecular progression to invasive disease. *World J Urol.* 1994;12:89–95.

Simoneau AR, Spruck CH III, Gonzalez-Zulueta M, et al. Evidence for two tumor suppressor loci associated with proximal chromosome 9p to q and distal chromosome 9q in bladder cancer and the initial screening for GAS 1 and PTC mutations. *Cancer Res.* 1996;56:5039–5043.

Sinik Z, Alkibay T, Ataoglu O, et al. Correlation of nuclear p53 overexpression with clinical and histopathological features of transitional cell bladder cancer. *Int Urol Nephrol.* 1997;29:25–31.

Slaton JW, Dinney CP, Veltri RW, et al. Deoxyribonucleic acid ploidy enhances the cytological predication of recurrent transitional cell carcinoma of the bladder. *J Urol.* 1997;158(3, pt 1):806–811.

Spruck CH III, Ohneseit PF, Gonzalez-Zulueta M, et al. Two molecular pathways to transitional cell carcinoma of the bladder. *Cancer Res.* 1994;54:784–788.

Stampfer DS, Carpinito GA, Rodriguez-Villanueva J, et al. Evaluation of NMP22 in the detection of transitional cell carcinoma of the bladder. *J Urol.* 1998;159:394–398.

Stavropoulos NE, Iachim-Velogianni E, Hastazeris K, et al. Growth fractions in bladder cancer defined by Ki67: association with cancer grade, category and recurrence rate of superficial lesions. *Br J Urol.* 1993;72:736–741.

Steiner G, Schoenberg MP, Linn JF, et al. Detection of bladder cancer recurrence by microsatellite analysis of urine. *Nature Med.* 1997;2:621–624.

Sugino T, Gorham H, Yoshida K, et al. Progressive loss of CD44 gene expression in invasive bladder cancer. *Am J Pathol.* 1996;149:873–882.

Sugiyama M, Woodman A, Sugino T, et al. Non-invasive detection of malignancy by identification of abnormal CD44 proteins in exfoliated cancer cells in urine. *J Clin Pathol Mol Pathol.* 1995;48:142–143.

Terrel RB, Cheville JC, See WA, et al. Histopathological features and p53 nuclear protein staining as predictors of survival and tumor recurrence in patients with transitional cell carcinoma of the renal pelvis. *J Urol.* 1995;154:1342–1347.

Tetu B, Fradet Y, Allard P, et al. Prevalence and clinical significance of HER-2/neu, p53 and RB expression in primary superficial bladder cancer. *J Urol.* 1996;155:1784–1788.

Theodorescu D. Commentary on genetic prognostic markers for transitional cell carcinoma of the bladder: from microscopes to molecules. *J Urol.* 1996;155:2.

Tiniakos DG, Mellon K, Anderson JJ, et al. c-jun oncogene expression in transitional cell carcinoma of the urinary bladder. *Br J Urol.* 1994;74:757–761.

Tsuji M, Kojima K, Murakami Y, et al. Prognostic value of Ki-67 antigen and p53 protein in urinary bladder cancer: immunohistochemical analysis of radical cystectomy specimens. *Br J Urol.* 1997; 79:367–372.

Turkeri LN, Erton ML, Cevik I, et al. Impact of the expression of epidermal growth factor, transforming growth factor alpha, and epidermal growth factor receptor on the prognosis of superficial bladder cancer. *Urology.* 1998;51:645–649.

Tut VM, Braithwaite KL, Angus B, et al. Cyclin D1 expression in transitional cell carcinoma (TCC) of the bladder: correlation with WAF1, P53 and Ki67 (Abstract). *J Urol.* 1998;159 (Suppl 5):281.

Uchida T, Wada C, Ishida H, et al. p53 mutations and prognosis in bladder tumors. *J Urol.* 1995;153:1097–1104.

Underwood M, Bartlett J, Reeves J, et al. C-erbB-2 gene amplification: a molecular marker in recurrent bladder tumors? *Cancer Res.* 1995;55;2422–2430.

Underwood M, Reeves J, Smith G, et al. Overexpression of p53 protein and its significance for recurrent progressive bladder tumors. *Br J Urol.* 1996;77:659–666.

Van der Poel HG, Van Balkenn MR, Schamhart DH, et al. Bladder wash cytology, quantitative cytology, and the qualitative BTA test in patients with superficial bladder cancer. *Urology.* 1998;51:44–50.

Vatne V, Maartmann-Moe H, Hoestmark J. The prognostic value of p53 in superficially infiltrating transitional cell carcinoma. *Scand J Urol Nephrol.* 1995;29:491–495.

Velthoven RV, Petein M, Oosterlinck WJ. The additional predictive value contributed by quantitative chromatine pattern description as compared to DNA ploidy level measurement in 257 superficial bladder transitional cell carcinomas. *Eur Urol.* 1996;29:245–251.

Vermeulen PB, Gasparini G, Fox SB, et al. Quantification of angiogenesis in solid human tumours: an international consensus on the methodology and criteria of evaluation. *Eur J Cancer.* 1996; 32A:2474–2484.

Vet JAM, Debruyne FMJ, Schalken JA. Molecular prognostic factors in bladder cancer. *World J Urol.* 1994;12:84–88.

Vet JAM, Bringuier PP, Schaafsma E, et al. Comparison of p53 protein overexpression with p53 mutation in bladder cancer: clinical and biologic aspects. *Lab Invest.* 1995;73:837–843.

Vet JAM, Witjes JA, Marras SAE, et al. Predictive value of p53 mutations analyzed in bladder washings for progression of high-risk superficial bladder cancer. *Clin Cancer Res.* 1996;2:1055–1061.

Vollmer RT, Humphrey PA, Swanson PE, et al. Invasion of the bladder by transitional cell carcinoma. Its relation to histologic grade and expression of p53, MIB-1, c-erbB-2, epidermal growth factor receptor, and bcl-2. *Cancer.* 1998;82:715–723.

Voorter C, Joos S, Bringuier PP, et al. Detection of chromosomal imbalances in transitional cell carcinoma of the bladder by comparative genomic hybridization. *Am J Pathol.* 1995;146:1341–1354.

Wagner U, Bubendorf L, Gasser TC, et al. Chromosome 8p deletions are associated with invasive tumor growth in urinary bladder cancer. *Am J Pathol.* 1997;151:753–759.

Wakatsuki S, Watanabe R, Saito K, et al. Loss of human E-cadherin (ECD) correlated with invasiveness of transitional cell cancer in the renal pelvis, ureter, and urinary bladder. *Cancer Lett.* 1996; 103:11–17.

Warren W, Biggs PJ, El-Baz M, et al. Mutations in the p53 gene in schistosomal bladder cancer: a study of 92 tumours from Egyptian patients and a comparison between mutational spectra from schistosomal and non-schistosomal urothelial tumours. *Carcinogenesis.* 1995;16:1181–1189.

Watanabe R, Tomiat Y, Nishiyama T, et al. Correlation of p53 protein expression in human urothelial transitional cell cancers with malignant potential and patient survival. *Int J Urol.* 1994;1:43–48.

Weidner N. Intratumoral vascularity as a prognostic factor in cancers of the urogenital tract. *Eur J Cancer.* 1996;32A:2506–2512.

Wright C, Thomas D, Mellon K, et al. Expression of retinoblastoma gene product and p53 protein in bladder carcinoma: correlation with Ki67 index. *Br J Urol.* 1995;75:173–179.

Xu X, Stower MJ, Reid IN, et al. A hot spot for p53 mutation in transitional cell carcinoma of the bladder: clues to the etiology of bladder cancer. *Cancer Epidemiol Biomarkers Prev.* 1997;6:611–616.

Yokogi H, Wada Y, Moriyama-Gonda N, et al. Genomic heterogeneity in bladder cancer as detected by fluorescence in situ hybridization. *Br J Urol.* 1996;78:699–703.

Yoshida Y, Sugino T, Tahara H, et al. Telomerase activity in bladder carcinoma and its implication for noninvasive diagnosis by detection of exfoliated cancer cells in urine. *Cancer.* 1997;79:362–369.

Zhang ZF, Sarkis AS, Cordon-Cardo C, et al. Tobacco smoking, occupation, and p53 nuclear overexpression in early stage bladder cancer. *Cancer Epidemiol Biomarkers Prev.* 1994;3:19–24.

Zhuang Y-H, Blauer M, Tammela T, et al. Immunodetection of androgen receptor in human urinary bladder cancer. *Histopathology.* 1997;30:556–562.

298

INDEX

Note: *t* indicates page contains a table; *f* is a figure.